Psychology for Nu
Health Care Profe

EDITED BY
DAVID MESSER AND CLAIRE MELDRUM

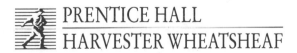

PRENTICE HALL
HARVESTER WHEATSHEAF

LONDON   NEW YORK   TORONTO   SYDNEY   TOKYO   SINGAPORE
MADRID   MEXICO CITY   MUNICH

First published 1995 by
Prentice Hall/Harvester Wheatsheaf
Campus 400, Maylands Avenue
Hemel Hempstead
Hertfordshire, HP2 7EZ
A division of
Simon & Schuster International Group

Typeset in 10/12pt Times
by Dorwyn Ltd, Rowlands Castle, Hants

Printed and bound in Great Britain by
T J Press Ltd, Padstow, Cornwall

Library of Congress Cataloging in Publication Data

Psychology for nurses and health care professionals/edited by David
    Messer and Claire Meldrum.
        p.   cm.
    Includes bibliographical references and index.
    ISBN 0–13–433178–8
    1. Clinical health psychology.   I. Messer, David J., 1952–
II. Meldrum, Claire.
    [DNLM: 1. Nursing Care—psychology.   2. Nurse–Patient Relations.
    3. Psychiatric Nursing.   4. Helping Behavior.   WY 100 P974 1995]
    R726.7.P7917   1995
    610.73—dc20
    DNLM/DLC
    for Library of Congress   94–40562
                                                              CIP

British Library Cataloguing in Publication Data

A catalogue record for this book is available from
the British Library

ISBN 0–13–433178–8

1 2 3 4 5   99 98 97 96 95

Psychology for Nurses and Health Care Professionals

Contents

Acknowledgements

Producing a book of twenty-five chapters is a relatively large enterprise and involves a good number of people. Our debt to all who have been involved is considerable. Both our families have provided support and have been tolerant of the work we have done to produce this volume, although in both families there often seemed to be the misguided assumption: 'I thought that was finished.' The contributors too have shown considerable patience with our suggestions for changes and amendments – all their hard work in drafting and redrafting the material has been greatly appreciated (in turn we think the editors showed a fair degree of tolerance when deadlines were not always strictly adhered to!).

Despite the occasional tribulation of the editing process we have had real pleasure in seeing the book grow in size and stature. We also appreciated the comments of the initially anonymous reviewers: Dr Elizabeth Clark, Distance Learning Co-ordinator, Institute of Advanced Nursing Education, Royal College of Nursing; Dr Christopher Eccleston, Lecturer in Health Psychology, University of Bath; and Marcia Worrell, Lecturer in Psychology, University of Luton. Their suggestions were very helpful and led to a number of important changes.

As always the secretarial staff in the Psychology Department of the University of Hertfordshire, Jean Thomas and Venetia Hussam, provided essential assistance when this was most needed, as did Don Pywell, who struggled with the disks.

The production of the book greatly benefited from the enthusiasm, advice and support of Farrell Burnett; our debt to her is large. We also owe a debt to Clare Grist and Nicola Horton for seeing us safely over the last hurdles.

Introduction

CLAIRE MELDRUM

Chapter outline

Psychology and its perspectives
Methods of study used in psychology
The work of psychologists
Organization and features of the book

There can be few statements more likely to raise the hackles of a psychologist than 'psychology is just common sense'. Not only is the statement false, it also implies that common sense is something that is both consistent and coherent. This is not the case. If common sense states that 'many hands make light work', then why does it also claim that 'too many cooks spoil the broth'? Common-sense sayings are highly inconsistent and are not based on any formal evaluation of their accuracy. Psychology, on the other hand, *is* concerned with testing whether ideas and theories about people are accurate.

Sometimes psychology's findings reinforce what people call their 'gut feelings' (intuitions), but on many occasions research produces counterintuitive results. Who could have predicted that 21 out of 22 nurses would comply with a telephone instruction to administer a drug to a patient that far exceeded the permitted dose and in direct contravention of a number of hospital rules? (See Chapter 3 for further revelations.)

Not so very long ago it would have been considered dangerously irresponsible to allow patients suffering pain to administer their own analgesia. But findings from nursing and psychophysiological research have once again proved counterintuitive: rather than take greater amounts of analgesia, patients actually take less. (See Chapter 13 for more information concerning pain and its management.)

Myth all too often masquerades as common sense. One of psychology's aims is to clarify, by the use of scientific methods, what is myth and what is reality concerning human behaviour and experience.

This book provides an up-to-date account of topics in psychology that are relevant to nurses, midwives, health visitors and other health care professionals. The chapters cover a wide range of issues, and links are made between theoretical and practical concerns. The editors strongly subscribe to the belief that psychology for health professionals should encompass their own psychology, the psychology of patients and the psychology of the environment in which they interact. By adopting this approach we have selected a broad and innovative range of topics. Unlike many existing health psychology texts, we have gone beyond the single consideration of patients/clients.

Many introductory psychology texts are available for those who have no prior acquaintance with the discipline. This book, however, is intended for readers who already have some rudimentary knowledge of psychology. The topics covered will be of particular interest to students studying on both pre- and post-registration courses in nursing, midwifery and health visiting and on other courses for health care professionals. The book focuses on the needs of nurses, and this term is often used rather than the more cumbersome phrase 'health care professional'. However, the use of the term 'nurse' does not mean that the material is designed exclusively for this group. Many other practising health care professionals, including midwives, occupational therapists and speech therapists, who are interested in the psychological aspects of their work will find much to stimulate them here.

At present, there is some difference of opinion about the appropriate use of the terms 'patient' and 'client'. For this reason, the contributors have chosen the expression they prefer, rather than the editors imposing an unnecessary uniformity.

For those who wish to familiarize themselves with the *perspectives*, *methods* and *work* of psychologists, an outline of each is provided in the following sections. The organization of the book is then described. Information about introductory psychology texts is given in the Further Reading at the end of this chapter.

Psychology and its perspectives

Atkinson *et al.* (1993) define *psychology* as the scientific study of behaviour and mental processes. This definition covers a wide range of topics and a glance at any modern psychology textbook will demonstrate the range. It includes, for example, the biological basis of behaviour, consciousness and perception, learning and remembering, language and thought, emotion, personality, abnormal behaviour and social behaviour. Knowledge of psychology, therefore, offers a better understanding of why people think and behave in the way they do. And this knowledge will extend to one's own thinking and behaviour.

Modern psychology can trace its roots as far back as the ancient Greek philosophers, but it was not until towards the end of the nineteenth century that psychology as a discipline in its own right was established, following the pioneering work of Wundt (e.g. 1905), James (e.g. 1890) and Ebbinghaus (e.g. 1890). These psychologists investigated the workings of the mind by using introspection whereby individuals reported and analyzed their own mental experiences. Although their techniques were very different from those used today, their findings produced some insights which are still of interest.

Perspectives

Topics in modern psychology tend to be studied within one or more of five of the following perspectives, each of which is briefly outlined:

1. The *neurobiological* perspective focuses on the role of biology and physiology in explaining behaviour and experience. The influence of the central nervous system is perceived as crucial. In the area of personality, for example, Eysenck (1982) claimed a biological basis for his theory of introversion–extraversion. (See Chapter 11 on brain damage for further insights into the neurobiological approach.)

2. Psychologists who use the *behaviourist* perspective study individuals by examining their overt, quantifiable behaviour. They believe that all behaviour is shaped by the environment in the form of reinforcements. The learning processes of classical and operant conditioning are seen as central to explaining human behaviour. (See Box 7.2, p. 137 for the behaviourist approach to personality). The application of the behavioural approach can be seen in the development of aversion therapy for addictive behaviours (see Chapter 12).

3. The modern *cognitive* perspective arose out of a dissatisfaction with the explanations offered by the behaviourist approach. Cognitive psychologists believe that the best way to understand human behaviour and experience is to understand the mental processes that occur during activities such as perceiving, remembering and problem-solving. Unlike their nineteenth-century predecessors, however, they do not use introspection, but have developed more objective means of focusing on particular behaviours. (Chapter 8 provides a discussion of memory, a topic of particular interest to cognitive psychologists.)

4. The *psychoanalytical* perspective was developed by Freud and views behaviour as largely determined by unconscious forces; that is, motivated by fears and desires of which we are unaware. Behavioural and emotional problems are seen as manifestations of unresolved conflicts, which have their origins in childhood. (Chapter 3 adopts a psychoanalytical perspective to explain the influence of groups.)

5. The *phenomenological/humanistic* perspective focuses on the subjective experience of individuals; that is, on their phenomenology or personal view of events. Unlike the other approaches, those using the phenomenological approach are interested in the inner life of people rather than in predicting how they will behave. The drive to self-actualize (achieve personal growth) is considered the main motivation for a person's behaviour. (Chapter 1 considers the importance of individual phenomenology.)

6. The *cultural/discursive* perspective arose out of the disillusionment some psychologists perceived with the scientific basis of psychological thinking and research. Psychologists such as Harré (1979) and Potter and Wetherell (1987), drawing on the fields of linguistics, sociology, anthropology and philosophy, have examined the explanations that people construct for the way they behave and the social/cultural forces that allow these explanations to make sense to us. This new psychology is sometimes known as discursive psychology because it focuses on the talk or discourse that people produce. For a good introduction to this perspective in health research, see Stainton Rogers (1991) in Further Reading.

Methods of study used in psychology

The psychologists whose work is discussed in this book use a variety of research methods. All methods have their limitations and these should always be borne in mind when evaluating any research findings. A brief outline of research methods is given.

Those psychologists who subscribe to the definition of psychology as the scientific study of behaviour and mental processes (see above) use methods that claim to be unbiased (not favouring one hypothesis over another) and objective (others who repeat their procedures will obtain the same results). Their aim is to be able to make predictions about behaviour based on research findings. Other psychologists reject this scientific method as inappropriate and advocate newer methodologies such as the phenomenological interview (Massarik, 1981) and discourse analysis (Potter and Wetherell, 1987). References for those who would like more information on these methods can be found in the Further Reading at the end of this chapter.

The most commonly used research methods employed by psychologists are outlined below.

The experimental method

In the language of the experimental psychologist a *variable* is anything that varies (can be different). For example, a person's weight and level of intelligence can be called variables because these can vary. Likewise, the number and type of questions a patient asks a doctor or the number of times a patient requests pain relief is a variable. An experimenter's aim is to discover which variables cause certain events.

In an experiment, researchers alter (manipulate) variables to see if this will produce a change in behaviour. The variable that is manipulated is called the *independent variable* and the behaviour measured is called the *dependent variable*. In the simplest experimental design, only one variable is manipulated. If the participants in the experimental condition, those who experience this manipulation, respond significantly differently compared to those who do not experience the manipulation (the control condition), then we claim that the manipulation caused the difference. For example, in the area of maternal bonding (see Chapter 18), Klaus and Kennell arranged for some mothers to have extra time with their newborn infants (experimental condition). That is, they manipulated the length of time allowed for mothers and babies to be together after the birth (independent variable). Subsequently, it was found that these mothers behaved differently towards their babies compared with mothers in the control condition who did not have the extra contact. The behavioural measures taken included the length of time breast-feeding continued and the number of kisses a mother was observed to give her baby. These measures are examples of dependent variables.

The experimental method is the only one that allows conclusions to be drawn about any cause and effect link between variables The assumption is that all other variables that might have confused (confounded) the results have been controlled. When a difference is found between the different conditions in an experiment, a decision has to be made about whether or not the difference is really significant or due merely to chance. This tells us whether we could expect the same result if the experiment was conducted again. A statistical test is carried out and the result is checked against a table value (critical value) to see if it reaches a level where there is a less than 5 per cent chance that the result is due to chance. If this is the case, then one can conclude that the manipulation caused the effect.

The experimental method has been criticized on many counts. Two of the most important of these relate to the artificiality of the method. The first states that the behaviour of people who know they are participating in an experiment may undergo changes relating to that situation. For example, they may try to be 'good' subjects to please the experimenter.

The second criticism has more to do with the location of the research. Many psychology experiments have been carried out in laboratories where it is relatively easy to control conditions. However, this is not always possible or even desirable and laboratory studies are often accused of lacking ecological validity (not being true to life). Psychologists have tried to overcome this problem by using real-life situations in which to embed their experiments. For example, the Klaus and Kennell study already mentioned was carried out in a hospital environment (see Chapter 18). It is, of course, difficult to exercise rigorous control over variables in such a real-life situation and this needs to be remembered when evaluating gains in ecological validity.

Another way that psychologists have responded to the criticism concerning the artificiality and narrowness of the experiment is by investigating human behaviour with the use of other methods. These include observations, case studies, surveys and correlational studies.

Observational studies

Often, for practical and ethical reasons, it would be inappropriate to use an experimental design. In the study of child development, for example, it has been the observational method that has dominated much research into attachment and childrearing. Some observational studies are conducted in a laboratory setting (e.g. Ainsworth's strange situation; see Chapter 18); others are carried out in the natural environment (naturalistic observation). As with the experimental method there is always the problem that people who know that they are being observed will behave differently. For this reason, covert observation is sometimes used where people are unaware that they are being observed. This can be done by the use of hidden recording devices within a laboratory type of setting or by having the observer participate with those whose behaviour is under study; that is, the observer works incognito. This technique, while raising ethical concerns, has sometimes been used by social psychologists when investigating the behaviour of groups/crowds (e.g.

Waddington, Jones and Critcher, 1987). Clinical observations also provide a valuable source of information. Freud's theory of personality development (see Chapter 3) was, in large part, derived from the clinical observations he made of his clients' problems.

Case studies

Case studies allow psychologists to study naturally occurring events. The method involves looking at single cases or events, usually an individual but sometimes a pair or small groups. Case studies of people with amnesia, for instance, have revealed interesting features about the process of memory (see Chapter 8). The case studies of stroke and head-injured patients have contributed much to knowledge about how the brain functions (see Chapter 11). The main limitation of the case study method relates to the question of how typical these cases are, and, therefore, the extent to which one can generalize from the findings.

Many case studies (e.g. Koluchova's (1972) study of twin boys found after seven years of extreme privation) involve reconstructing a biography of the person/people, usually based on available records and on what is remembered. This retrospective method has problems associated with it, as forgetfulness and distorted memories are common occurrences (see Chapter 8). Nevertheless, despite its limitations, the case study method has provided some startling insights into psychological processes and development.

Surveys

By the use of surveys based on structured questionnaires or interviews, psychologists are able to gather information about people which it would not be possible to acquire by any other means. Rather than observe a person's behaviour, one can simply ask if the behaviour is practised. Of course, there are no guarantees that the answer will be an accurate reflection of the behaviour. Individuals may try to present themselves in a favourable light, especially if the survey is conducted by having the investigator administer the questions in person, rather than using a postal questionnaire. This method improves the response rate compared to postal surveys, but is liable to bias effects. Nevertheless, the use of questionnaires has revealed much of interest about people's attitudes and beliefs as well as about their behaviour. See Chapters 5 and 6 for further examples.

Correlational studies

Correlational studies look at relationships between variables; for example, the relationship between certain behaviours and health outcomes. (See Box 7.3, p. 138

for further information about correlations.) If one wanted to use an experimental design to establish whether or not cigarette smoking really caused lung cancer in humans, one would run into considerable ethical and practical difficulties. At least two groups of people would be required. They would need to be matched on all potentially confounding variables, such as health status and age. The control group would not smoke while the experimental group(s) would be required to smoke a fixed number of cigarettes per day. For how long should such an experiment run before one reached a conclusion about the link between smoking and lung cancer? How could one control for all the other factors that might affect a person's susceptibility to the disease, e.g. environmental pollutants, passive smoking? Obviously, this type of investigation is impracticable. Correlational studies, however, have shown that people who smoke are more likely to develop lung cancer than those who do not, and that the heaviest smokers are most at risk. Nevertheless, the fact that these findings are correlational – that is, they show a relationship (not a cause and effect link) between smoking and lung cancer – allows tobacco companies to say there is no conclusive proof that smoking causes cancer in humans. Findings from animal studies have, however, demonstrated this causal link in several non-human species. For this reason, and because of the evidence from studies of the distribution and determinants of disease in human populations (that is, epidemiological studies), the link between smoking and cancer has been established to the satisfaction of most people.

Attempts to establish whether there is a relationship between levels of aggressive behaviour and watching violence on television is another area where correlational studies have been employed. The direction of the causal link, should one exist, continues to provoke debate among media pundits and psychologists alike. You might consider the problems that would arise if one tried experimentally to test the hypothesis that there is a causal link between watching television violence and levels of aggressive behaviour.

Meta-analysis

You will notice that, in some areas of psychology, studies produce conflicting results. In order to see if there is a general pattern discernible among the many sets of quantitative data, a set of statistical techniques may be used to detect trends. In this way, the results of independent studies are statistically integrated into what is called a meta-analysis. Ajzen and Fishbein (1977), for example, used meta-analysis in their work on attitudes and behaviour (see Chapter 5).

Qualitative methods

Some psychologists have preferred to use qualitative rather than quantitative methods. Quantitative methods produce numerical data. However, some human experiences would lose their meaning if one tried to reduce them to a set of numbers. For instance, the way people experience hospitalization might be better understood by using an open-ended interview, rather than asking them to tick boxes on a structured questionnaire or respond to structured questions in an interview. During such a procedure, interviewees are allowed to reveal *their* way of seeing things without the interviewer imposing any preconceived framework on how the interview should proceed. This type of interviewing requires sensitivity and skill. For more information on this technique and other qualitative methods, including participant observation, see Seale (1994). See also pp. 5–6 above.

Most psychologists consider it useful to gain evidence by employing a variety of methodologies. Since no method is entirely free of criticism, the skill of the psychologist involves trying to minimize the problems rather than trying to eliminate them.

The work of psychologists

Only the briefest of outlines is given here about the work that psychologists do. For a more thorough account see the British Psychological Society (1988, 1989).

The majority of people graduating with a psychology degree do not become professional psychologists. The knowledge and transferable skills acquired while studying psychology equip one for a variety of careers. Many psychology graduates can be found, for example, in teaching, nursing and management consultancy. For those who do become professional practitioners, the most common occupation is clinical psychologist. In the course of your work as a health care professional, this is the group you are most likely to encounter. Professional psychology specialisms are described below.

Professional psychologists

Clinical, counselling and health psychologists apply their knowledge to problems associated with health and illness. Most, but by no means all, clinical psychologists are employed in the National Health Service and work with people who are mentally ill or who have learning difficulties. They often work in multidisciplinary teams and use their understanding of behaviour to adopt a problem-solving approach to help clients deal with their difficulties. Health psychologists are typically more concerned with the role of psychological factors in physical health and illness. To date, the professional status of clinical psychology is different from that of health psychology as its training route is more established. The work of counselling psychologists overlaps that of clinical psychologists, although usually it is concerned with less serious problems. Commonly, counselling psychologists will deal with vocational, personal or academic problems.

Educational psychologists are concerned with the problems and wellbeing of children and young people. They are usually employed by local education authorities. Their work includes assessing children who are thought to have special educational needs, counselling children and their parents, devising behaviour modification programmes and advising teachers on issues related to curriculum planning and school organization.

Occupational psychologists are interested in how people perform at work and how organizational systems affect employees' behaviour. Their aims are to increase an organization's effectiveness and to raise the level of job satisfaction for the employee. Occupational psychologists may work in organizational consultancy, assessment and training and in ergonomics, health and safety. Both the public and the private sector employ occupational psychologists.

Criminological and legal psychologists (sometimes called forensic psychologists) may undertake a number of different jobs. These may include doing therapeutic work with offenders, participating in the running of a prison or other secure establishment, providing expert testimony about a person's level of impairment in a court case to fix compensation following an accident, carrying out research into what psychological factors underlie different types of offence, helping the police to 'profile' a suspect. Forensic psychologists usually work within the prison department, in special hospitals or in secure units. Some work in academic departments in universities.

Teaching and research psychologists work in universities, colleges and schools. Their work involves preparing and teaching psychology on many different courses and carrying out research. At higher education level, most academic psychologists have specialist interests and many are professionally qualified to practise.

Organization and features of the book

This is a topic-based text with free-standing chapters which may be read in any order. However, frequent cross-references between chapters are made, enabling readers to follow up particular topics. The twenty-five chapters are organized into five parts and each part begins with a short introduction.

Part I focuses on the different roles of health professionals. Part II examines the way in which psychological concepts can be applied to the nursing situation. Life processes and events that are relevant to health care professionals are discussed in Part III. Part IV considers topics that will be of particular interest to those who work with children. Those who work with elderly people will be particularly interested in Part V.

A major feature of this book is its up-to-date treatment of a wide range of areas in psychology allied to a depth of coverage seldom found in texts written for non-psychologists. Nevertheless, one must acknowledge that the psychological literature does not adequately address all the issues that are of current concern. Much research in psychology has tended to be presented as culture-free, as though the historical period in which it was conducted, or the ethnic identity of its participants, were irrelevant. It is important that nurses recognize the limitations as well as the strengths of the psychological literature when they are evaluating its findings within today's heterogeneous society.

The contributors to this volume believe that psychology has much to offer those who work in health care. Not only do they hold to the belief that those studying to become health care professionals will benefit from knowing about many aspects of psychology, but they also believe that there is a need to avoid superficial treatment of these areas. Frequently, in their roles as teachers, the contributors have found a demand for more detailed psychological material relating to health care than is available in most psychology texts written for this group of students. It is hoped that this book will satisfy that demand. By its breadth and depth of coverage, the book aims to increase students' and health professionals' awareness of how a knowledge of psychology can contribute towards a better understanding of their practice.

To facilitate this process, each chapter contains Discussion Points to encourage reflection on the material and how it applies to practical health care concerns. Likewise, Seminar Questions are included to help students and tutors make optimum use of the material covered. Throughout the text, links between theory and practice are made explicit. Within each chapter, new technical terms are highlighted and defined. The use of Boxes to provide additional or special interest material, along with illustrative figures and tables, is intended to enhance the reader's understanding.

At the beginning of each chapter there is a Chapter Outline and at the end there is a Summary. It is hoped that these two features will enable the reader to peruse the contents of each chapter quickly. The Index will help readers locate issues of particular interest. At the end of each chapter, in addition to the References, a list of annotated Further Reading is provided, so that the reader who wishes to pursue a topic in more detail can obtain accessible information. Tutors as well as students may find this useful.

Further reading

For a good introduction to psychology it is still difficult to better R.L. Atkinson *et al.* (1993) *Introduction to Psychology*, 11th edition. New York: Harcourt Brace. For those who prefer a text written by a British author, then two, published for the A level market, provide sound accounts: N. Hayes (1994) *Foundations of Psychology: An introductory text*. London: Routledge and R. Gross (1992) *Psychology: The science of mind and behaviour*, 2nd edition. London: Hodder & Stoughton.

Another useful book for those interested in the different approaches and methods of psychology is M.W. Eysenck (1994) *Perspectives on Psychology*. Hove: Lawrence Erlbaum. This text is a lucid account of the current approaches and historical roots of psychology, its research methods and some of the major issues that have engaged psychologists, such as free will versus determinism and nature versus nurture.

For those who wish to know more about qualitative research methods, a good starting place is C. Seale (1994) 'Qualitative methods in sociology and anthropology', in K. McConway (ed.) *Studying Health and Disease*, 2nd edition. Milton Keynes: Open University Press. This chapter clearly describes the ethnographic methods of participant observation and qualitative interviewing. An introduction is also given into how qualitative researchers might analyze and report their findings.

Another excellent account of many research techniques, including chapters on meta-analysis and qualitative research, is provided by C.M. Judd, E.R. Smith and L.H. Kidder (1991) *Research Methods in Social Relations*, 6th edition. New York: Holt, Rinehart & Winston.

A good introduction to cultural/discursive psychology in the health area is given by W. Stainton Rogers (1991) *Explaining Health and Illness*. Hemel Hempstead: Harvester Wheatsheaf.

References

Ajzen, I. and Fishbein, M. (1977) 'Attitude–behaviour relationships: A theoretical analysis and review of empirical research', *Psychological Bulletin* **84**, 888–918.

Atkinson R.L., Atkinson, R.C., Smith, E.E. and Bem, D.J. (1993) *Introduction to Psychology*, 11th edition. New York: Harcourt Brace.

British Psychological Society (1988) *Career Choices in Psychology.* London: BPS.

British Psychological Society (1989) *How about Psychology? A guide to courses and careers.* London: BPS.

Ebbinghaus, H. (1885) *Memory: A contribution to experimental psychology*, rev. edition 1964. New York: Dover

Eysenck, H.J. (1982) *Personality, genetics and behaviour.* New York: Praeger.

Harré, R. (1979) *Social Being.* Oxford: Basil Blackwell.

James, W. (1890) *Principles of Psychology.* New York: Holt.

Koluchova, J. (1972) 'Severe deprivation in twins: A case study', *Journal of Child Psychology and Psychiatry* **13**, 107–14.

Massarik, F. (1981) 'The interviewing process re-examined', in P. Reason and J. Rowan (eds.) *Human Enquiry: A source book of new paradigm research.* Chichester: John Wiley.

Potter, J. and Wetherell, M. (1987) *Discourse and Social Psychology: Beyond attitudes and behaviour.* London: Sage.

Seale, C. (1994) 'Qualitative methods in Sociology and anthropology', in K. McConway (ed.) *Studying Health and Disease*, 2nd edition. Milton Keynes: Open University Press.

Waddington, D., Jones, K. and Critcher, C. (1987) 'Flashpoints of public disorder', in G. Gaskell and R. Benewick (eds.) *The crowd in contemporary Britain.* London: Sage.

Watson, J.B. (1913) 'Psychology from the standpoint of a behaviourist', *Psychological Review* **20**, 158–77.

Wundt, W. (1905) *Grundriss der Psychologie.* Leipzig: Engelmann.

The roles of
health care professionals

Many people are involved in providing health care, some paid to do so, others providing their services voluntarily. Those who work as health care professionals are often employed by large organizations and they are involved in a number of different roles with patients or clients and with each other. Working alongside other people brings its satisfaction and its frustrations. Inevitably, there will be differences of opinion. The health professional, however, will always need to work cooperatively with patients, clients and colleagues to ensure that good care is provided. Part I addresses topics relevant to this issue.

Chapter 1 begins with an examination of some models of organization and how these relate to health care situations. In this way a wider context is established for the remaining topics in this part of the book. Chapter 2 focuses on the way we form impressions of others and the way in which these impressions may influence interactions between health professionals and their clients. The importance of group influences and processes are discussed in Chapter 3, which proposes a psychodynamic approach as a means of accounting for the research findings that are discussed. When considering the role of health professionals in providing care, it is important to remember that the family has a crucial part to play. Chapter 4 reminds us that we need to take account of their role if we are to understand fully the nature of illness and people's reactions to it. Attention is drawn to the diverse nature of what is covered by the term 'family'.

There is now considerable agreement among health professionals that factors such as attitudes and beliefs make significant contributions in determining whether people will adopt healthy behaviours and how they will respond to illness. Health professionals need to understand these processes to be effective in their interaction with patients or clients. Chapters 5 and 6 consider these issues. Chapter 5 also examines the extent to which the techniques for changing attitudes might be useful to the health professional; while in Chapter 6, Harris and Middleton widen the discussion to explore the roles of intention, self-efficacy and optimism in adopting and maintaining healthy behaviours. They provide a critical analysis of selected social cognition models of health.

CHAPTER 1

Models of organization for nursing practice

JOANNA DODD

Chapter outline

Introduction
Organizations as conceptual entities
Models and approaches to organizations in psychology
Organizations as functional structures
Organizations as accountability relationships
Organizations as cultures
Summary: models of organization in nursing practice

Introduction

While studying as a student and when employed as a nurse, you will have to deal with large organizations. These will have a considerable impact on what you are required to do and are able to achieve; they will also have an effect on your sense of wellbeing and satisfaction. All of you will experience organizations where you feel comfortable and those in which you feel uncomfortable, even when the jobs are similar.

Chapters 14 and 15 deal with particular aspects of motivation, stress and anxiety at work. The aim of the present chapter is to offer some general insights into some of the models used by organizational psychologists to understand and explain the day-to-day consequences for the individual of working in a complex organization. The contribution of social science in health organizations is becoming increasingly relevant as 'caring for the carers' is recognized as an important factor in the wellbeing of patients.

The aim of organizational psychology is to understand and solve problems at work. The metaphor underpinning this is that, like people, organizations can be healthy or 'diseased'. In people parts of the body become dysfunctional; in organizations 'disease' can be seen in the way the relationships within them operate. The assumption is that effective organizations have healthy relationships whereas ineffective organizations have working relationships that have broken down in some way. We have all experienced directly or heard accounts of failure of communication at work or personality clashes. These are signs that a working relationship has broken down. Therefore, diagnosing difficulties in these relationships is the path to 'curing' the problem and helping all the people in an organization perform more effectively. The perspective of this chapter is that organizational psychology is a 'technology' (Hollway, 1984). That is to say, it is an applied field, rather like engineering in the physical sciences. Hence its effectiveness must be judged by its applications. Knowledge in this area is significant in the way it contributes to the understanding of specific and immediate situations in the workplace. The different models which will be outlined later provide a resource for generating different explanations. It is not appropriate to present theories in isolation without describing actual problems, since discussing these can illuminate how a theoretical idea can aid understanding. Therefore, throughout this chapter relevant examples from consultancy will be used to describe the models used.

One of the central assumptions to psychology is that people differ in their attitudes, skills, knowledge and in the way they take in and process ideas and information (see Chapter 7). One aim of psychology is to understand and account for these differences. The various branches of psychology deal with this issue in different ways. Organizational psychology focuses on the implications of these differences for behaviour at work; specifically, the differences between people in the way they 'construct' their ideas about their workplace and the different contributions each individual makes to the organization in which they work. The term 'construct' is widely used in psychology to describe how people act like 'scientists', gathering information from experience, which they build into 'models', from which they make predictions about future events. Although it is assumed that all people process experience in this way, the ideas or 'constructs' that are produced can differ widely, even though people may appear to have had the same experience.

The differences between people in terms of their skills, knowledge and their ways of understanding and explaining problems is a tremendous resource for an organization. For example, it is difficult to imagine one person trying to fulfil all the roles needed if a community drug team is to operate effectively. However, these important differences can also be a source of disagreement, confusion and misunderstanding. All too often when such differences occur an attempt is made to blame one person for the mistake or to argue that one person's assessment of a situation was incorrect. This can lead to the process of scapegoating – rather than solving the problem, the blame is attached to one individual. Organizational psychology, on the other hand, aims to locate problems in the nature of relationships rather than in individuals. After reading this chapter, I hope you will be encouraged to try to understand the problems you experience at work in a way that focuses on organizations rather than individuals, so you can begin to find lasting solutions to the difficulties you may face at work in the future. (See also Chapter 25 for a discussion of the systems approach to health care.)

Organizations as conceptual entities

Organizations used to be understood as physical phenomena with goals and characteristics which could be investigated, rather in the way you might investigate the behaviour of a fish or the physical nature of a tree. Now it is increasingly being recognized that organizations are conceptual entities. (See Mangham, 1987; Morgan, 1986; Silverman, 1971.) This is based on the theory that people need to make sense of the situations they find themselves in, and, in doing so 'construct' situational models to help them predict what responses are likely to be elicited by each of their actions. This also happens in the workplace. However, we can never have direct experience of all parts of an organization, so we have to use our imagination, together with our preconceptions and experiences, to complete the picture. The resultant picture serves as a framework when we make decisions about how to operate at work and is constructed from the interaction with the parts of an organization that we can have contact with: the people, the policies, the products. Therefore, when we talk about the characteristics of the organization we work for, we are describing what our imagination has created from our expectations and experiences. All people employed by an organization or who have contact with it are involved in the same process. This is as true for an organizational psychologist as it is for a community psychiatric nurse. This means that for any one place of employment, no two people will necessarily have created the same 'conceptual entity'.

Morgan (1986) has discussed the different metaphors that people can use in interpreting events within organizations. He suggests that we are all involved in 'reading' the organizational situations we find ourselves in, but that some people are more skilled than others:

> Effective managers . . . have become skilled in the art of 'reading' the situations that they are attempting to organize or manage. This skill usually develops as an intuitive process, learned through experience and natural ability. . . . For this reason it is often believed that effective managers and problem solvers are born and not made. If we take a closer look at the processes used however, we find that this is often based on an ability to develop deep appreciation of the situations being addressed. (Morgan, 1986: 11)

Morgan goes on to suggest that the key to this skill is a diversity of possible frameworks or metaphors at an individual's disposal. Mangham (1987) extends this idea by suggesting that it is not just skill at reading situations which influences how we respond; rather, we improvise our behaviour in the light of the context we have created. We struggle to make sense of things and take action in the context we have created. Nevertheless, we can never know that others have constructed a similar context. People frequently do not create the same understanding when working in the same environment, and organizational development consultants are often called in to help clarify the problems that result from misunderstandings. The exercise in Box 1.1 is designed to illustrate the points we have made about different understandings as a source of confusion. It allows you to begin to apply this approach in your own work/learning situation. (For supporting texts, see Grint, 1991; Hassard and Pym, 1990; Mangham, 1987; Morgan, 1986.) This diversity in explanation is as evident in the literature on organizational psychology as it is in day-to-day work.

BOX 1.1 **UNDERSTANDING YOUR IMMEDIATE ORGANIZATION**

The purpose of this exercise is to begin to recognize that when we state that organizations are conceptual entities, the implication is that to identify and solve problems we need to explore the understanding that each individual has generated. To do this, we have to accept that these are all valid interpretations of the situation. Frequently, when problems arise in the workplace, one particular person, or one particular task is blamed. However, difficult situations in the workplace are usually much more complicated than this, with many different factors playing a part.

   My first activity when working as a consultant to an organization with a problem is to try to understand how each individual constructs and explains a problem. It is worth attempting a similar exercise yourself by acting as a 'consultant' attempting to understand how you 'construct' ideas at work, school or home. Start by thinking about one situation you found difficult to deal with last week and explore the factors that were involved in making it a problem and in resolving the problem. For example, it could be a difficulty in understanding a new procedure or dealing with a 'difficult' patient or a conflict with a classmate or family member. Do this by taking the following steps:

1. Describe the situation and how it developed.
2. State what you expected to happen at each key point, whether or not your expectations were met and how having your expectation met, or not met, influenced how the situation then developed.
3. Use this information to describe the 'constructs', the problem and its context which made you expect certain things and not others. For example, if it was a new procedure, did you expect it to be easy or difficult? If it was a 'difficult' patient, did you expect to be supported by your colleagues?
4. Identify how many other people you had to relate to about this event. Examples of the types of relationships to think about are those you have with the people involved in your work; your patients or clients, your boss, your immediate colleagues and members of other departments, your parents, your spouse, your children.
5. If you wish to take this a little further, consider what other 'constructs' are used. Take each of the individuals you have identified in (4) above and try to describe the 'constructs' about this problem each used.

(See also Morgan, 1986.)

Models and approaches to organizations in psychology

Problems arising in the workplace are understood in organizational psychology in many different ways. This is evident in the range of models that have been proposed, each built up from experience in work contexts. Although all the models claim to provide a comprehensive explanation, in fact they tend to provide insight into some problems but not others. An analogy can be drawn with the growing interest in alternative or complementary medicine: the way the body is visualized by an acupuncturist is very different from the way it is seen by conventional, Western doctors; however, each view has its advantages and access to both offers a greater resource for understanding health and disease processes.

As this is an introduction to a large field, three models only have been chosen to illustrate the diverse ways that organizations are viewed by organizational psychology (see Morgan, 1986). The first allows us to diagnose and solve problems between departments in organizations; the second allows the diagnosis and solution of manager–subordinate problems; and the third allows us to understand the ways in which habitual patterns of behaviour are maintained within social groups. The three models are as follows:

1. *Organizations as functional structures.* Mintzberg's (1979, 1983) *Structure in Fives* sees organizations as comprising different functional components. For example, the different functions that Mintzberg might identify within the health service would be: treating patients, the managing of budgets and the administration of records. The purpose of this model is to provide a way of describing the organizational structure needed to integrate separate functions and the types of coordinating mechanisms used.
2. *Organizations as accountability relationships.* Jaques's (1986, 1989) Jaques and Clements (1991) stratified systems theory identifies a general pattern of levels of work found in all organizational hierarchies. This model suggests that, as a consequence of individual differences in capability, there are well-balanced and imbalanced managerial relationships.
3. *Organizations as cultures.* This approach looks at the social processes within organizations which produce the same patterns of behaviour even though the individuals employed change. Interest here has grown from a concern to explain the observed resistance to change in many organizations. This is one of the approaches to organizations which focus on processes at work within organizations and how organizational systems are arranged to permit or inhibit the flow of information, people or products (Hollway, 1991; Morgan, 1986).

Organizations as functional structures

In *Structure in Fives*, Mintzberg (1983) suggests that organizations exist to achieve more complex work than an individual can achieve working alone (see Payne, in Warr, 1987). He divides organizations into different sections and identifies different functions which need to be coordinated. The aim is: (1) to produce a comprehensive description of all organizations with a minimum number of categories; (2) to relate the structure of these different parts to the function each fulfils; and (3) to apply this classification to all organizations. This last aim is a difficult task as there are so many different types of organizations: a local tennis club, a regional health authority and a multinational corporation are all organizations, but they have widely different structures.

   In addition to describing the structure, Mintzberg has produced a method of classifying the ways in which collective human activity can be coordinated, in terms of
mechanisms of communication. By combining an understanding of the different parts
of organizations and the different coordinating devices, he hoped to identify which
approaches to coordination work most effectively with which types of organization.
His model describes five basic parts to an organization, five coordination devices and
five types of organization. Three of the five parts concern the delivery of goods and
services (1–3 below); the other two (4–5) provide support to the central core.

1. *The strategic apex* (i.e. the top of the organization) is where decisions are taken
   and communicated about the direction of the organization and where resources
   will be allocated. In health care this comprises, for example, the chief executive
   of a trust and the board of directors of the various services.
2. *The middle line* has the responsibility for ensuring that the decisions made by
   the strategic apex are executed. This comprises day-to-day management. In a
   hospital this would include those who manage budgets for various aspects of
   health care and those who are responsible for ensuring that all the necessary
   resources for the efficient running of the services are available.
3. *The operating core* actually undertakes the day-to-day work of ensuring that
   the goods or services are delivered. In health care this comprises those nurses,
   doctors and others who take responsibility for the direct care of patients. It is
   through these people that the purpose of the organization is realized.
4. *The support structure* consists of those functions which provide the
   'housekeeping' services, e.g. building maintenance, cleaning, laundry and
   management of accounts. One important example from health care is the
   department responsible for the maintenance of patient records and the
   notification of appointments.
5. *The technostructure* comprises those professionals or technical specialists with
   knowledge relevant to the delivery of specialist services. In health care, as in many
   other organizations, one of the key functions in this category is the personnel and
   training support who co-ordinate the selection and development of staff.

   Different organizations have different arrangements for these parts. Mintzberg
describes these as different types of organization and suggests that these exist
because of the relative importance of different functions in differing endeavours.
Each of these five structures are given below:

1. *Simple structures* describe those organizations with a predominantly strategic apex
   and operating core. An example in health care would be a voluntary organization
   which has a central office and many regional projects run by volunteers.
2. *A professional bureaucracy* is mainly comprised of an operating core of self-
   managing professional staff with a small strategic apex and some support
   structure. The technostructure may well be bought in on a consultancy basis
   when necessary. Many doctors' practices are run along these lines, with doctors
   in partnership sharing the support costs of their work.

3. *A machine bureaucracy* has a balanced contribution from all the parts described above. A regional health authority is an example of this type of organization.
4. *A divisionalized form* is predominantly a middle line and operating core, with all the other parts retained in a separate 'parent' organization. The move away from coordinating regional health authorities towards self-governing trusts reporting to outposts of the NHS management executive represents an example of this in health care.
5. *An adhocracy* describes those organizations where the operating core is separated from other parts of the organization as rapid response to changing conditions is necessary. This is seen increasingly in teaching environments, where multiple changes continuously overturn patterns of work.

The coordination of the various parts into a coherent whole is extremely complex. To help understand this, Mintzberg has produced a classification which identifies five coordination devices: two (1–2) involve interpersonal interaction and three involve employing standards (3–5):

1. *Mutual adjustment* is the approach we all use in our day-to-day lives; for example, chatting with others to exchange relevant information and modifying our actions and intentions accordingly.
2. *Direct supervision* involves a similar activity, but is undertaken more formally, usually with a manager ensuring that information is passed, in the form of briefing sessions, say, and that the consequent actions are monitored.
3. *Standardizing the input* involves establishing a base line of education and training requirements. Nursing education, examinations and registration are good examples of this as they help ensure that new personnel have the necessary knowledge and skills.
4. *Standardizing the process* tends to be applied to coordinating repetitive work by drawing up sets of rules designed to standardize the way in which tasks are performed, e.g. the procedure established for the insertion of a drip.
5. *Standardizing the output* concentrates on prescribing an acceptable quality of service or goods and then monitoring to ensure that this is achieved.

These issues and concepts are explored in Box 1.2.

Organizations as accountability relationships

In this section, I shall consider Jaques's (1986) model of hierarchy in organizations (Jaques, 1986; Whittington and Bellaby, 1979). Jaques's model starts with a similar question to that underpinning Mintzberg's (1979) work. How can people best be organized for organizations to succeed in their complex objectives? However, whereas Mintzberg (1979) focused on categorizing the different functions in an organization, Jaques's (1986) model seeks to categorize the levels in hierarchies and to describe the necessary features of manager–subordinate relationships. His

---

BOX 1.2 CHANGES IN ORGANIZATIONAL STRUCTURE

For reasons of confidentiality, this case does not describe any one specific organization, but is constructed out of material gained from various consultancy activities.

In the early 1990s all the providers of mental health care in one district in London succeeded in their bid for trust status. To become a trust, a 'critical mass' of services needed to be incorporated to be able to cover the costs of managing the necessary systems for fulfilling the requirements of the new funding arrangements. The management of this new trust had acquired funding for community and inpatient psychiatric care. They had also secured funding for various counselling and outreach services for drug users and people with alcohol problems. This had taken two years and considerable effort on the part of the mental health executive of the district health authority.

To achieve this, a new organization had been established. The trust was headed by a chief executive to whom senior managers from nursing, community nursing, psychiatry, psychology, medical and development reported. The development function included sections responsible for managing contract information and quality assurance. This latter function was seen as essential as the executive recognized that when new contracts were allocated, it would be necessary to account for expenditure, quantity and quality of provision. In recognition of this, increased budget and resourcing responsibilities were allocated to the managers of wards and community services. In the past, each ward had limited accountability for expenditure and the freedom to use their own, frequently undocumented, quality assurance procedures. Now standardized systems for budgeting and quality assurance were identified as crucial. Recruitment was also passed to this level. In addition, the administrative staff were cut in an effort to reduce overheads.

- What parts of an organization can you identify in the above description?
- What type of organization do you think this new trust is?
- What type of organization do you think it has changed from to become a trust?
- What coordination devices are needed within and between these parts to ensure that the new organization can function effectively?

(See also Warr, 1987: ch. 14.)

---

observations made in many different contexts (for example, health care, business and the armed forces) led Jaques (1986) to suggest that a repeated pattern of seven levels of work exists, regardless of the type of work undertaken by the organization. These levels differ according to the complexity of the work required. The first four are outlined in the summary descriptions in Box 1.3.

Jaques (1986) argues that the existence of hierarchies across different employment organizations is an expression of fundamental differences between people in their ability to handle complexity. Evidence for such differences led Jaques (1986) to suggest that the reason people produce hierarchies is that hierarchies meet the needs of most people to have others who are more able to handle complexity working at a level higher in the hierarchy than themselves.

BOX 1.3 **DESCRIPTIONS OF LEVELS OF WORK**

Level I

Description: The output from such work and the methods and resources for this work can be completely specified beforehand. This work comprises concrete tasks which may be prescribed. An example of creativity at this level might be the care a hospital porter takes not to knock a stretcher against a wall.

Responsibilities: To work on one task at a time to achieve a specific goal. To follow instructions until a task is complete or a problem does arise; if a problem arises, to follow a previously learned solution or report back.

Level II

Description: The output of the work cannot be specified precisely, but has to be judged according to the needs of each situation as it arises. Work at this level involves serving people working at level I by supporting their work and ensuring safe working conditions. In addition, it involves providing a service to customers, or in the case of health care to people with illnesses, and in sensitively assessing and responding to their needs. An example from health care is the work of a community nurse diagnosing the changing needs of an elderly patient living at home and ensuring that appropriate services are provided at the appropriate times, or the work of a staff nurse explaining a procedure or observation to a student nurse.

Responsibilities: To deal with each situation and resolve it; to improve practice by making it explicit and discussing the way work is done; to explain why work is done in a particular way; to demonstrate how a specific task needs to be undertaken.

Level III

Description: To construct, implement and fine-tune systems that can cope with the fluctuating resource demands of a given area of work. An example from health care is the construction and running of the system for allocating duties to ensure that all staff are given an adequate balance of work and rest to be effective, while at the same time ensuring that the ward is adequately staffed.

Responsibilities: To imagine all the possible practices and systems that might be used and select those that maintain the efficiency of the current situation but are flexible enough to respond to changing conditions; to make the best possible use of all the resources available including people, finances and technologies in getting the work done.

Level IV

Description: The work is to manage the relationship between the future viability of the organization and the current operational practices. An example from health care is the work of the director of the development function in a trust.

Responsibilities: To set the framework for existing work by allocating resources; to manage the development of new systems and practices; to integrate new developments with established procedures; to close departments and stop work that is no longer viable. Following Baker and Stamp (1992).

BOX 1.4 **MANAGERIAL RELATIONSHIPS IN NURSING**

I described in Box 1.2 a shift from district health authority organization to trust organization. One aspect of these changes involved reviewing the status and grading of nurses on an acute psychiatric ward. To gain trust status, the staff from two wards had been combined which meant that there were three G grade charge nurses (the highest grade on this ward) allocated to this ward, four F grades and the remaining were E grades (the lowest grade on this ward).

Various problems had been identified by key personnel:

1. The trust executive were concerned that there were too many higher grade nurses employed on these wards.
2. The E grade nurses complained that they were unclear about what distinguished them from F grade nurses in terms of their responsibilities.
3. The F grade nurses also said that they were unclear about their role in relation to E grade nurses. They did not feel that they had been given adequate scope to supervise staff.
4. All staff nurses complained that they were unclear about whom they had to take instruction from on those occasions when two G grade nurses were present on a shift.
5. They all complained of one G grade nurse, who, when in charge, tended to focus on giving complicated instructions on therapeutic interventions, while not dealing with the day-to-day running of the ward.

It was decided that this would be investigated as an issue of confused line management relationships. The wards had been merged with no consideration for the staff involved, but only for the contractual requirements of the trust application. Investigation of this situation using the levels of work model gave some possible causes of the problems and some options for action.

An analysis of the work of staff psychiatric nurses suggested that the work is at level II – that is, deciding on particular responses to individual patients. This work was being undertaken by all E and F grade nurses. Looking at the current staffing, it could be seen that the E grades were all in appropriate situations for their capability. However, the structure above them was very unclear, with the result that they were not receiving an adequate level of managerial support. For three F grade nurses this same level of work was also appropriate. Their F grade was an acknowledgement of their long experience; it did not mean that they should have a supervisory role.

The running of the ward involved staff allocation, quality assurance and other administrative functions to ensure the most efficient use of ward resources. The requirements of the trust had made this level III role much clearer. This was the work of the G grade nurses. However, one of the F grade nurses was clearly capable of undertaking level III work and was very frustrated by the lack of opportunity. Occasionally, she was allocated charge nurse duties as her capability was recognized, but more often she tried inappropriately to take charge when working as a staff nurse.

Two G grade nurses were appropriately employed but the one identified as problematic, was capable of level IV work. This was expressed in her interest in the research and development of alternative therapeutic options rather than managing the ward. This meant that when she was on duty, the staff felt abandoned as the operational management was overlooked.

Using the levels described above and the rules about successful managerial relationships discuss what could be done to resolve this situation by:

1. Drawing an appropriate organizational chart.
2. Making recommendation about possible developments for individuals.

(See also Jaques, 1986: esp. chs. 4, 6 and 8; Whittington and Bellaby, 1979.)

The term 'capability' describes the individual decision-making involved in choosing, from the many different possible courses of action, the one most appropriate to the actual circumstances. It is the number of different variables which need to be manipulated and the duration of the uncertainty about the choices which contribute to the complexity of the work. Jaques (1986) argues that hierarchical forms help to 'manage' the uncertainty inherent in working. Hierarchies need to be designed so that individuals in different levels are coordinated through appropriate managerial relationships. These relationships have two necessary conditions to be effective.

First, those who have managerial authority over others must also have managerial accountability for the work of their subordinates. (See Evans (1979) for a detailed account.) Briefly, a manager can only have the authority to delegate work to someone else if the manager is then accountable to more senior people in the organization for the output of that person. Problems frequently arise when an employee is required to do something by another person, but where that other person has no responsibility for the outcome and so is free to make unreasonable demands.

Second, the manager must hold a position at one level above their subordinates: individuals working at level I in Box 1.3, must be managed by someone at level II, and so on. Employees can have other types of working relationship with people of *any* level, but the *managerial* relationship must be at one level above. (Situations often arise where the capability of an individual does not match the level of work he or she has been given. However, for the purposes of this discussion, we are assuming that the demands of the level of work and the individual capability are matched.) If the manager works at the same level, then their subordinates will feel crowded; on the other hand, if the manager works at more than one level away, subordinates will feel abandoned. These issues are explored in Box 1.4.

DISCUSSION POINT
Discuss the similarities and differences between Mintzberg's *Structure in Fives* and Jaques's *Levels of Work*.

Organizations as cultures

This approach is an attempt to explore organizations from the perspective of processes within them; it therefore contrasts with the two previous approaches which focus on structure. The original models which looked at organizations in this way used the metaphor of organizations as biological systems. The more recent models apply the study of social processes in other contexts to organizations. For example, as a concept, 'culture' has been widely used to describe the collective characteristics of a social group (see Morgan, 1986: ch. 5). It has become increasingly common in recent years to apply this notion to employment organizations (Hollway, 1991). There are two reasons for using the concept of culture to investigate organizations. First, it focuses on 'meaning' or the interpretations that individual members of an organization put upon events. The importance of this is highlighted by Martin (1992: 3):

> as individuals come into contact with organizations, they come into contact with dress norms, stories people tell about what goes on, the organization's formal rules and procedures, its informal codes of behaviour, rituals, tasks, pay systems, jargon, and jokes only understood by insiders, and so on. These elements are some of the manifestations of organizational culture. When cultural members interpret the meaning of these manifestations, their perceptions, memories, beliefs, experiences and values will vary, so interpretations will differ – even of the same phenomena. The patterns or configurations of these interpretations, and the ways they are enacted, constitute culture.

Second, it provides a useful way of exploring change, resistance to change and performance in organizations.

The study of organizations as cultures has its roots in two broad strands of social science. These are (1) anthropology, which is the study of the ways different groups of people in different parts of the world act, and (2) the psychological study of work, which has recently been seeking broader explanatory principles than those already discussed. The two have been combined to produce a growing field of investigation. The reason for looking at employment organizations in this way is outlined by Handy (1981: 176) thus:

> organisations are as different as the nations and societies of the world. They have differing cultures – sets of values and norms and beliefs – reflected in different structures and systems. The cultures are affected by the events of the past and by the climate of the present, by the technology and the type of work, by their aims and the kind of people that work in them.

The phenomenon called 'culture' functions as an 'adaptive-regulatory mechanism' (Smircich, 1983) uniting individuals into social processes which are consistent over time, regardless of changes to the membership of the group (see Chapter 3).

However, it is a mistake to assume that any one company or organization operates with a single homogeneous culture. To illustrate this, consider the jokes and criticisms that abound between the different professions that contribute to health care when, for example, the doctor's way of approaching a problem may contrast sharply with the charge nurse's assumptions. Fragmentation often exists, characterized by a multiplicity of subcultures. This has been highlighted by Smircich (1983) in her investigation of an American insurance company. She showed that earlier in its history the company had encountered difficulties, and this experience had created two separate subcultures. The first incorporated the original staff; the second a new group of professionals. Although not immediately obvious, there was an undercurrent of tension between these two groups. Many parallels from health care could be cited, particularly in times of rapid and frequent change.

One of the most interesting observations is that an organization's culture remains more or less stable regardless of who is employed in the organization. There are various practices within the organization that act to maintain this by giving the employees similar experiences. Many of the human resource practices within an organization can reinforce its culture. For example, selection procedures, performance evaluation, pay systems, training and development practices and promotion criteria all ensure that those hired are incorporated into the existing culture. If organizational culture can be said to refer to the common beliefs and values held by individuals within an organization, it follows that the greater the similarity there is between an individual's beliefs and values and those expressed by the organization through documents and actions, the better will be the person–job fit. It is these sets of values, norms and beliefs that are the focus for this kind of organizational analysis.

However, getting information about such things is not straightforward. Geertz (1973: 15) has suggested that 'man is an animal suspended in webs of significance he himself has spun. I take culture to be those webs, and the analysis of it to be therefore not an experimental science in search of law, but an interpretive one in search of meaning.' Hence we return to the points raised at the beginning of this chapter, that participation in organizational life is a conceptual exercise where we struggle to make sense of the situations we find ourselves in. What the study of organizations as cultures allows us to do is to find data about the way sense is made of organizational life. Deal and Kennedy (1982) suggest a wide variety of cultural indicators which can be studied: physical settings, publicity material, annual reports, promotion principles and qualification processes. One of the clearest examples of this within health care environments is the way that clothing conveys messages about the role and status of staff. Consider the way artefacts in your organization serve a symbolic function as well as a practical one. Think about the way clothes are used within health organizations to segregate different groups or to bring them closer together. Focus your discussion on:

- What message does the wearing of theatre greens give to other professionals? To patients?
- What message does the wearing of white coats give to other professionals? To patients?
- What impact do nurses wearing uniforms make? Or their own clothes?
- What impact does the use of different sorts of uniform have on the status of different jobs?

- What message does patients wearing day clothes in psychiatric wards and night clothes in medical wards give?
- Think of other ways that clothes are used, either to segregate or group people together.

A final area of interest when considering organizations as cultures concerns the management of change. Over the last twenty years many organizations have come to realize that, in order to survive, they need to be able to respond to rapid and dramatic changes in the environment. Implementing such changes involves understanding the 'culture' of an organization so that the new goals can be achieved through its members. This is not an easy task, however. Peters and Waterman (1982) claim that culture cannot be changed; while Bibeault (1982) argues that culture change can be achieved only by making significant changes in personnel. Others, such as Williams, Dobson and Walters (1989), argue that culture change is possible and desirable in many circumstances, but accept that it will be resisted because culture provides the security necessary to function effectively at work.

Most of the studies that have investigated organizational change have found that a critical incident, such as severe economic difficulties, has preceded such change. These studies have identified five strategies which facilitated the change (Williams, Dobson and Walters, 1989):

1. Changing people in key positions helps change the pattern of beliefs and behaviours within an organization.
2. Reshuffling people with different skills and experiences into different positions.
3. Increasing participation, management education and formal communication processes.
4. Reviewing systems of reward, budgeting and other key systems.
5. Changing the corporate image.

All five focus on the established patterns of interaction that constitute culture and allow new patterns to develop. Understanding the culture of an organization helps in recognizing the established patterns and how they need to be handled sensitively when adopting these strategies. If this is ignored, Schein (1990) believes that entrenched resistance to the proposed changes can result.

Summary: models of organization in nursing practice

This chapter has introduced the importance of the organizational context to workers in health care environments. It argues that organizations are the product of the imagination based on experience, conceptual entities. This is the case for people working in organizations and for organizational psychologists; however, the latter are presented as theoretical texts. Three of these models have been discussed: Mintzberg's (1979) model of organizations as functional structures, Jaques's (1986) model of organizations as accountability relationships, and the growing literature which views organizations as cultures (Hollway, 1991; Morgan, 1986). These models are applied to different kinds of organizational problem within health care through the use of specific exercises.

Seminar questions

1. By using the exercises in the Boxes or drawing on your own experience, discuss how the changes from regional health service organization to trust arrangements have (a) changed the type of organization health care workers function within by using the 'Structure in Fives' model, or (b) influenced the accountability relationships in the organizations using the 'Levels of Work' model.
2. Discuss how patients/clients are assimilated into a health care environment and what structures and processes are necessary to ensure they receive the right treatment. In what ways could (a) the functional structure, (b) the managerial relationships, or (c) the cultural and subcultural patterns in a hospital contribute to a patient receiving the wrong treatment?
3. We have explored the idea of culture in organizations. Drawing on your experience and reading, discuss how financial and medical cultures differ. Identify what the main problems will be in trying to change medical responsibilities to include financial decision-making.

Further reading

Silverman (1971) presents one key argument for this view. A background discussion of organizations as conceptual entities can be found in Morgan (1986: ch. 1) and Mangham (1987: ch. 1). An introduction to the different ways that theorists have made sense of organizations is covered in Grint (1991: ch. 4) and is argued for in Hassard and Pym (1990).

Morgan (1986: ch. 10) describes a case study which illustrates the differences between individuals in the way they make sense of organizational situations. Many other theoretical approaches are introduced in a very accessible way in Morgan (1986).

A very accessible account of Mintzberg's work is given by Payne in Warr (1987: ch. 14).

For more details of levels of work, see Jaques (1986, esp. Chapters 4, 6 and 8). The main critique of this approach is given by Whittington and Bellaby (1979).

Morgan (1986: ch. 5) describes the approach to organizations using the metaphor of 'culture'.

Beyer and Trice (1987) suggest that an understanding of the culture underpinning everyday behaviour can be of practical help to managers.

References

Baker, J. and Stamp, G. (1992) *The Nature and Experience of Employment Work and the Levels of Work and Capability.* IOC course material. Uxbridge, Middx: Brunel University.

Beyer, J.M. and Trice, H.M. (1987) 'How an organization's rites reveal its culture', *Organization Dynamics* **15** (4), 5–24.

Bibeault, D.B. (1982) 'Corporate turn-around: How managers turn losers into winners', in J.D. Edwards and Kleiner, S. (eds.) (1988) 'Transforming organisational values and culture effectively', *Leadership and Organisational Development Journal* **9**, 1.

Deal, T. and Kennedy, A. (1982) *Corporate Cultures.* Reading, Mass.: Addison-Wesley.

Evans, J.S. (1979) *The Management of Human Capacity.* Bradford: MCB.

Geertz, C. (1973) *The Interpretation of Cultures.* New York: Basic Books.

Grint, K. (1991) *The Sociology of Work.* Cambridge: Polity Press.

Handy, C.B. (1981) *Understanding Organizations.* Harmondsworth: Penguin Books.

Hassard, J. and Pym, D. (1990) *The Theory and Philosophy of Organizations.* London and New York: Routledge.

Henriques, J., Hollway,W., Urwin, C., Venn, C. and Walkerdine, V. (1984) *Changing the Subject.* London and New York: Methuen.

Hollway, W. (1984) 'Fitting work: Psychological assessment in organizations', in J. Henriques *et al.* (eds.) *Changing the Subject.* London and New York: Methuen.

Hollway, W. (1991) *Work Psychology and Organizational Behaviour: Managing the individual at work.* London: Sage.

Jaques, E. (1986) *A General Theory of Bureaucracy.* Aldershot: Gower.

Jaques, E. (1989) *Requisite Organization.* Arlington, VA: Cason Hall.

Jaques, E. and Clements, S.D. (1991) *Executive Leadership.* Cambridge, Mass.: Blackwell and Cason Hall.

Mangham, I.L. (1987) *Organization Analysis and Development: A social construction of organizational behaviour.* Chichester: John Wiley.

Martin, J. (1992) *Cultures in Organizations: Three perspectives.* New York and Oxford: Oxford University Press.

Mintzberg, H. (1979) *The Structuring of Organizations.* Englewood Cliffs, NJ: Prentice Hall.

Mintzberg, H. (1983) *Structure in Fives.* Englewood Cliffs, NJ: Prentice Hall.

Morgan, G. (1986) *Images of Organization.* Beverly Hills, Calif: Sage.

Payne, R. (1987) 'Organizations as psychological environments', in P. Warr (ed.) *Psychology at Work.* Harmondsworth: Penguin Books.

Peters, T.J. and Waterman, R.H. (1982) *In Search of Excellence.* New York: Harper & Row.

Schein, E. (1990) 'Organizational culture', *American Psychologist* **45** (2), 109–19.

Silverman, D. (1971) *The Theory of Organizations.* London: Heinemann.

Smircich, L. (1983) 'Concepts of culture and organisational analysis', *Administrative Science Quarterly* **28** (3), 339–58.

Warr, P. (1987) *Psychology at Work.* Harmondsworth: Penguin Books.

Whittington, C. and Bellaby, P. (1979) 'The reasons for hierarchy in social services departments: A critique of Elliott Jaques and his associates', *Sociological Review* **27** (3), 513–37.

Williams, A., Dobson, P. and Walters, M. (1989) *Changing Culture.* London: IPM.

CHAPTER 2

Interacting with patients/clients

Impressions, attributions and adhering to medical advice

DENISE KNIGHT

Chapter outline

Introduction

Before reading this chapter consider the following:

- To what extent do you feel that the prior information you receive about a patient/client's personality influences your subsequent interaction with that individual?
- Do you think that your practice is influenced in any way when you believe that the patient/client has contributed to his/her condition, e.g. by not following health advice or engaging in risk-taking behaviour?
- How do you feel you can help a patient/client to remember and act on your instructions concerning his/her medication?

This chapter concerns the main theories that describe and explain psychological processes in relation to the situations described above. These include:

1. *Impression formation* – the way we form impressions of other people and the way impressions can be affected by features of the individual (e.g. perceived attractiveness) and by our own expectations.
2. *Causal attributions* – the way we make judgements about the causes of an individual's behaviour and the way those judgements might be distorted.

3. *Non-adherence to medical advice* – the extent and nature of the problem and the ways in which adherence might be improved.

It should be borne in mind that this chapter does not offer a complete account of *all* characteristics of the nurse–patient/client interaction. It aims rather to enable readers to gain an informed, critical perspective on those features of the interaction that the practitioner ordinarily has little awareness of, but which often exert a significant effect on the quality of subsequent interaction.

Forming impressions of others

Research into *social perception* concerns such matters as how impressions are formed, whether initial impressions are accurate and how we explain others' behaviour. Two main approaches are found in the study of social perception: (1) The *data-driven* or *structuralist* approach is concerned with the influence that the characteristics of a 'target' has on perceptions. (2) The *constructivist* or *theory-driven* approach concentrates on the ways in which pre-existing theories and concepts influence the impressions of a perceiver. Thus impressions are not formed entirely on the basis of facts but are also influenced by what we expect or want to see.

Both approaches will be examined, together with a discussion of the literature relating to nurses' perceptions of their patients/clients. It is important to remember that interaction is a two-way process and that the patient/client will also be forming impressions of the nurse. For this reason common perceptions of nurses will also be examined.

Influence of target individual on impressions formed

Several physical characteristics of the target individual have been shown to influence social perceptions. It is generally believed, for example, that redheads are tense and excitable, blondes are delicate and weak-willed, while those with brown hair are seen as dependable and sincere (Lawson, 1971). Many other physical characteristics have been found to influence the impressions formed. For example, height, a youthful gait and infantile features such as a large forehead and eyes generally lead to favourable impressions (Montepare and Zebrowitz-McArthur, 1986).

Physical attractiveness may create a *halo effect* so that all other characteristics of the individual are viewed positively, an effect which is found in both Western and non-Western cultures (Zebrowitz, 1990). We can see this effect in studies of the way attractive clients/patients are treated by nurses. Corter *et al.* (1978) found that nurses gave better intellectual prognoses to attractive premature infants, and Nordholm (1980), in a large study of health professionals, reported that nurses judged physically attractive adult patients to have more motivation for improvement and to be more intelligent. Similarly, Bordieri, Solodky and Mikos (1985) found that nurses judged that attractive female paediatric patients were less likely to be responsible for a hypothetical disturbance in hospital and to have fewer behavioural problems.

Non-verbal characteristics also influence impressions. Doctors, for example, are liked best by patients when they hold their arms in an open position and nod their heads to indicate agreement (Harrigan and Rosenthal, 1983). Touch is another important non-verbal cue. In some contexts, it creates a positive impression of warmth and caring, but in other contexts may yield a less favourable impression. In a hospital or geriatric setting touch is often used only for task-related purposes and so gains negative connotations for patients (Kreps and Thornton, 1984). Oliver and Redfern (1991) also suggest that touch is used mainly for instrumental purposes. Readers might like to consider the effect of instrumental touch on patient/client impressions and ways in which communicative touching might be increased.

Perceiver influences on impression formation

The assumptions we make about others often go beyond the objective data, suggesting that the perceiver's characteristics also play a part in the impressions that are formed. These assumptions are examples of the different *theories* that we hold about people, e.g that certain personality characteristics such as intelligence and industriousness tend to coexist in individuals. The term *implicit personality theory* (Bruner and Tagiuri, 1954) is used to describe such mental representations. One type of implicit personality theory is the *stereotypes* we have about certain groups of individuals so that, for example, we may assume that an elderly person possesses certain characteristics simply by being a member of the elderly group (see Chapter 23).

Implicit personality theories and stereotypes thus represent the means by which people actively organize incoming data about individuals in order to make sense of the world and to make this information appear more manageable (Fiske and Taylor, 1984). These processes are, of course, not entirely objective. Their use can often lead to *biases* in that attention may be directed towards information which supports the theory only, thus ignoring other information (see Chapter 5). The persistence of negative stereotypes of certain groups, despite contradictory evidence, forms the basis of prejudice.

A number of influential perceiver biases have been identified in the formation of impressions. These include expectancy effects, central traits and group stereotypes.

Expectancy effects
These occur when the perceiver holds certain expectations about the target person. Langer and Abelson (1974) found that therapists expecting to interview a 'patient' evaluated the individual as more disturbed than therapists who expected to see a 'job applicant'.

A more profound effect was found in a study by Rosenthal and Jacobson (1968). They identified to teachers a number of 'late bloomers' who were supposedly likely to show a marked improvement in their academic performance. The pupils in fact had been randomly selected. On testing a year after their teachers' expectations were raised, the 'late bloomers' indeed showed a greater increase in their IQ scores than those of their peers. This has been interpreted as an example of the *self-fulfilling prophecy* where an event, experience or behaviour occurs because of an expectation that it will occur. Many studies have demonstrated this effect (e.g. Skrypnek and Snyder, 1982). Later research has not, however, always supported the existence of expectancy effects or the self-fulfilling prophecy (see Fiske and Taylor, 1991 in Further Reading).

Central traits
Prior information about certain personality traits or characteristics of a target person may have a particularly significant effect. Asch (1946), in a series of twelve studies, asked people to form an impression of an individual based on a list of personality traits supposedly possessed by that individual. One group were told about someone who was 'intelligent, skilful, industrious, warm, determined, practical and cautious' (before reading on, you might like to briefly examine your impression of somebody who possesses these characteristics). A second group were told of an individual who had the same characteristics, except 'cold' was substituted for 'warm' (again, examine your impression of somebody with these characteristics and compare your impressions of the two individuals). Asch's subjects believed that the first individual was 'wise' while the second individual was seen as 'calculating'. Wishner (1960) has suggested that the personality trait 'warm–cold' acts as a *central trait* because it is closely related to many other characteristics of the individual and

---

BOX 2.1   PRIOR INFORMATION AND CENTRAL TRAITS: A POTENT INFLUENCE ON INTERACTIONS?

Kelley (1950) gave a group of psychology students prior information about the characteristics of a visiting lecturer. All students were given the same information about the individual except that one half of the group were told that he was a warm individual while the remainder were told that he was cold. All students then attended the same lecture. Following the lecture, students' perceptions of the lecturer varied consistently with the prior information they had received about him. Students who had been led to believe that the lecturer was a warm individual rated him more positively on a number of characteristics such as being sociable, popular, good-natured, considerate of others, etc.

More significant, however, is the finding that students who believed the lecturer possessed the central trait 'warm' also behaved more positively towards the lecturer in class. They asked more questions, responded more and were more likely to approach the lecturer after the class. Thus the students' expectations about a central trait was a powerful influence on their behaviour.

thus has a very strong influence on the impression formed. Kelley (1950), in a real-life setting, obtained similar findings (see Box 2.1).

These findings have implications for the nurse's interaction with patients/clients. A first meeting with a patient/client may take place after the nurse has already received information about the person (e.g. from hospital records for a newly admitted patient, discharge records for a patient requiring further care in the community, or a verbal report from a nurse or midwife transferring a patient/client). In verbal reports particularly, information is also given about the patient/client's characteristics, e.g. 'She's a lovely woman', 'He can be difficult at times', etc.

DISCUSSION POINT
How might health professionals guard against the formation of biases when they need information about patients?

Group stereotypes

A number of studies have investigated the role of group stereotypes in impression formation, particularly in relation to race and gender. For example, after viewing a videotape showing a heated discussion in which one individual pushed the other, the push was interpreted as 'playful' when the perpetrator was white, but 'aggressive' when he was black (Duncan, 1976). Men are generally perceived as more competent than females (e.g. Goldberg, 1968), although a contrast effect is shown in that incompetent males are perceived as less competent than women who are of equal competence (e.g. Deaux and Taynor, 1973).

Several explanations have been proposed for group stereotypes. These include favouritism towards the *ingroup* of which one is a member (Brewer, 1979) and assumptions of homogeneity among the *outgroup*, i.e. the erroneous belief that all members of an outgroup are the same (Park and Rothbart, 1982). Evaluations of outgroup members may also be more extreme. Hence gifted black law students were rated more positively than an equally gifted white student, while a weak black student was rated less favourably than a comparable white student (Linville and Jones, 1980).

Stereotypes of group members may lead to behaviour confirming those stereotypes and to self-rejection and self-devaluation by individuals in the stereotyped group (Levine and Campbell, 1972). Stereotypes may be overcome by repeated occurrences of behaviours which do not confirm the stereotype held (Krueger and Rothbart, 1988).

Ganong, Bzdek and Manderino (1987) point out that nurses also hold stereotypes and that these may compromise their ability to deliver individualized care to all patients/clients and to show them acceptance and respect. In a review of thirty-eight studies of stereotyping by nurses and nursing students, they found evidence that nurses hold stereotypes of patients on the basis of age, gender, diagnosis, social class, personality and family structure. Very few studies have, however, investigated the effects that such stereotypes have on nurses' behaviour or on nurse–patient/client interaction. The value of the studies is further limited by poor sampling techniques and by the use of non-standardized questionnaires. (See Chapter 5 for a discussion of the link between attitudes and behaviour.) Bowler (1993), in a small, ethnographic study of midwives' stereotypes about Asian women, suggests that these relate to four main themes: communication problems, failure to comply with care, making a fuss about nothing and a lack of normal (Western) maternal instinct. Bowler points to several instances where care was less than optimal because the midwives relied on their stereotypes of the women. Thus, after observing the deliveries of six Asian women, Bowler noted that only one was offered pain relief. She suggests that the midwives may have found it too difficult to explain pain relief options to women who spoke little English, or perhaps they thought that the 'women did not need (or deserve) pain control because of their known "low pain thresholds" ' (Bowler, 1993: 13).

DISCUSSION POINT
How might health care professionals ensure that assessment of patient/client need is not influenced by group stereotypes?

Several common stereotypes of nurses are held, particularly within the media. All female, the stereotypes portray the nurse as a ministering angel, a battle-axe, a naughty nurse or as a doctor's handmaiden (Salvage 1986). Bridges (1990) suggests that the stereotypes are derived from the historical roots of nursing but persist because of few attempts to challenge them, particularly by nurses themselves. Readers might wish to consider the effect that such stereotypes have on the patient/ client's impressions of the nurse and how such stereotypes might be overcome.

Several models have been developed which attempt to explain the way in which people form an overall impression, i.e. the way in which information from data-driven and theory-driven processes is integrated. Linear combination models suggest that the different items of information are 'added' together or averaged to form an impression. Anderson (1981) suggests that certain information is weighted according to its importance to the perceiver. However, the predictive power of this model is limited since the weighting for a certain item of information may well vary from one situation to the next (Zebrowitz, 1990). Other models suggest that data-driven and theory-driven processes play separate roles in impression formation. Initial impressions are largely theory-driven, with data-driven processes occurring if the target is personally relevant or interesting to the perceiver (Brewer, 1988; Fiske and Neuberg, 1990).

Impressions are therefore influenced by many characteristics of the target person as well as the theories, expectations and stereotypes held by the perceiver. It is important for health care professionals to be aware of the ways in which impressions formed can influence both their behaviour and that of the patient/client in any given interaction.

Causal attributions

Our beliefs about why people behave in the way that they do are another important influence on our perceptions of others and on our interactions with them. *Attributions* are the causal explanations given for a certain event or behaviour (Kelley and Michaela, 1980). Causal attributions have been found to influence both the individual's response to health matters and the practitioner's response to that individual. For example, Brewin (1984) found that pre-clinical medical students were more likely to advise psychotropic medication if they felt that the events leading to a depressed person's illness lay outside the patient's control.

Correspondent inference theory (Jones and Davis, 1965) and *covariation theory* (Kelley, 1967) attempt to explain how people make judgements about the cause of events and behaviour. Both theories suggest that people act rationally so that the cause of an event or behaviour must lie either within the situation or within some characteristic of the individual. Attributions may thus be *situational* or *dispositional*.

Jones and Davis's (1965) model provides details about the way in which we make dispositional attributions following observation of somebody's action and its associated effects. The model suggests that people make judgements as to whether or not a person knew what the *consequences* of the action would be, whether there was a *choice* in carrying out the action and the *ability* to carry out the action. A positive response to each of these questions will lead to a dispositional attribution. However, if it is judged that the action is socially desirable or behaviour typically associated with a role, a situational attribution will follow. Thus you may decide that a colleague who spends time with an uncommunicative patient is doing so because of his/her role as a nurse, while if a patient did the same thing you might decide that he/she was a warm, caring person.

BOX 2.2   DETECTING COVARIATION: AN ILLUSTRATION OF KELLEY'S (1967) MODEL

You are working with a patient one day when you hear the ward manager telling a junior colleague that she is lazy and stupid. Kelley's model suggests you go through the following decision-making process in reaching a decision as to whether the manager's behaviour is due to the situation or says something about the ward manager:

Observations

Nobody thinks the nurse is lazy and stupid. (Low consensus)

The ward manager always makes negative comments about the nurse. (Low distinctiveness)

The ward manager is usually negative in her comments about everybody junior to her. (High consistency)

Decision reached

Dispositional attribution made, e.g. the ward manager is the cause of this situation since she is bad-tempered and usually negative.

Kelley (1967) suggests that we look at how behaviour *covaries* with particular causes. We therefore make attributions only after several observations of behaviour, following which we make judgements about the *distinctiveness, consistency* and *consensus* of the behaviour. Thus we make decisions as to whether the behaviour occurs only in one situation (distinctiveness), whether the individual always acts in this way (consistency) and whether other people also behave in this way (consensus). Kelley maintains that the pattern of responses to these questions determines whether situational or dipositional attributions are made (see Box 2.2).

DISCUSSION POINT
Consider the situation in Box 2.2. What observations might lead to a situational attribution being made?

Bias in the attribution process

The rational, objective nature of attributions has been questioned by later studies. It is posited that people take shortcuts when making inferences about the causes of other people's behaviour and these can lead to biases in our judgements of causality. However shortcuts also lead to the efficient processing of a great deal of incoming information, even if not entirely accurately (Fiske and Taylor, 1984).

There appear to be three main biases in the attribution process:

1. *The fundamental attribution bias* describes a tendency to underestimate the impact of situational factors and overestimate the effects of a person's characteristics (Ross, 1977).
2. *The actor–observer bias* suggests that, within a given situation, the actor or target person is more likely to judge the situation as the cause of his or her behaviour while an observer of the same situation would attribute the behaviour to characteristics of the actor. House, Pendleton and Parker (1986) found, for example, that physicians were more likely to view diabetic patients' difficulties with their diet as due to motivational problems in the patient but the same patients were more likely to cite external causes.
3. *The self-serving bias* is particularly relevant to the attribution processes of health care professionals. It suggests that individuals are more likely to attribute the cause of their success to internal factors such as ability, while failures will be attributed to external factors such as other people, etc. (Zuckerman, 1979). Marteau and Johnston (1986), in a study of doctors' attributions for failure in collecting blood samples from diabetic children, found that 84 per cent of attributions cited some feature of the child as the reason for failure. Gamsu and Bradley (1987) found that doctors and nurses were more likely to attribute good diabetic control to medical intervention and poor diabetic control to the patient.

Attributions and the patient

Many studies have shown that the cause of their illness is an important consideration for many patients. In one such study (Greenberg *et al.*, 1984), patients reported that the cause of their illness was the most important piece of information given to them by their doctor at the time of diagnosis. Several studies have shown that months and even years after diagnosis, a causal explanation of their illness remains important to patients (DuCette and Keane, 1984). Attributions about illness may also affect the uptake of preventive health behaviours (Rothman *et al.*, 1993) and the response to treatment (e.g. Affleck *et al.*, 1987).

Several studies have examined the role of patients' beliefs about *control* over their illness or health-related behaviours. Control involves a number of related constructs as identified in Box 2.3.

It has been suggested that a sense of personal control will have a positive impact on health. Rodin and Langer (1977) found that steps to increase control, such as letting nursing home residents choose which night to attend a film or giving them a plant to care for, led to an increased sense of wellbeing and better intellectual functioning.

Health education programmes that emphasize the individual's personal control in reducing coronary heart disease have been found to increase the uptake of preventive health behaviours (Rothman *et al.*, 1993). Wallston *et al.*, (1989) suggest that a sense of personal control influences health by mitigating the harmful effects

---

BOX 2.3 **PERCEIVED CONTROL AND HEALTH**

Beliefs about control and health may focus on perceived control over past health-related behaviours or events. Thus, an individual may believe that work stress was the major cause of his duodenal ulcer and that he had little control over this factor. Wallston *et al.* (1989) point out that perceived control also involves the following:

■ *Perceived locus of control (LOC)* Rotter (1966) refers instead to *perceived expectancies about future outcomes*. Individuals with an internal LOC therefore perceive that outcomes are determined by their own behaviour rather than by chance or other people. Many studies have suggested that an internal LOC leads to improved health outcomes in the individual (Strickland, 1978). Wallston *et al.* (1989), however, point out that a simple internal–external dimension is not valid for health beliefs and suggest a multidimensional construct involving chance and powerful others, as well as beliefs about personal control.

■ *Self-efficacy* refers to the expectancy that the individual is able to engage in a specific behaviour, i.e. that he/she has control over the behaviour (Bandura, 1982). Somebody could, therefore, believe that a particular behaviour might produce a certain outcome but might not believe that he/she is capable of carrying out that behaviour, i.e. low self-efficacy.

of stress and by increasing the likelihood of engaging in one or more protective health behaviours. A perceived lack of control could, they suggest, also be stressful in its own right. (See Chapter 6 for a discussion of the role of other cognitive factors.)

DISCUSSION POINT
Tom Matthews has recently suffered a heart attack. He is anxious to do everything he can to improve his health but feels it will be impossible since he has tried in the past to 'live more healthily'. He blames his stressful job.

- What beliefs about control does Tom have?
- How might you help him adopt more positive health behaviours?
- Examine your own perceptions about personal control of health and illness.

Attributions and the health care professional

We have seen that the attributions of health professionals are subject to a self-serving bias. Attributions about a patient's illness may, however, also influence the practitioner's attitudes towards that patient and, potentially more seriously, may also affect the treatment of the patient. As already discussed, Brewin (1984) found that medication was more likely to be recommended if the cause of the illness was judged to be outside the patient's control. Brewin (1984) interprets these results through the *attributional model of helping behaviour*, which suggests that a belief that a negative event was not under an individual's control leads to feelings of pity. These in turn mediate helping behaviour (Weiner, 1980).

Curbow, Andrews and Burke (1986), however, found that registered nurses tended to feel that many cancer patients were responsible for their illness, but that these attributions did not lead to negative attitudes or behaviour on the part of the nurses. Curbow, Andrews and Burke (1986) suggest that nurses are socialized in their role to act with 'compassion and nurturance' and thus, unlike college students, they do not behave negatively towards patients who have brought about their own illness. Marteau and Riordan (1992), on the other hand, found that patients who had not followed the health behaviours appropriate for their illness were rated more unfavourably on a number of dimensions by nurses. Nurses judged that these patients were likely to be less concerned about their condition, less likely to follow any instructions and were likely to be less rewarding to work with. Knight (1993) also found that district nurses and health visitors showed significantly less favourable attitudes towards a patient/client with coronary heart disease when healthier behaviours were not adopted. They were, however, more likely to engage in giving advice and support regarding stopping smoking, dietary change, etc., when they perceived the individual as responsible for his or her condition.

The small number of studies in this area suggests that the attributions made by health professionals can influence the attitudes held about patients and may influence professional actions. Gillespie and Bradley (1988) point out that attributional discrepancies between the patient/client and professional might lead to recommendations about treatment that are not appropriate for the true cause of the individual's illness and which are therefore unlikely to be followed. (See also Box 6.2, p. 122).

DISCUSSION POINT
How might attributions about illness be incorporated into treatment/care plans to the benefit of patient outcomes?

Adhering to medical advice

Satisfaction with interaction with a practitioner appears to be an important influence on compliance and adherence with advice or treatment (Ley, 1988). The terms 'adherence' and 'compliance' are often used interchangeably. However, the term adherence is to be preferred since compliance suggests that the practitioner is authoritarian (Turk, Salovey and Litt, 1986).

The extent and nature of the problem

Both practitioners and patients appear to over-report the extent of adherence to medication (DiMatteo and DiNicola, 1982). In a study of cancer patients receiving allopurinol to protect their kidneys from cytotoxic therapy, Richardson *et al.* (1987) found that 77 per cent of patients showed total non-adherence to recommendations. i.e. *none* of the drug was detected in their blood. A further 8 per cent were not taking as much medication as prescribed. Adherence to short-term medication appears to be about 78 per cent, dropping to about 50 per cent with long term medication (Sackett and Snow, 1979). Adherence to lifestyle changes is generally variable and often low (Cluss and Epstein, 1985).

Factors influencing adherence

Adherence to the medication prescribed or advice offered is affected by many factors (see also Chapters 5 and 6). Stanton (1987) identifies four factors that influence adherence to medical advice and treatment:

1. Patient-provider communication
Our information processing channels are limited and patients/clients are unable to retain a great deal of information, particularly if they are anxious when they receive it. Boyd *et al.* (1974) found that patients retained only 10 per cent of verbal information, 20 per cent of visual information, but 65 per cent of information transmitted in both ways. Ley (1988) suggests that the contents of the message should

be structured or categorized so that the patient/client is able to retrieve information easily using 'markers' provided by the practitioner, e.g. 'I want to tell you about your raised blood pressure and why it is important that it is treated properly, what medicines you must take and changes you can make to your lifestyle to try to reduce the problem happening again.' This gives structure for the information and should increase recall.

Patient knowledge of the treatment regime appears quite low and is not improved by the practitioner's use of medical terms and jargon. Samora, Saunders and Larson (1961) found that patients were likely to remember only 56 per cent of the technical terms used. Patients' knowledge of their own bodies and disease processes may also be limited. For example, patients may not know that the stomach secretes acid (Roth, 1979) or that a coronary thrombosis involves the heart (Ley and Spelman, 1967).

Satisfaction with the practitioner has also been shown to influence adherence. Several studies show that patients generally are not satisfied with the communication they have with medical staff (e.g Korsch, Gozzi and Francis, 1968). Patients prefer a medical practitioner who is empathetic, who listens carefully and who explains their illness and its treatment clearly. Many studies, however, show that this form of interaction rarely occurs. Doctors appear to spend only 10 per cent of the time explaining the patient's condition (DiMatteo, 1985) and even less time, if any, on explaining the treatment (Svarstad, 1976).

DISCUSSION POINT
How might the patient/client's understanding and recall of medical information be improved?

2. Internal locus of control
Stanton (1987) suggests that patients with an internal locus of control or those who are encouraged to believe that they can influence their health are more likely to adhere to health advice. As already discussed, Rothman *et al.* (1993) have found that health messages emphasizing an individual's control over a health problem encourage the uptake of preventive health behaviours.

Other aspects of the health beliefs which can influence adherence include beliefs about whether the condition is a threat to health and whether any action by the individual will be effective. Examination of an individual's health beliefs might therefore prove to be an effective strategy in improving adherence.

3. Perceived social support
Many studies have demonstrated the importance of social support from family and friends in ensuring continued adherence to long-term medication or lifestyle changes. Rosenstock (1985) suggested that the involvement of the family in the treatment recommendations is to be encouraged. Support and encouragement in the form of periodic reviews and/or telephone reminders from medical and nursing staff will also increase patient/client adherence (Haynes, 1976).

4. Treatment disruption to lifestyle

Adherence is reduced when the patient perceives that the treatment disrupts his or her lifestyle unacceptably. Factors that influence this include the complexity of the recommended treatment and its duration. Long-term medication schedules and lifestyle changes show poorest adherence. The inconvenience and expense of any treatment are also important in determining adherence (Kirscht and Rosenstock, 1979). Several strategies have been suggested to minimize these difficulties. Frequent follow-up visits should occur so that feedback and encouragement is given (Ley, 1988). Lifestyle change can be achieved over a longer time frame with small changes only being introduced one at a time. In this way, the patient/client will be motivated by demonstrated success which is reinforced by the practitioner. Wherever possible, complex drug schedules should be incorporated into regular daily activities to minimize inconvenience. Several strategies, therefore, may be used in

---

BOX 2.4   STRATEGIES TO INCREASE ADHERENCE

Ensure patient-centred communication

- Empathetic manner.
- Listen to individual actively.
- Encourage discussion of individual perceptions of illness and expectations and feelings about treatment or lifestyle change.

Increase understanding and memory

- Avoid jargon, explain relevant physiology.
- Be specific, e.g. instructions 'to cut down' are too vague.
- Repeat important statements.
- Structure information.
- Provide written and/or visual supplementary material.

Increase support

- Enlist cooperation of family and significant friends.
- Arrange for periodic review of individual's progress.
- Give praise and encouragement where appropriate.
- Use telephone and/or written reminders.
- Suggest support group if available.

Be aware of individual's health beliefs (see also Chapter 6)

- Perceptions of cause of illness/condition.
- Perceptions of personal control over outcome.
- Perceptions of self-efficacy.
- Perceptions of seriousness of and vulnerability to condition.
- Family's health beliefs are also important.

order to enhance adherence to drug treatments or lifestyle changes. These are summarized in Box 2.4.

Finally, it is important to examine whether patients/clients have a 'right' to non-adherence. Becker and Rosenstock (1984: 200) discuss circumstances in which 'intelligent non-compliance' (sic) might act in the patient's favour as, for example, when their chronic condition has changed, altering their treatment requirements. Donovan and Blake (1992) suggest that such decisions should be viewed from the patient's viewpoint. It is likely, they suggest, that patients carry out a cost–benefit analysis of recommended treatments, taking their own personal and social circumstances into account. They claim non-adherence is often very rational when examined from the patient's perspective.

DISCUSSION POINT
Examine your own and colleagues' views of the patient's right to non-adherence.
What does the UKCC Code of Professional Conduct (UKCC, 1992) suggest about the professional's role in this situation?

Summary

This chapter has examined two aspects of our social perceptual processes: impression formation and making causal attributions. Our information processing strategies appear to be flawed in that they lead to several biases in the decisions reached. They do, however, represent a very efficient means of dealing with the vast amount of data which we receive about the people with whom we interact. The impressions we form of others can have widespread effects on other decisions we make about them and also on the way they behave. The attributions patients and clients make about health related issues may exert a significant effect on their health–illness experience. Professional attributions made about the patient's/client's illness can affect attitudes held about the individual and professional action towards that individual. Adherence with medical advice depends, to a large extent, on patients'/clients' satisfaction with their interaction with the health professional. Non-adherence on the part of patient/clients is a significant problem. Ways to address this include increasing patient/client satisfaction with the communication, structuring the message and ensuring the patients' perspective is taken into account.

Seminar questions

1. Re-examine the reponses you made to the questions posed at the beginning of the chapter. Do you feel it necessary to revise them?
2. What strategies would you recommend to the manager of an acute elderly care unit to overcome the negative stereotypes of people who are elderly which are frequently expressed by staff on his/her unit.

3. A 38-year-old man with insulin-dependent diabetes has been admitted several times with his diabetes poorly controlled. He listens with little interest as you talk to him about managing his diabetes, finally blurting out: 'It's no good. Nothing I do has any effect, it's just a complete waste of time. The doctors ought to be doing more.' What do these statements reveal about his perceptions of control? How might you help him to achieve a more stable diabetic condition?

Further reading

Fiske, S.T. and Taylor, S.E. (1991) *Social Cognition.* New York: McGraw-Hill.
An examination of the literature relating to impression formation and attribution theory. Recommended for those who wish to further their understanding of theoretical issues in these areas.
Ley, P. (1988) *Communicating with Patients: Improving communication, satisfaction and compliance.* London: Chapman & Hall.
An excellent review of the literature relating to patient adherence and the many factors associated with this issue.
Marteau, T.M. (1989) 'Health beliefs and attributions', in A.K. Broome (ed.) *Health Psychology: Processes and applications.* London: Chapman & Hall.
A critical examination of the relationship between cognitions, behaviour and health outcomes.
Saks, M.J. and Krupat, E. (1988) *Social Psychology and its Applications.* New York: Harper & Row.
Examines many areas within social psychology. Contains a comprehensive account of social perception, written in an easy to understand style.

References

Affleck, G., Tennen, H., Croog, S. and Levine, S. (1987) 'Causal attribution, perceived control and recovery from heart attack', *Journal of Social and Clinical Psychology* **5**, 356–64.
Anderson, N.H. (1981) *Foundations of Information Integration Theory.* New York: Academic Press.
Asch, S. (1946) 'Forming impressions of personality', *Journal of Abnormal and Social Psychology* **41**, 258–90.
Bandura, A. (1982) 'Self-efficacy mechanism in human agency', *American Psychologist* **37**, 122–47.
Becker, H.M. and Rosenstock, I.M. (1984) 'Compliance with medical advice', in A. Mathews and A. Steptoe (eds.) *Health Care and Human Behaviour.* London: Academic Press.
Bordieri, J.E., Solodky, M.L. and Mikos, K.A. (1985) 'Physical attractiveness and nurses' perceptions of paediatric patients', *Nursing Research* **43** (1), 24–6.

Bowler, I.M.W. (1993) 'Stereotypes of women of Asian descent in midwifery: Some evidence', *Midwifery* **9**, 7–16.

Boyd, J., Covington, T., Stanasczk, W. and Cousons, R. (1974) 'Drug defaulting – Part 1: Determinants of compliance', *American Journal of Hospital Pharmacy* **31**, 362–4.

Brewer, M.B. (1979) 'In-group bias in the minimal intergroup situation: A cognitive-motivational analysis', *Psychological Bulletin* **86**, 307–24.

Brewer, M.B. (1988) 'A dual process model of impression formation', in T. K. Srull and R.S. Wyer Jr (eds.) *Advances in Social Cognition*, Vol. 1. Hillsdale, NJ: Lawrence Erlbaum.

Brewin, C. R. (1984) 'Perceived controllability of life events and willingness to prescribe psychotropic drugs', *British Journal of Social Psychology* **23**, 285–7.

Bridges, J.M. (1990) 'Literature review on the images of the nurse and nursing in the media', *Journal of Advanced Nursing* **15**, 850–4.

Bruner, J.S. and Tagiuri, R. (1954) 'The perception of people', in G. Lindzey (ed.) *Handbook of Social Psychology,* Vol. 2. Reading, Mass.: Addison-Wesley.

Cluss, P.A. and Epstein, L.H. (1985) 'The measurement of medical compliance in the treatment of disease', in P. Karoly (ed.) *Measurement Strategies in Health Psychology.* New York: John Wiley.

Corter, C., Trehub, S., Boukydis, C., Ford, L., Celhoffer, L. and Minde, K. (1978) 'Nurses' judgments of the attractiveness of premature infants', *Infant Behaviour and Development* **1**, 432–9.

Curbow, B., Andrews, R.M. and Burke, T.A. (1986) 'Perceptions of the cancer patient: Causal explanations and personal attributions', *Journal of Psychosocial Oncology* **4** (1/2), 115–34.

Deaux, K. and Taynor, J. (1973) 'Evaluation of male and female ability: Bias works two ways', *Psychological Reports* **32**, 261–2.

DiMatteo, M.R. (1985) 'Physician–patient communication: Promoting a positive health-care setting', in J.C. Rosen and L.J. Solomon (eds.) *Prevention in Health Psychology.* Hanover, NH: University Press of New England.

DiMatteo, M.R. and DiNicola, D.D. (1982) *Achieving Patient Compliance: The psychology of the medical practitioner's role.* New York: Pergamon.

Donovan, J.L. and Blake, D.R. (1992) 'Patient non-compliance: Deviance or reasoned decision-making?' *Social Science and Medicine* **34** (5) 507–13.

DuCette, J. and Keane, A. (1984) 'Why me? An attributional analysis of a major illness', *Research in Nursing and Health* **7**, 257–64.

Duncan, S. L. (1976) 'Differential social perception and attribution of intergroup violence: Testing the lower limits of stereotyping of blacks', *Journal of Personality and Social Psychology* **34**, 590–8.

Fiske, S.T. and Neuberg, S.L. (1990) 'A continuum of impression formation from category-based to individuating processes: Influences of information and motivation on attention and interpretation', in M.P. Zanna (ed.) *Advances in Experimental Social Psychology*, Vol. 23. New York: Academic Press.

Fiske, S.T. and Taylor, S.E. (1984) *Social Cognition.* Reading, Mass.: Addison-Wesley.

Gamsu, D.S. and Bradley, C. (1987) 'Clinical staff's attributions about diabetes: Scale developments and staff vs patient comparisons', *Current Psychological Research and Reviews* **6**, 69–78.

Ganong, L.H., Bzdek, V. and Manderino, M.A. (1987) 'Stereotyping by nurses and nursing students: A critical review of research', *Research in Nursing and Health* **10**, 49–70.

Gillespie, C.R. and Bradley, C. (1988) 'Causal attributions of doctors and patients in a diabetes clinic', *British Journal of Clinical Psychology* **27**, 67–76.

Goldberg, P.A. (1968) 'Are women prejudiced against women?' *Transaction* **4**, 28–30.

Greenberg, L.W., Jewett, L.S., Gluck, R.S., Champion, L.A.A., Leikin, S.F., Altieri, M.F. and Lipnick, R.N. (1984) 'Giving information for life-threatening diagnosis: Parents' and oncologists' perceptions', *American Journal of Diabetes Care* **138**, 649–53.

Harrigan, J.A. and Rosenthal, R. (1983) 'Physician's head and body position as determinants of perceived rapport', *Journal of Applied Social Psychology* **13**, 496–509.

Haynes, R.B. (1976) 'A critical review of the "determinants" of patient compliance with therapeutic regimens', in D.L. Sackett and R.B. Haynes (eds.) *Compliance with Therapeutic Regimens.* Baltimore, MD: Johns Hopkins University Press.

House, W.C., Pendleton, L. and Parker, L. (1986) 'Patients' versus physicians' attributions of reasons for diabetic patients' non-compliance with diet', *Diabetes Care* **9** (4), 434.

Jones, E.E. and Davis, K.E. (1965) 'From acts to dispositions. The attribution process in person perception', in L. Berkowitz (ed.) *Advances in Experimental Social Psychology*, Vol. 2. New York: Academic Press.

Kelley, H.H. (1950) 'The warm–cold variable in first impressions of persons', *Journal of Personality* **18**, 431–9.

Kelley, H.H. (1967) 'Attribution theory in social psychology', in D. Levine (ed.) *Nebraska Symposium on Motivation*, Vol. 15. Lincoln: University of Nebraska Press.

Kelley, H.H. and Michaela, J.L. (1980) 'Attribution theory and research', *Annual Review of Psychology* **31**, 457–501.

Kirscht, J.P. and Rosenstock, I.M. (1979) 'Patients' problems in following recommendations of health experts', in G.C. Stone, F. Cohen and N.E. Adler (eds.) *Health Psychology: A handbook.* San Francisco: Jossey Bass.

Knight, D.A. (1993) 'Attributions for illness: Their relationship to community nurse attitudes and actions.' Unpublished MSc dissertation, Middlesex University.

Korsch, B.M., Gozzi, E.K., and Francis, V. (1968) 'Gaps in doctor–patient communication: 1. Doctor–patient interaction and patient satisfaction', *Pediatrics* **42**, 855–71.

Kreps, G.L. and Thornton, B.C. (1984) *Health Communication.* New York: Longman.

Krueger, J. and Rothbart, M. (1988) 'Use of categorical and individuating information in making inferences about personality', *Journal of Personality and Social Psychology* **55**, 187–95.

Langer, E. and Abelson, R.P. (1974) 'A patient by any other name . . . clinician group differences in labeling bias', *Journal of Consulting and Clinical Psychology* **42**, 4–9.

Lawson, E. (1971) 'Hair colour, personality and the observer', *Psychological Reports* **28**, 311–22.

Levine, R.A. and Campbell, D.T. (1972) *Ethnocentrism: Theories of conflict, ethnic attitudes and group behavior.* New York: John Wiley.

Ley, P. (1988) *Communicating with Patients: Improving communication, satisfaction and compliance.* London: Chapman & Hall.

Ley, P. and Spelman, M.S. (1967) *Communicating with the Patient.* London: Staples Press.

Linville, P.W. and Jones, E.E. (1980) 'Polarised appraisals of outgroup members', *Journal of Personality and Social Psychology* **38**, 689–703.

Marteau, T.M. and Johnston, M. (1986) 'Doctors taking blood from children: A suitable case for treatment', *British Journal of Clinical Psychology* **25**, 159–60.

Marteau, T.M. and Riordan, D.C. (1992) 'Staff attitudes to patients: The influence of causal attributions for illness', *British Journal of Clinical Psychology* **31**, 107–10.

Montepare, J.M. and Zebrowitz-McArthur, L. (1986) 'The influence of facial characteristics on children's age perceptions', *Journal of Experimental Social Psychology* **42**, 1014–24.

Nordholm, L. (1980) 'Beautiful patients are good patients: Evidence for the physical attractiveness stereotype in first impressions of patients', *Social Science and Medicine* **14**, 81–3.

Oliver, S. and Redfern, S.J. (1991) 'Interpersonal communication between nurses and elderly patients: Refinement of an observation schedule', *Journal of Advanced Nursing* **16**, 30–8

Park, B. and Rothbart, M. (1982) 'Perceptions of out-group homogeneity and levels of social categorisation: Memory for the subordinate attributes of in-group and out-group members', *Journal of Personality and Social Psychology* **42**, 1051–68.

Richardson, J.L., Marks, G., Johnson, C.A., Graham, J.W., Chan, K.K., Selser, J.N., Kisbaugh, C., Barranday, Y. and Levine, A.M. (1987) 'Path model of multidimensional compliance with cancer therapy', *Health Psychology* **6**, 183–207.

Rodin, J. and Langer, E.J. (1977) 'Long-term effects of a control-relevant intervention with the institutionalised aged', *Journal of Personality and Social Psychology* **35**, 897–902.

Rosenstock, I.M. (1985) 'Understanding and enhancing patient compliance with diabetic regimens', *Diabetes Care* **8**, 610–16.

Rosenthal, R. and Jacobson, L. (1968) *Pygmalion in the Classroom.* New York: Holt, Rinehart & Winston.

Ross, L. (1977) 'The intuitive psychologist and his shortcomings: Distortions in the attribution process', in L. Berkowitz (ed.) *Advances in Experimental Social Psychology*, Vol. 10. New York: Academic Press.

Roth, H.P. (1979) 'Problems in conducting a study of the effects on patient compliance of teaching the rationale for antacid therapy', in S.J. Cohen (ed.), *New Directions in Patient Compliance.* Lexington, Mass.: Lexington Books.

Rothman, A.J., Salovey, P., Turvey, C. and Fishkin, S.A. (1993) 'Attributions of responsibility and persuasion: Increasing mammography utilisation among women over 40 with an internally-oriented message', *Health Psychology* **12**, 39–47.

Rotter, J.B. (1966) 'Generalised expectancies for internal vs external control of reinforcement', *Psychological Monographs* **90**, 1–28.

Sackett, D.L. and Snow, J.C. (1979) 'The magnitude of compliance and non-compliance', in R.B. Haynes, D.W. Taylor and D.L. Sackett (eds.) *Compliance in Health Care.* Baltimore, MD: Johns Hopkins University Press.

Salvage, J. (1986). *The Politics of Nursing.* London: Heinemann Nursing.

Samora, J., Saunders, L. and Larson, R.F. (1961) 'Medical vocabulary knowledge among hospital patients', *Journal of Health and Human Behaviour* **2**, 83–9.

Skrypnek, B.J. and Snyder, M. (1982) 'On the self-perpetuating nature of stereotypes about women and men', *Journal of Experimental Social Psychology* **18**, 82–113.

Stanton, A.L. (1987) 'Determinants of adherence to medical regimens by hypertensive patients', *Journal of Behavioural Medicine* **10**, 377–94.

Strickland, B.R. (1978) 'Internal–external expectancies and health-related behaviours', *Journal of Consulting and Clinical Psychology* **6**, 1192–211.

Svarstad, B. (1976) 'Physician–patient communication and patient conformity with medical advice', in D. Mechanic (ed.) *The Growth of Bureaucratic Medicine.* New York: John Wiley.

Turk, D.C., Salovey, P. and Litt, M.D. (1986) 'Adherence: A cognitive-behavioural perspective', in K.E. Gerber and A.M. Nehemkis (eds.) *Compliance: The dilemma of the chronically ill.* New York: Springer.

United Kingdom Central Council for Nursing, Midwifery and Health Visiting (1992) *Code of Professional Conduct for the Nurse, Midwife and Health Visitor*, 3rd edition. London: UKCC.

Wallston, K.A., Wallston, B.S., Smith, S. and Dobbins, C.J. (1989) 'Perceived control and health', in M. Johnston and T.M. Marteau (eds.) *Applications in Health Psychology*. New Brunswick, NJ: Transaction Publishers.

Weiner, B. (1980) 'A cognitive (attribution) emotion-action model of motivated behaviour: An analysis of judgments of help-giving', *Journal of Personality and Social Psychology* **31**, 186–200.

Wishner, J. (1960) 'Reanalysis of "Impressions of personality"', *Psychological Review* **67**, 96–112.

Zebrowitz, L.A. (1990) *Social Perception*. Milton Keynes: Open University Press.

Zuckerman, M. (1979) 'Attribution of success and failure revisited, or: The motivational bias is alive and well in attribution theory', *Journal of Personality* **47**, 245–87.

CHAPTER 3

Working with groups

MARY HORTON

Chapter outline

Introduction

Because nurses work as members of teams and groups, an understanding of the nature of group processes is crucial for effectiveness. Equally important is an understanding of the possibilities and limitations of using groups with patients and colleagues – to inform, promote insight, change behaviour or alleviate suffering. Nurses work alongside psychologists, social workers and group and family therapists to achieve these aims.

Most social psychology textbooks discuss group behaviour, but few attempt to show the relationship between the usual cognitive approach and the psychodynamic approach to groups used by many therapists. This chapter confronts this large task. In the first section we review social psychological work on group influence. Next we consider the various explanations provided by cognitive social psychology and suggest that a model from psychodynamic theory might subsume them. Finally, we look at some applications of the ideas described in the first two sections, thereby providing an overall perspective.

The social psychology of group influence

Introduction

That people are social beings and open to each other's influence is a truism, but the depth and nature of these exchanges are often unrecognized. The 'messages' may be unconscious or deliberate, verbal or non-verbal, and we may be aware or un-aware that we are receiving them. But social psychologists argue that these influ-ences structure our perceptions and attitudes and underpin our beliefs about the social world. Such influences form part of professional training and are largely beneficial. But unquestioning acceptance of all received 'wisdom' can be harmful. For example, to accept that 'Mrs X in bed 3 is a troublemaker' may blind you to the distress of a dying woman. Too ready agreement with a colleague's interpretation of an ambiguous set of symptoms could lead to a wrong diagnosis. In this section, we shall consider some of the work on social influence, in order to help students recognize these processes and 'choose their teachers wisely'.

Unobtrusive Influence

In *ambiguous* situations people will tend to accept each other's judgements in the absence of evidence about what is really there. But these norms, once formed are hard to change. Sherif's (1936) classic study tested the hypothesis that others are used as reference points in the emergence of norms. He instructed people to judge, in each other's presence but without discussion, the degree of apparent movement of a single light-point in a dark room. Although subjects were unaware of it, such perceived movement is illusory, being caused by random eye movements. None the less, successive judgements of individuals in the group converged – the blind having led the blind – thus confirming Sherif's prediction. When tested individually after-wards, as expected, subjects did not diverge from the previously established group average or norm. Sherif proposed that this process of using others as an anchor for one's own perceptions could explain the emergence of all social norms from 'a common need to define a common reality'. Although we may now consider his generalization too sweeping, Sherif's conclusion stands – that in the absence of other information, people tend to use each other to define a reality, which then may grow to have the status of an external given.

Second, in *unambiguous* situations, individuals may succumb to majority press-ure if they find themselves the single dissenter, even when the majority position is clearly wrong. In Asch's (1956) seminal studies, groups of 7–9 male American college students were shown a white card with a vertical black line, and a second card with three lines of varying lengths. They had to choose which of the three lines best matched the standard and give their answers aloud. All the subjects except one were confederates of the experimenter, secretly primed to lie. Nearly one-third of the lone naive subjects made wrong statements on more than half the trials in order to fit in with the majority. Asch had expected far fewer people to deny the blatant evidence of their own eyes and concluded that those who consistently succumbed to 'wrong-headed' majority pressure, did so because of a personality defect – an excessive need for dependence.

Asch's paradigm has been repeated many times but with growing divergences from the original findings. Nicholson, Steven and Rocklin (1985) conducted a replication with British and American students. None of the British and only 14 per cent of the Americans made false judgements on more than half the trials. Asch (unpublished correspondence, quoted in Perrin and Spencer 1980) explained the change in terms of Western culture becoming more supportive of independence of mind.

DISCUSSION POINT

Think of a situation when you felt under pressure to agree with a decision of your peers against your better judgement. Did you succumb? What were the characteristics of the situation which led you to agree or to refuse to agree with the others? How might group pressure be resisted?

Overt group pressure

Many social psychologists have studied the influence of the authority structure on the behaviour of people in groups. Recent work on leadership has found there are no personality traits or working styles that show leadership 'quality', but the best leaders are those who can adapt their styles to changing group or external conditions (Fiedler, 1967).

Milgram (1974) posed a different question. What are the limits of influence of a *malign* authority? In his experiments he pitted the (presumed) moral norm of his subjects – that of not inflicting unnecessary pain on another human being – against the tendency to obey orders seen as coming from a legitimate authority. Milgram used adult volunteers for an experiment at Yale University, ostensibly about learning, which involved them as 'teachers' inflicting electric shocks of increasing severity on a 'learner' as a punishment for errors. The volunteers obeyed the experimenters although they were neither forced nor threatened. Milgram, like Asch, was surprised by his results. About two-thirds obeyed until told to stop even though the levers they were pulling were labelled 'DANGER – SEVERE SHOCK'. The experiment was a deception, the 'learner' was not really shocked, but Milgram's findings *were* shocking.

Why is the tendency to obey so strong? Milgram proposed what he called '*the agentic state*'. An innate or early learnt sensitivity to cues defining another person as an 'authority' will create an internal change so that a previously independent individual will become 'the agent of the other' in response to such stimuli. In the initial experiments the authority cues were thought to be the prestigious reputation of Yale, the 'scientific' laboratory environment and the experimenter's dress and manner. Variations of setting showed that 'total obeying' was reduced when authority's prestige or proximity were reduced, but even when overt status cues were removed, the tendency remained. The situation itself, of having voluntarily entered a role relationship entailing putting oneself under the orders of another, seemed sufficient to induce the agentic state and to absolve subjects from responsibility for their actions.

Milgram's findings may help to explain why some bogus doctors, in the hierarchical hospital environment, are able to escape detection for alarmingly long periods. A study by Hofling *et al.* (1966) gives a striking example of the strength of the agentic state in the role relationship between doctor and nurse. Nurses in an American hospital received telephone instructions from an unknown 'doctor' to give twice the maximum daily dose of a drug to a patient. Twenty-one of the 22 nurses agreed to give the dose. The hoax was revealed before the drug was administered. Although there are ethical and methodological criticisms of this experiment, the point it demonstrates remains.

DISCUSSION POINT

Do you think nurses sometimes experience pressure to obey orders that conflict with their personal values or professional judgement? Under what circumstances, if any, should nurses disobey instructions?

Group membership

That people can influence us to a greater extent than we might have imagined has been demonstrated. But two related questions remain. First, what is the nature of the attraction towards group membership that opens us to the possibility of being both influenced and influential? Second, what effect has our group membership on our perception of and behaviour towards non-members?

In answer to the first question, Asch suggested the 'need for dependence' to explain why some people may be susceptible to influence. The answer to the second question may help nurses to become more aware of their reactions to patients and colleagues who come from different social groups from their own. Social psychology has always been concerned with the problem of prejudice, defined as the making of faulty and inflexible negative attributions to others simply on the basis of their group memberships ('All doctors are . . .'). Prejudice also involves the tendency to behave towards these others in a manner consistent with these negative attributions.

Early explanations (Adorno *et al.*, 1964) were made in terms of personality differences. People who were more rigid and authority conscious and less self-aware were more likely to be prejudiced. This may be partly the case, but Tajfel

(1970) has proposed an explanation in terms of the general human propensity to seek to belong to groups and to value these memberships. That is, Tajfel is saying we are all 'prejudiced', to some extent, against outsiders, but we can learn to understand and counter this tendency. Tajfel's Social Identity Theory (1981) suggests that the search for personal identity and self-esteem, which is the motivation for joining groups, becomes linked to the need to maintain group or social identity once membership has been attained. The social identity of groups is created by a process of social categorization which simplifies the social world by 'clumping' it into discrete categories. The fundamental social categorization, Tajfel suggests, is into 'us' and 'not us' or 'them' (e.g. patients and staff.) Social identity is then maintained by *discrimination*; that is, behaviour designed to establish or to increase the difference between 'us' and 'them'.

Tajfel's seminal Minimal Group Experiments (1970) were designed to discover whether the simple fact of social categorization was sufficient to invoke discrimination against the out-group or whether further positive in-group attributes were necessary before such 'loyal' behaviour could be produced. A sample of 14-year-old boys was randomly divided into two groups. Each boy in isolation was asked to choose amounts of money to be given to pairs of other boys differentiated only by their categorizations into 'my group', and 'not my group'. It was found that the boys awarded the money so that the *difference* between the amount given to 'my group member' and 'not my group member' tended to be as large as possible, even when this meant that less money in total would accrue to 'my group'.

Tajfel's hypothesis was thus supported. Social categorization was, in itself, sufficient to produce discriminatory behaviour. The paradigm has been repeated many times with different people in different situations and the findings appear to be robust, although the artificiality of the design has been criticized.

DISCUSSION POINT
What, if anything, do you find difficult when caring for patients from a different race or class from of your own? How do you deal with these difficulties?

There is an important corollary to social identity theory. A distinction is made between the social categories we choose (for example, by training as a nurse) and those into which we are born, such as race, religion, nationality and gender. These qualities are already present in the social world as *stereotypes* and they may not always be positive. What happens if a category into which you are placed by birth, such as race or gender, is predominantly negative, that is, when you have a *negative social identity*? Tajfel suggests you have four survival possibilities: 'accepting', 'exiting', 'passing' or 'voicing'. An example may clarify.

In countries with a white majority, black people are generally given a negative social identity. These attributions can (but need not) be *accepted* or adopted by the individual. On the other hand, s/he may choose to *exit* and move to another country or to a community composed entirely of black people. A third possibility is to *pass* by adopting the habits and attitudes of the white majority and trying to be one of 'them'. A final possibility is to voice the black identity as positive (the slogan 'black is beautiful' is an example). By 'voicing', Tajfel suggests, black people increase their self-esteem, enabling them to compete with the white group and perhaps eventually change the negative black identity held by white groups. (See Chapter 2 for more information on sterotyping.)

DISCUSSION POINT
Most social identities are neither all positive nor all negative. What social identity do you think you have as a health professional? That is, how do you think you are seen by others? Would you like to change aspects of this identity? If so, which aspect and how?

Social identity theory goes beyond the small group and looks at the psychology of society. By defining the group as a division into 'us' and 'them', it has highlighted the fact that the group cannot exist in a social vacuum. Finally, it provides us with a radically new explanation for the age-old phenomena of prejudice and discrimination. In all, it provides useful ways to help us be more effective when 'working with groups'.

The group dynamic approach to the understanding of group processes

Introduction

We have seen that when in a group our behaviour is affected by others through the roles and categories we accord ourselves and them. Explanations for this pheno- menon have been many. These explanations do not necessarily contradict one another, but there are many, and it may be difficult to see how they can explain certain aspects of group behaviour that they do not directly address.

The question now is: Is there any approach to the understanding of group pro- cesses that can encompass all these explanations? Psychodynamic theory may be able to do so. Although this section is largely theoretical, it provides the means for a return to practical issues of working with groups in the final section.

What is psychodynamic theory?

Freud is generally known through his clinical work in understanding and treating neuroses, but his life's aim was to develop a theory of the human mind that could account for *all* behaviour of individuals, groups and institutions.

There are three main tenets to Freud's theory. The first is that of *two primary motives*. Freud (1930) named these two motives the pursuit of pleasure and the avoidance of pain – a profound if not entirely original proposal. These two motives are, at times, in conflict. That is, we must sometimes bear pain (such as that of waiting) to get pleasure; and some pleasures (such as over-indulgence) lead to pain.

The second tenet is that of the *unconscious*. To Freud, the unconscious is not simply a repository for what we do not remember. It is a repressive force, preventing awareness of painful memories or desires that would conflict with our conscious goals. However, these unconscious fears and wishes inform our actions so that we may behave, not necessarily irrationally, but from motives deeper than we realize. The unconscious makes itself known through our small mistakes, such as forgetting or slips of the tongue, through jokes, dreams and neurotic symptoms.

The third tenet is the fundamentally *social nature* of the human mind. We internalize and identify with aspects of those who are important to us, such as our parents, whom we both love and fear. Freud used the terms *ego* and *superego* to describe the different levels at which the mind incorporates the social world. Freud describes the ego as largely preconscious (not entirely repressed) and in direct contact with the outside world through the sensory receptors. Through the ego, we imitate and learn, influence and are influenced, throughout our lives. The superego is a more archaic, less malleable structure, deeply unconscious, where our early internalized parental 'images' are metaphorically 'laid down', forming our conscience. This is not the adult conscience of sophisticated moral argument, but a jumbled collection of prohibitions and ideals, accessible to our adult awareness only as the 'pricking of conscience' when we may be on the point of transgressing an early learned rule. None the less Freud sees the primitive superego as the basis of our 'social being'.

I can now return to my main argument, that the motives put forward by social psychologists to explain behaviour can be subsumed under one or other of Freud's two primary motives. Psychodynamic theory suggests that, as the baby develops, the simple *pain-avoidance* motive becomes that of the avoidance of anxiety, which is the anticipation or fear of pain. This feared pain can be of physical or psychological events such as the fear of the loss of self-esteem (cf. Tajfel) or the loss of the comfort of supportive others (cf. Asch's dependency motive). It can simply be the fear of the unknown itself. This fear can be realistic or simply imagined. But by avoiding even the anxiety of envisaging it, we fail to discover which of the two it is.

Primitive *pleasure-seeking*, the impulse for self-gratification, also undergoes modification into what Klein (1928) calls knowledge-seeking or the motive to understand ourselves (cf. Tajfel's need for personal and social identity) and the outside world (cf. Sherif's need to define a 'common reality'). The seeking of knowledge can be used in the service of the avoidance of anxiety. For example, we seek scientific knowledge partly to predict and avert unpleasant environmental change, as well as for the benefits it brings. However, just as they conflict in their primitive modes, the two more 'adult' motives sometimes conflict: the knowledge that we seek may be of the unknown that we fear. The study of social psychology, or the search for knowledge of ourselves as 'social beings', may itself be an example of that conflict.

To summarize: the motivational bases for group behaviour provided by traditional social psychology can be subsumed in terms of two basic motivations posited by psychodynamic theory – the fear of harm and the desire for knowledge. Because these motivations are conceived as being in conflict, psychodynamic theories of group behaviour, such as those of Freud and Bion (to follow, pp. 57–8; pp. 58–9), can be more deeply explanatory than those theories described above, each of which posits a single, if different motivational base. I am not suggesting that these cognitive explanations are thereby negated; rather, that they can be more clearly understood when included in the perspective provided by psychodynamic theory.

Freud's group theory

Freud (1933: 99) gave the following definition of a group:

> A psychological group is a collection of individuals who have introduced the same person (i.e. the leader) into their *superego*, and on the basis of this common element have *identified* themselves with one another in their *ego*.

What Freud is saying here is that for a psychological group to emerge from a collection of individuals, there must first be a potential leader. The potential followers unconsciously choose this leader by identifying with him or her at a deep level, replacing the parental images in their superego with the image of the leader. Having *all* done this, they have something fundamental in common and can identify with each other at the more surface level of the ego, as if they were siblings. However, although Freud introduces the analogy of the family, he was talking about groups of unrelated adults and he clearly differentiates the two types of group. Whereas the feelings and behaviour of the child in the family form part of a natural developmental progression, those of group members in Freud's model are regressive. By becoming part of a group, the adult member is, in part, regressing to an earlier life stage.

DISCUSSION POINT
Do you think all groups need a leader? Do you think people tend to act childishly when in a group?

There are difficulties posed by Freud's group theory (De Board, 1978). But there are also some inferences we can draw which may deepen our understanding of current thinking. The first concerns the relation between follower and leader. Freud says this involves the replacement of personal conscience by the internalized image of the leader, so that the follower can perform actions 'in the service of' the leader which might otherwise be personally abhorrent. This is reminiscent of the 'agentic state' proposed by Milgram to explain the behaviour of his subjects in his obedience experiments. Milgram (1974) himself links his explanation with Freud's ideas, suggesting the tendency to obey comes from the depths of our social being.

Second, the state of mutual ego-identification of group members, involving a common shared attachment, might be seen as similar to Asch's dependency motive, used to explain the phenomenon of conformity. It suggests that the motive itself (though not its excessive manifestation in Asch's experiments) may be a general one.

Third, Freud (1921) suggests that when groups are formed, a barrier of what might be called 'personal space' is broken between individuals who have now

Figure 3.1 *Model of Freud's group types*

	Primitive	*Secondary*
Natural	A religious cult	The Amish community
Artificial	A research team in a university	A management committee in a hospital

become members. This barrier has previously been maintained by a natural am-bivalence (or conflict of hostility and liking). When the group forms, hostility towards other members disappears and ties are made without ambivalence. Hos-tility is now directed towards outsiders, the 'personal space' barrier having become a 'group space' barrier. In this way, Freud's theory could explain some of the findings of Tajfel's minimal group experiments if we accept Tajfel's conclusion – that his boys were socially primed to react to minimal group cues by defining themselves as members.

Perhaps we can understand Freud's group theory further, by considering his thinking as applied to actual groups (Freud, 1921; see Figure 3.1). He distinguishes between what he calls *primitive* groups with an actual leader (e.g. a street gang or a religious cult with an actual, living leader) and *secondary* groups led by an abstrac-tion (e.g. a rule-book, which lays down procedures for who will be appointed to the chair and the conduct of the group). He also distinguishes between a *natural* group, held together entirely by the internal forces he has described (e.g. the Amish community in Pennsylvania, who are tolerated by, but live independently from, the wider society) and an *artificial* group, held by both internal and external social forces. Examples are a committee appointed in a hospital, or a higher level organ-ization such as a hospital existing within the NHS.

It is apparent that the types of group we have been considering, as well as those we shall look at in the final section, and the groups to which the reader may belong in a professional role, can be either 'primitive' or 'secondary' in Freud's sense, but they are all 'artificial' or embedded in the social matrix.

DISCUSSION POINT
Do you find Freud's group theory helps you to understand the way in which the groups to which you belong function? In what ways is it useful or not useful?

Bion's group theory

The psychoanalyst Bion (1961) disagreed with some of Freud's ideas – in particular, the importance of the emergent leader in the formation of the group. Bion's ideas have been tested on many volunteer groups from the general public in Britain and the United States (De Board, 1978), albeit this testing is an experiential rather than an experimental process. An example are the study groups described in the next section.

Like Freud, Bion designed his theory so that it could be generalized to the understanding of all groups and institutions in society. But the model on which it is based is that of small, face-to-face, 'secondary' and 'artificial' groups with boundary rules (of time, space, role and task) set in the context of a larger institution. Bion sees the group as operating on two levels: the conscious work-group trying to fulfil the group task and a simultaneously existing set of unconscious 'myths' about what the group goals are and how they can be achieved. These group myths operate when the task of the work-group becomes too difficult, such as when the responsibility of decision-making creates too much anxiety. The myths act as a defence against anxiety by deflecting the group away from the task. Bion thinks these basic assumptions are jointly held, unconscious beliefs which can be sensed in the emotional content of the atmosphere they engender. Like Freud, he thinks the group in basic assumption mode tends to regress to child-like thinking and sometimes behaviour.

There are three unconscious basic assumptions in Bion's theory and these are used as a defence against reality. They are: dependency, fight-flight and pairing. The myth of '*dependency*' is that the group is meeting so that a leader on whom it depends absolutely should satisfy all its needs. The feeling is one of helplessness and then despair when (inevitably, in time) the leader fails to live up to these ideal expectations. A group of anxious nursing students, working under the supervision of a 'powerful' and 'wise' experienced nurse, easily fits this picture.

The myth of *fight–flight* is that there is an external enemy who must be attacked or avoided if the group is to survive. The group finds an emergent or unofficial 'leader' who will take them into aggressive 'fight' or panic 'flight'; and the feeling is one of fear and hate. Sometimes the enemy is found within the group and scape-goating can ensue. Teams of nurses who work in emergency situations such as large-scale accidents are trained to conduct themselves professionally and not to succumb to such panic leaders. But in the quieter atmosphere of the meeting or the ward round, antagonism toward an 'unfeeling' management or 'irresponsible' juniors may cloud the group's judgement.

The myth of *pairing* is that the future will solve all present problems. The group often focuses on two members who are seen as the prophets from whom the solution to the group task will be born. The underlying atmosphere is of unrealistic hope, often expressed in vague generalizations: 'Things will be better in the spring/ when we get more money/when the management reorganizes us.' But addressing the here-and-now task that the work-group has met to consider (e.g. to cover the next shift with an inadequate number of staff) is avoided.

In the life of any group, according to Bion, unconscious 'myths' (or basic assumptions) will alternate, but only one myth can operate concurrently with the conscious 'work-group'. The basic assumption groups have emergent leaders, unconsciously chosen by the group. However, unlike Freud's leaders, they are not psychologically the 'strongest', but are often those least able to resist the unconscious group pressure to re-enact the 'myth'. The externally appointed chair, on the other hand, is distinguished from the group by his or her role, which may or may not be matched by greater skill and knowledge.

DISCUSSION POINT

Bion thought that unconscious 'basic assumption thinking' could occur in all types of groups at any time. Are there any groups to which you belong in your professional role where you think that basic assumptions may have clouded rational discussion or decision-making?

Working with groups: some applications of theory

Introduction

We have now reviewed some of the major approaches to the understanding of group processes. In this final section we shall look at ways of applying both cognitive and psychodynamic approaches to our practice when working with groups.

Training groups

These are experiential learning groups under the guidance of a qualified facilitator or consultant. They are face-to-face groups with fixed membership, meeting for a set time of at least 10–15 hours, but often longer. Learning is either 'massed' into two or three days, or 'spaced' across months. Although the specific aims will differ according to the group's theoretical orientation, the overall purpose is to increase group interaction skills. The *Johari Window* (so named after its inventors, Joe and Harry) gives a diagrammatic picture of the learning potential provided by experiential training groups (Figure 3.2).

In a training group the aim is to help trainees change such public behaviour (cell 1) that might be agreed to be maladaptive; to increase awareness of behaviour to which they might be blind (cell 2); to encourage people to disclose thoughts and feelings they keep hidden (cell 3), but only if this openness is appropriate to the group task. The interpretation of unconscious processes (cell 4) is the aim of study groups (these are training groups run on Bionian lines) where the aim is to bring to the group's awareness the blocks to effective task performance created by processes such as 'basic assumption' thinking. This latter objective is not usually present in T-groups or training groups based on the work of Lewin (De Board, 1978).

Figure 3.2 *Johari social behaviour window*

	Known to Self	*Unknown to Self*
Known to Others	PUBLIC (1)	BLIND (2)
Unknown to Others	HIDDEN (3)	UNCONSCIOUS (4)

DISCUSSION POINT

As a teacher, I am sometimes made aware of mannerisms by feedback from a class. Can you think of any feelings or behaviour to which you may have been blind, until made aware of them in a group?

The criterion for success of a training group is usually the self-evaluation of the learner, sometimes combined with assessment by trainers, other group members and work colleagues. Testing the outcome of some groups may be thought anti-thetical to their experiential purpose, and rigorous testing of training groups is difficult because of the lack of appropriate controls and sensitive change measures (Oatley, 1984). But a large-scale study by Lieberman, Yalom and Miles (1973), which did use matched controls and compared ten group styles, showed that, six months later, 39 per cent of participants, compared with 17 per cent of controls, thought they had made lasting positive changes in their social relationship skills.

Both T-groups and study groups are used in professional and management training. A study by Geitgey *et al.* (1966) showed that student nurses were judged more positively by nurse tutors and by patients after the students had completed T-group training.

Therapy and counselling groups

In contrast to training groups, therapy and counselling groups are designed to offer professional help to patients or clients in emotional distress or with behavioural problems. They can be used as an alternative or adjunct to individual therapy or counselling. However, the conduct of any of the three types of group (training, therapy or counselling) necessitates the acquisition of specific professional qualifications by the group leader. These groups are thus distinct from the types of group-work which nurses and other health professionals should be competent to conduct without further training. A brief summary of the main types of therapy and counselling groups is given here, as it seems important for practitioners to know what to choose from should they wish to train as group therapists or counsellors in order to add a valuable skill to their professional competence.

There are numerous approaches to *group therapy* (Aveline and Dryden, 1988). They can be seen as fitting into three categories according to their theoretical orientation: the psychodynamic, the cognitive behavioural and a middle group using a humanistic approach (see Box 3.1).

Group counselling reflects the same theoretical orientations as group therapy, but in practice it is more eclectic. Training for both individual and group counselling is under the general direction of the British Association for Counselling. Often groups are organized to deal with specific areas of distress, such as groups for the bereaved, for disaster survivors, for adult survivors of child abuse or groups for marital counselling. Community nurses sometimes conduct counselling groups.

BOX 3.1   SOME GROUP THERAPIES AVAILABLE IN BRITAIN

1. *Psychodynamic*
   (a) *The Tavistock approach* is influenced by Bion's work (1961). The focus is on the group as a whole, rather than the individual in the group. Training is centred in the Tavistock Clinic (London).
   (b) *Group analysis* was developed by Foulkes (Foulkes and Anthony (1957)). It focuses on the individual in the context of the group, looking at the development of *transference relationships* (patterns of interpersonal behaviour which unconsciously re-enact past patterns). Members are helped to become aware of these patterns within the matrix of the group. Training is through the Institute of Group Analysis (London).

2. *Cognitive-Behavioural*
   (a) *Social skills training (SST)* was developed from the work of Argyle (Trower *et al.*, 1978) As a group therapy it transfers to the group ideas about social learning drawn from individual psychology. It is used, for example, with physically or mentally disabled patients to help them develop the abilities and confidence to live in the community. Practitioners are social and clinical psychologists, psychiatric nurses and social workers. *Assertion* and *anger management* training are specific forms of group therapy using the SST approach.
   (b) *Anxiety Management Training (AMT)* applies the principles of cognitive therapy (Aveline and Dryden, 1988) for use in groups of anxious or neurotic patients. It is used by clinical psychologists. Training for psychiatric nurses to lead AMT groups has been developed at the Maudsley Hospital (London).

Many of these groups are private and fee-paying, but some NHS hospitals provide therapy for in- and/or outpatient groups. Intensive group-work, mainly from a psychodynamic base is used in psychiatric hospitals or clinics using the *therapeutic community* approach (Kennard, 1988).

Outcome studies of group therapy, like those of training groups are difficult to conduct, and many studies do not use controls. Parloff and Dies (1977) reviewed research from 1966 to 1975 and found mixed results. Perhaps the most important conclusion to be drawn is the need to match the type of patients to the type of group.

Group-work by health professionals

There are many situations where it is appropriate for health professionals to conduct group-work with patients. Much of the literature concerns groups for people who are mentally ill; and the use of nurses as group facilitators in therapeutic communities is well documented (Kennard, 1988).

For the group transmission of health-related information, see Chapter 6. But McCaughan (1980) gives a practical guide to group organization, which can be adapted for use by health professionals. In group formation, care should be taken in the selection of members so that there are enough differences for useful comparison processes to be undertaken, but not so many that cohesion is difficult to achieve or that scapegoating may occur. The boundaries of time and space need to be clearly delineated. Groups can either have a fixed time limit and membership (like many training groups) or a changing membership and no fixed ending (like many therapy groups). More intensive work can be done with fixed groups, but they should end at the time stipulated. Psychodynamic theory would suggest that it is only after the group's loss has been mourned that the former members can internalize and use the learning achieved.

Other types of group, such as reminiscence groups in the care of the elderly, where those able to do so can be encouraged to exchange life stories, will have, by definition, a changing membership. But the aim of such groups is to give comfort rather than to promote learning.

DISCUSSION POINT

Have you attended, or helped to run, a patient group? What was the group's purpose? Have you found the points made here useful or not when looking back at your experience? In what ways?

Group processes and the nursing culture

In the 1950s Menzies (Menzies Lyth, 1985), in a study of a London teaching hospital, showed that organizational measures designed by nursing staff ostensibly to reduce the high anxiety levels engendered by daily confrontation with suffering and death, were in fact increasing anxiety because the projective processes had become fixed in a vicious circle and, by its very existence, the social defence system had broken down.

The organizational measures (or social defences) used to protect the nurses from direct contact with the patients' pain were, first, splitting the nurses' work into discrete tasks (i.e. bed-making) performed on many patients, thus minimizing relationships with any individual patient. Second, the patients were deindividuated into exemplars of their illness category ('the pneumonia in bed 15'), and the nurses were deindividuated into grade and skill categories. The final measure was the teaching of detachment and lack of feeling as prime attributes of a good nurse. The defensive organizational measures used to protect nurses from the anxiety of the daily responsibility of making life-or-death decisions were a rigid demarcation upward of responsibility, combined with obscuring the formal distribution of responsibility at senior nursing levels. This resulted in a reprojection downward of the attribute of irresponsibility onto student nurses, who thus found themselves holding the unconsciously enforced and somewhat contradictory roles of being both 'unfeeling robots' and 'irresponsible children'. The reality of suffering and death on the wards still faced them, but nurses in their enforced unconscious roles of robots and children now felt even less competent to cope. Anxiety and drop-out rates increased.

The resistance to change, predicted by the theory of institutional defence systems, prevented early acceptance of Menzies' analysis of the nursing culture. But today, many of the changes suggested in her report are being introduced, together with other changes in nurse education as embodied in Project 2000.

DISCUSSION POINT
Do you think Menzies' analysis of the nursing culture in the 1950s applies to hospitals in the 1990s? In what ways is it the same? In what ways has it changed?

Summary

The purpose of this chapter has been to show how the practice of working with groups in nursing and other health professions can be better understood and improved by greater comprehension of the theories underlying particular ways of working. I have tried to show that cognitive and psychodynamic approaches to the understanding of small groups and organizational cultures need not be seen as either contradictory or each applying to a separate area of practice; but that the ideas in terms of the understanding of the motivational bases of group behaviour can be seen to complement each other. This knowledge can help us to develop our competence and skills, by allowing us to utilize a greater range of techniques and ideas.

Seminar questions

Compare the contexts of hospital and community nursing when considering the following:

1. Should patients/clients be coerced into obeying advice or instructions? If so, under what circumstances, and by what means? If not, why not?
2. How might knowledge about the factors involved in group influence be useful to the practising nurse?
3. How might health professionals use group-work to address their own stereotypes and prejudices?

Further reading

Abraham, C. and Shanley, E. (1992) *Social Psychology for Nurses*. London: Edward Arnold.
A comprehensive and up-to-date text. Chapter 8, 'Working and changing in groups', is particularly relevant. Social identity theory is discussed in Chapter 3.
Aveline, M. and Dryden, W. (eds.) (1988) *Group Therapy in Britain*. Milton Keynes: Open University Press.

A useful source book. The papers by Kennard on therapeutic communities and Miller on organizational dynamics are both relevant.

De Board, R. (1978) *The Psychoanalysis of Organisations*. London: Tavistock.

Chapter 2 on Freud's group theory and Chapter 4 on Bion give extended coverage to the ideas in this chapter, as do his Chapter 7 on T-groups and Chapter 9 on social defence systems.

References

Adorno, T.W., Frenkel-Brunswik, E., Levinson, D. J. and Sanford, R.N. (1964) *The Authoritarian Personality*. New York: John Wiley.

Asch, S. E. (1956) 'Studies of independence and conformity: A minority of one against a unanimous majority', *Psychological Monographs* **70** (9) (whole No. 416).

Aveline, M. and Dryden, W. (1988) *Group Therapy in Britain*. Milton Keynes: Open University Press.

Bion, W.R. (1961) *Experiences in Groups and Other Papers*. London: Tavistock.

De Board, R. (1978) *The Psychoanalysis of Organisations*. London: Tavistock.

Fiedler, F.E. (1967) *A Theory of Leadership Effectiveness*. New York: McGraw-Hill.

Foulkes, S.H. and Anthony, E.J. (1957) *Group Psychotherapy. The psycho-analytic approach*. Harmondsworth: Penguin Books.

Freud, S. (1921) 'Group psychology and the analysis of the ego', in S. Freud (1985) *Civilisation, Society and Religion*, Vol. 12, Pelican Freud Library. Harmondsworth: Penguin Books.

Freud, S. (1930) 'Civilisation and its discontents', in S. Freud (1985) *Civilisation, Society and Religion*, Vol. 12, Pelican Freud Library. Harmondsworth: Penguin Books.

Freud, S. (1933) 'Dissection of the psychical personality', in S. Freud (1973) *New Introductory Lectures in Psychology*, Vol. 2, Pelican Freud Library. Harmondsworth: Penguin Books.

Geitgey, D.A. *et al.* (1966) 'A study of some effects of sensitivity training on the performance of students in associate degree programmes of nursing education', Dissertation *Abstracts* **27B**, 2000–1.

Hofling, C.K., Brotsman, E., Dalrymple, S., Graves, N. and Pierce, C.M. (1966) 'An experimental study in nurse–physician relationships', *Journal of Nervous and Mental Diseases* **143**, 171–80.

Kennard, D. (1988) 'The therapeutic community', in E. Aveline and W. Dryden, *Group Therapy in Britain*. Milton Keynes: Open University Press.

Klein, M. (1928) 'Early stages of the Oedipus conflict', in M. Klein (1975) *Love, Guilt and Reparation*. London: Hogarth Press.

Lieberman, M.A, Yalom, I.D. and Miles, M.B. (1973) *Encounter Groups: First Facts*. New York: Basic Books.

McCaughan, N. (1980) 'The purposes of group-work in social work', in P.B. Smith (ed.) (1980) *Small Groups and Personal Change*. London: Methuen.

Menzies Lyth, I. (1988) *Containing Anxiety in Institutions: Selected essays*. Vol. 1, London: Free Association Books.

Milgram, S. (1974) *Obedience to Authority*. London: Tavistock.

Nicholson, N., Steven, C.G. and Rocklin, T. (1985) 'Conformity in the Asch situation: A comparison between contemporary British and U.S. university students', *British Journal of Social Psychology* **24**, 59–63.

Oatley, K. (1984) *Selves in Relation: An introduction to psychotherapy and groups. New Essential Psychology.* London: Methuen.

Parloff, M.B. and Dies, R.R. (1977) 'Group psychotherapy outcome research 1966–1975', *International Journal of Group Psychotherapy* **27**, 281–319.

Perrin, S. and Spencer, C. (1980) 'The Asch effect: A child of its time?' *Bulletin of the British Psychological Society* **32**, 405–6.

Sherif, M. (1936) *The Psychology of Social Norms.* New York: Harper & Row.

Stogdill, R.M. (1974) *Handbook of Leadership: A survey of theory and research.* New York: Free Press.

Tajfel, H. (1970) 'Experiments in Intergroup Discrimination', *Scientific American* **223** (5), 96-102.

Tajfel, H. (1981) *Human Groups & Social Categories.* Cambridge: Cambridge University Press.

Tajfel, H., Flament, C., Billig, M. and Bundy, R. (1971) 'Social categorisation and intergroup behaviour', *European Journal of Social Psychology* **1**, 149–78.

Trower, P., Bryant, B. and Argyle, M. (1978) *Social Skills and Mental Health.* London: Methuen.

CHAPTER 4

Nursing the family

PAUL MARCH

Chapter outline

Introduction

The nursing profession has become increasingly interested in holistic care (Owen and Holmes, 1993), which is based on considering a person's physical, mental and environmental conditions together (see Seminar Questions). The assumption that a person's physical and mental wellbeing constitute a mutually dependent system (see Chapter 15) appears to have been accepted within nursing (Jacono and Jacono, 1994; Owen and Holmes, 1993). However, the influence of the family on health has not been emphasized (Doherty, McDaniel and Hepworth, 1994). The aim of this chapter is to draw attention to the role of the family in relation to illness. As Campbell, McDaniel and Seaburn (1992) point out, there are four reasons why it is useful for a health professional to concentrate upon the family:

1. The family is the primary source of many health beliefs and information.
   Individuals will usually ask the opinions of other family members before

seeking outside help. As such, the family is an important gatekeeper to health care.

2. Individuals experience a variety of family-related stressors over time: births, deaths, marriages, etc., and these can be associated with increased levels of illness.

3. A physical illness, while distressing to the individual, may provide a useful function when the whole family is considered. For example, as we shall see, a child with asthma may provide two, otherwise distant parents with a joint concern and so help them to avoid the realization that they are growing apart.

4. In the community, health professionals rarely provide treatment. Rather, they recommend a treatment which is then provided by the patient or other family member and the family may support or sabotage the treatment. Moreover, an individual is likely to change unhealthy behaviour only with the encouragement and support of his/her family (see Chapter 5).

Forty years ago it was easier to describe a 'normal' family. Parsons (1955) had no difficulty defining the family as being an independent nuclear unit of husband, wife and children. Since the 1950s the nature of families has changed radically and it is no longer possible to provide an uncontroversial definition (Cheal, 1991; see also the following Discussion Point). For this chapter, the family is defined as mother and/or father and children. The parent/s may be step-parents and the families may be reconstituted. Pairs or groups of adults who live together on a stable, long-term basis are seen as equivalent. (This definition is an Anglo-Saxon one; other cultures define the family differently; see p. 72.)

In this chapter I shall begin by considering the effects of illness on family members and their relationships. I shall then consider whether a family's reaction to illness can influence the course of an illness. Evidence will be reviewed which suggests that stress on one or more individuals can trigger illness in other family members. The notion that an illness can play an adaptive role in a family will also be discussed. I conclude with a checklist to help nurses assess whether the treatment of a patient might benefit from family intervention.

DISCUSSION POINT

Think about the experiences of chronic illness in your own family. How does your family react, cope and change when confronted by illness?

The effects of illness on the family

The effects of illness on couples

In a variety of chronic medical conditions, the level of a spouse's distress is of the same magnitude as that of the patient (Coyne and Fiske, 1992). Although patient and spouse face different challenges, their success in overcoming them is correlated; demoralization and distress in the spouse is associated with poorer recovery by the

---

BOX 4.1   **CASE STUDY: MR AND MRS G**

Mr and Mrs G were both in their early seventies. Mr G was referred to a clinical psychologist by his GP, prompted by Mrs G's concern that her husband was making little effort over rehabilitation six months after a heart attack.

Mr and Mrs G were seen together. Mr G said that he knew he should be exercising and picking up his interests again but felt incapable of doing so. Mrs G added that she had suffered from cancer a few years before and believed that the only way to deal with life-threatening conditions was to refuse to succumb to the disease. She had fought her condition with complete success and was worried that Mr G was not following her example.

When Mr G had his heart attack he found himself to be, secretly, much more frightened than he had expected. He could not throw himself into the fight. His wife encouraged him to return to his old life as soon as possible and her indomitable spirit contrasted with his hidden fears and lowered his self-esteem even further. A vicious circle emerged in which the more Mr G's self-esteem decreased, the more difficult it was for him to fight. Mrs G would then take on more and more of the responsibility for his rehabilitation programme, which left him feeling even more useless. In this case the vicious circle began to unravel when Mr G let his wife know how frightened he was and she reacted with understanding rather than hostility.

---

patient. For example, patients who are disturbed by their spouse's anxiety may discontinue their rehabilitation programmes in order to spare their spouse the sight of their difficulties and pain. (See Box 4.1 for an illustration of this.)

Nurses treating adults with a chronic illness need, therefore, to take the following factors into account: (1) that distress felt by the patient's partner about the patient's condition may be as great as the distress of the patient; (2) that the partner may need emotional support to cope with the illness and concrete support to cope with the day-to-day tasks; (3) the partner, rather than the patient, may be instrumental in implementing lifestyle changes recommended by the nurse and/or may be as involved in the treatment regime as the patient. So couples may need to be considered as equal partners in the treatment programme and given equal access to information and support. (See Chapter 2 for adherence to treatment.)

The effect of a child's illness on the rest of the family

Beresford (1994) is critical of earlier models which attempt to explain the reactions of families to children's chronic illness or disablement. This is because these models do not emphasize that parents are attempting to cope with an objectively stressful experience, but concentrate on the vulnerabilities of families. Instead, Beresford suggests that by focusing on coping mechanisms, one can concentrate on families' strengths.

She uses Lazarus's (1966) coping model to explain how parents are likely to react when caring for a disabled child. Childhood illness is seen as a potential stressor for parents, the impact of which is determined by the parents' appraisal of the situation. The impact of the illness will depend on three factors:

1. *Socio-ecological coping resources.* The availability of social support is partly determined by the parents' social skills. Formal support (i.e. from health professionals) is seen as a potential source of stress (as well as of support), either because of the effort needed to obtain the support in the first place or because of its inadequacy.

2. *Parents' coping resources and parents' belief about the situation.* Beresford (1994) highlights the parents' physical health as an important personal resource, but also notes the interactive relationship between this resource and coping. For example, the parents' physical wellbeing is frequently used as a measure of how well they are coping as well as being a resource to help them to cope. Moreover, the strain of caring for a disabled child results in relatively poorer parental physical health and so reduces the availability of this resource.

   Beresford found the following beliefs to be associated with families who were coping well: religious or spiritual beliefs, the ability to be flexible about previously held values, an optimistic outlook that avoided wishful thinking, an internal locus of control concerning day-to-day problems and an external locus of control with regard to cause of illness or disability (see also Chapter 5).

3. *Parents' problem-solving skills and coping style.* There is obviously an overlap between parental beliefs and parental coping strategies. It appears that problem-oriented, solution-focused and positive self-appraisal are more associated with parental wellbeing than strategies aimed at coping with the emotional impact of stress. However, there are methodological reasons why such a finding is not surprising. Many of the parental coping questionnaires use the expression of emotions such as 'crying' or 'getting angry' as indications of poor coping, despite there being no valid reason for doing so. The acceptance of some aspects of a chronic condition may be very similar to a grief reaction. In this context, weeping or expressions of anger and sorrow should not be seen as maladaptive. Rather, they are indications that the family are facing up to their predicament. In these situations, it does appear that men have a greater tendency than women to react by becoming distant rather than emotional. This male way of coping is likely to increase the strain on the mother, who has to shoulder the extra burden.

Beresford's model gives a good overall picture of the various factors involved in shaping parents' coping response. Families who are coping with the care of a chronically ill or handicapped child will undoubtedly find it a stressful experience, especially at first. In order to cope, families will need to change their lifestyle. Those who cope well appear to become problem-oriented, organized, routine-based and so relatively inflexible. Far from being seen as coping well, to the onlooker these families may appear pathological in the apparently rigid way in which they tackle the world. But the onlooker is in danger of committing a common human mistake, known as the *fundamental attributional error* (Ross, 1977; see also Chapter 2).

When applied to families with problems, this means that we may wrongly perceive family behaviour as due to some basic family pathology rather than as a reaction to stressful circumstances.

The health professional can help families to cope with chronic illness by helping them develop their problem-solving skills using, for example, D'Zurilla's (1990) problem-solving techniques, cognitive-behavioural strategies or modelling (see Chapter 15). By definition, there are aspects of chronic conditions that cannot be solved, so that the only reaction available is an emotional one. Professionals can assist by helping parents to understand that an emotional response it not a sign of collapse and by looking at ways in which the involvement of all family members can be increased.

The effects of ill parents on children

There has been very little work done in this area. One study by Peters and Esses (1985) compared the experiences of adolescent offspring of a parent who had multiple sclerosis (MS) with those of a control group. The offspring of those with MS reported higher levels of family conflict and lower levels of family cohesion, fewer joint activities and less emphasis on cultural, intellectual and religious matters. Peters and Esses suggest that these families may feel less cohesive, partly because the nature of the disability makes joint activities more difficult and partly because the parents may respond to the illness by withdrawing emotionally from the rest of the family. Finally, Peters and Esses suggest that the higher levels of conflict are understandable in a household that needs to renegotiate the responsibilities for many family tasks.

The course of illness and its interaction with the family lifecycle

The family lifecycle

The impact of an illness or disability on a family will be influenced by lifecycle changes. A number of family lifecycle models have been formulated and all present the family as needing to evolve and develop in response to external influences and internal maturational changes. Many of these influences are predictable and so the models divide the family cycle into separate stages. For instance, Carter and McGoldrick (1989) identify six stages:

1. The unattached young adult.
2. The newly married couple.
3. The family with young children.
4. The family with adolescents.
5. Launching children and moving on.
6. The family in later life.

Carter and McGoldrick's model is based on the lifecycle of a middle-class American family. Families of other backgrounds are likely to follow different patterns. According to McGoldrick (1989), different cultures have different definitions of family. For example, in the United States, white Anglo-Saxon Protestants (WASPs) see the family as comprising a mother, father and children – the nuclear family. Italian Americans' notion of the family is wider and includes grandparents, uncles, aunts and cousins. The Chinese notion of an extended family includes ancestors. The black American concept of family includes a wide, informal network of kin and community, where friends become family members and blood relatedness is less important.

McGoldrick also suggests that different cultures place different emphases on different stages in the lifecycle. Crucial to Irish and Black American culture is the funeral and wake. The Italians and Polish particularly celebrate weddings and Jews celebrate Bar Mitzvah. She concludes that certain lifecycle changes have greater significance for some cultures, so problems are likely to emerge at different stages of the lifecycle. For example, WASP families are very concerned that their young adults become independent. This can result in some adolescents feeling isolated from their families. She also suggests that WASP families may find it relatively more difficult to cope with having a family member with a mental handicap who cannot easily become independent. At the other extreme is Greek and Italian culture where independence is not highly valued. Young Greeks and Italians may find it difficult to negotiate an emotional distance from their family without breaking with them altogether.

McGoldrick's work is useful in that it highlights the danger of a dominant culture imposing its norms on minority groups, but she does not cite any evidence to support the cultural distinctions that she makes. Without good, carefully collected evidence, these distinctions risk becoming indistinguishable from racial stereotypes (see also the following Discussion Point).

DISCUSSION POINT
How can we take account of ethical and cultural differences without creating stereotypes?

Anxiety and the family lifecycle

Carter and McGoldrick (1989) classify the anxieties experienced by a family into vertical and horizontal stressors. The vertical stressors are those that are passed down through the generations – family belief systems, taboos, etc. The horizontal stressors are those that the family meets over time in the form of external (e.g. child reaches school age) and internal (e.g. child reaches puberty) stressors. Carter and McGoldrick expect vertical and horizontal stressors to interact to produce greater anxiety than the sum of the two. For example, there are a number of horizontal stressors associated with a child becoming an adolescent, e.g. the onset of puberty, increasing involvement with peers. The family will need to make some changes to

---

BOX 4.2 **CASE STUDY: NIGEL**

Nigel, aged 9, was an only child. His parents were separated and he lived with his mother. His father occasionally and unpredictably returned to live in the family home for unspecified lengths of time. Because Nigel found he could not rely on his father, he led a rather anxious life. His mother responded to Nigel's predicament by trying to be reliable and always available for him. But her increased reliability meant that there was less need for the father to be a steady presence and so he became more unreliable. Eventually, an equilibrium formed between the mother's reliability and the father's unreliability.

Nigel then broke his leg and spent two weeks in hospital. Following this he understandably needed to feel especially secure and his mother tried to comfort him. But soon after his return home he began suffering from panic attacks on arrival at school. His mother responded by trying to ensure that she never let Nigel down and the panic attacks subsided after a few weeks. In a less vulnerable family, his mother would then have been able to become less attentive to Nigel as he regained his confidence. In this family there was a danger that his mother's efforts at reliability would be counterbalanced by new levels of unreliability from his father. His mother was therefore committed to providing this new level of support for Nigel, which left her near breaking point.

This case demonstrates how illness can interact with stressors that are already present to reduce the family's ability to cope, both with the present and whatever stressors arise in the future.

---

accommodate these horizontal stressors. The impact of these stressors will be greatly influenced by the beliefs of the family (the vertical stressors). If the family believes that all children change into ungrateful rebels when they reach adolescence, then any attempt by the adolescent to spend more time away from home will be seen as confirmation of ingratitude and rebellion. As a result, adjusting to the horizontal stressors will become more difficult.

Events occurring at unexpected times in the lifecycle are more likely to be traumatic. Families are primed to expect certain changes, such as the death of a grandparent. From this perspective, the serious illness of a child is likely to be very traumatic and difficult to cope with because it is a major departure from the natural cycle. In addition, as McCubbin and Figley (1983) point out, a family's efforts to adapt to such catastrophic events puts a major strain on family members' emotional and material resources. This may leave the family unable to overcome concurrent but more mundane events. (For an example of this, see Box 4.2.)

But it is not only the onset of illness that causes problems. Reiss and Kaplan-Noir (1989) suggest that, as an illnesses runs its course, it will present the family with qualitatively different challenges and tasks. They describe illness as having an acute phase, a chronic phase and, sometimes, a terminal phase. The acute phase is associated with concerns over diagnosis, overcoming the shock of bad news and coping with series of tests and medical procedures. The role of the family during this stage is comparatively reactive and passive. As the illness becomes chronic, family members become important in a more practical sense as they may become involved in treatment and in lifestyle changes. There may be increased conflict as new roles are negotiated. For some patients, it will become increasingly unlikely that they will survive. The families' concerns then change to their impending loss (see Chapter 17).

To summarize, we have considered the relationship between the course of an illness and the stage in the family lifecycle at which the illness is occurring. Families find illness more difficult if it appears at a developmentally abnormal time in the lifecycle or at a time when the family is trying to cope with other stressful changes. When nursing a patient, it is worth considering what else is happening in the patient's family. Moreover, different sorts of help are needed by families at different stages in the course of an illness.

The effects of families on illness

We shall next consider whether the course of an illness may be influenced by the family's ability to adapt to it. In the following three examples we shall see that it is surprisingly difficult to disentangle the influences of illness and of family and to identify an ultimate cause.

Diabetes

In a controversial study, Minuchin, Rosman and Baker (1978) identified a number of differences between families of children with poorly controlled diabetes and normal families. We have already considered one explanation for such a difference: that the difficulty of coping with a child with diabetes has resulted in a change in family structure. Minuchin, Rosman and Baker set out to demonstrate that there is a strong causative link in the other direction – that family pathology results in difficulties in the control of diabetes.

Minuchin, Rosman and Baker compared families with children who had (1) poorly controlled diabetes, (2) well-controlled diabetes, and (3) either asthma or anorexia nervosa. All families were interviewed and set a discussion task in which the parents were asked to discuss a recent area of conflict. The identified patient would watch his/her parents' discussion via a one-way screen. A therapist would then join the parents and exacerbate the conflict by focusing on areas of difference. At the height of the argument the therapist would leave and the child would join the parents.

From the interviews and from observation of the families in discussion, Minuchin *et al.* found that the families of children with psychosomatic symptoms (e.g. uncontrolled diabetes, anorexia, asthma) had four characteristics in common:

1. *Enmeshed.* Every family member knew everyone else's business. There was no privacy.
2. *Overprotective.* Family members were highly sensitive to each others' distress, bodily symptoms and physical wellbeing.

3. *Rigid.* They were unable to adapt to changing circumstances and would attempt to solve problems in a stereotypical way irrespective of whether their solutions were successful.
4. *Afraid of conflict.* They had difficulty in addressing issues of potential conflict and avoided doing so by a series of distracting devices. For example, as a conflictual situation became more unbearable, attention would shift to concern about physical symptoms and the conflict would soon be forgotten.

What makes this study particularly interesting and influential is that Minuchin *et al.* also looked at the physiological changes in families with a child with diabetes. During the family discussion task, intravenous blood sampling units were used to gain regular measures of free fatty acid (FFA) levels in both parents and child. FFA levels are an indicator of emotional arousal. The results of the FFA analysis demonstrated that children with well-controlled diabetes showed no increase in physiological arousal, either when watching their parents' discussion from behind the one-way screen or when introduced into the room. The children with poorly controlled diabetes, on the other hand, showed a dramatic increase in FFA levels, which continued throughout the interview. This is evidence that the children with poorly controlled diabetes were emotionally involved in their parents' discussion in a way that the other children were not. Furthermore, another interesting difference emerged. In the families with a 'normal' diabetic there was no significant increase in FFA in either parents or child during the discussion. However, in the parents of a child with poorly controlled diabetes the emotional arousal of the both the child and the parents increased up to the point when the child was introduced into the interview room. At this point, the emotional arousal of the parents immediately dropped and continued to drop, whereas the arousal of the child continued to rise. This appears to provide strong support for Minuchin *et al.*'s hypothesis that the symptomatic child plays an important role in the avoidance of conflict within the family.

This experiment is a vivid portrayal of the link between childhood illness and family dynamics, but it is not without its problems. Most importantly, Coyne and Anderson (1988) highlight a flaw in the experimental design. The child joins the parental discussion at the same time as the therapist leaves. This means that the drop in parental anxiety levels may be connected with the therapist leaving rather than with the child entering.

As an alternative to Minuchin's explanation of events, Coyne and Anderson suggest that children with poorly controlled diabetes become anxious as they watch their parents discuss their serious medical condition. When they join the discussion, their anxiety continues to rise. The parents' anxiety increases during their discussion partly because of the seriousness of the situation and partly because the therapist is antagonizing them. When the therapist leaves, their anxiety diminishes. Such a pattern is not found in the control families for two reasons. First, they were not experiencing a medical crisis, so the family members were not frightened in the way the families of the uncontrolled diabetics were. Second, the therapists of the parents of uncontrolled diabetics may have been more antagonistic to those families by implying the problem was a result of family difficulties. Coyne and Anderson provide evidence to suggest that the differences between children with uncontrolled diabetes and well-controlled diabetes lies not within their families but within their physiology.

In summary, Minuchin *et al.* have not claimed that family pathology causes childhood illness; rather, the analysis attempts to show that family psychopathology can influence the extent to which physiology dysfunction is expressed. Minuchin *et al.*'s analysis also raises other issues. Family members might have conflicting needs and requirements and a family might be attempting to attend to a number of tasks concurrently. Under these circumstances, a family may, quite unwittingly, live under an illusion that they are attending to one task – curing an illness – when in fact they are attending to another – ensuring family stability by avoiding conflict.

Schizophrenia

In the 1950s, Bateson *et al.* (1956) proposed that individuals become schizophrenic in response to a particularly confusing family environment. In such families the communication patterns between family members are characterized by what Bateson *et al.* called 'double binds' (known in common usage as Catch 22 situations), e.g. 'You don't really love me, you are just pretending that you do' or 'Don't do what I tell you, just be yourself.' These communications put their recipient in a no-win situation because whatever the person does, they are vulnerable to criticism. Under circumstances where such communications pervade the family, an understandable response is to go mad. Bateson *et al.*'s suggestions have never received empirical support (Mishler and Waxler, 1968), but have remained influential as a basis for socio-environmental explanations of schizophrenia.

Nevertheless, later studies have shown that family atmosphere is predictive of remission and relapse. When schizophrenic patients return from hospital to families in which there are high levels of emotional involvement (similar to Minuchin *et al.*'s concepts of enmeshment and over-involvement) and where a high number of hostile comments are made about the patient, they are more likely to be readmitted to hospital than patients who return to a more supportive environment (Brown, Birley and Wing, 1972). A large number of studies have since confirmed the link between these so-called 'high expressed emotion' (high EE) families and relapse. Furthermore, Lebell *et al.* (1993) have shown that the degree of disparity between the patient's view of the family environment and that of other family members predicts outcome. High EE has since been used to predict the recovery from a variety of physical and mental conditions (Lask, 1994).

The model for schizophrenia proposed by those working in the field of expressed emotion is very similar to the psychosomatic model proposed by Minuchin *et al.* (1978). A primary organic dysfunction leads to the onset of schizophrenia, and its course is in part determined by family atmosphere. The argument about whether schizophrenia has a primary organic or socio-environmental genesis continues (see, for example, Carpenter 1993); but, there is strong evidence to suggest that specific family factors contribute to relapse.

Chronic pain

Chronic pain (see Chapter 13) is a good example of how the search for the ultimate cause can become fruitless. Most recent psychological models of chronic pain describe how symptoms form circular rather than linear patterns of influence. For example, the existence of pain is likely to reduce sexual activity if such activity increases pain. In a couple experiencing sexual difficulties, this reduction in sexual activity might provide a welcome relief from the sense of failure, guilt and poor self-esteem that often accompanies sexual difficulties. The pain then begins to serve a function for the couple and becoming pain-free means that the sexual difficulties may re-emerge.

There are a number of family characteristics of patients with chronic pain (Norfleet et al., 1982; Norfleet and Payne, 1986). There is increased marital disharmony, partners of pain patients experience higher than normal levels of pain themselves and chronic pain appears to last up to three times longer than in patients who have a solicitous spouse (Shovelar and Perkel, 1990). Whether these characteristics are a cause or an effect of chronic pain is uncertain. A more useful way forward might be to bypass this question and look for patterns of circular relationships between symptoms and the systems in which they arise. In the instance of chronic pain, the evidence suggests that the symptom (pain) influences and is influenced by the patient's partner and family. It is therefore appropriate to consider treatments aimed at the patient and family. Such treatments for chronic pain are beginning to emerge (see Norfleet et al., 1982; Moore and Chaney, 1985).

In this section we have considered the notion that family behaviour patterns influence the course of illness. It seems clear that illness affects families and families affect illness. In order to gain a better understanding of this relationship it is useful to consider a transactional perspective.

A transactional perspective

The term 'transactional perspective' comes from a paper by Sameroff and Chandler (1975), although similar approaches have been suggested by a variety of authors. All these models are systemic; that is, they differ from the traditional medical, psychiatric and psychological approaches in that they take as their focus an interacting system of people and environment rather than an individual (see also Chapter 25). The transactional model was originally applied to child development, but has since been applied to family illness by Fiese and Sameroff (1989).

Let us assume that children's environments influence their development to a greater or lesser extent. Fiese and Sameroff (1989) add the notion that children also influence their environments so that, at any point in time, a child and his/her environment together are a product of the results of all their previous interactions.

If a child suffers from a chronic illness, then the child and the illness together create a particular family environment which in turn influences the course of the illness (and the child's development). For example, Hauser *et al.* (1986) found that families where diabetes was newly diagnosed interacted in different ways from families of acutely ill children. Like the families of children with other chronic illnesses (Beresford, 1994) these families engaged in more problem-solving, solution-focused and facilitating interactions than the acutely ill families. Hauser *et al.* explain the difference by suggesting that, in response to a child's chronic illness, family members, and particularly the mother, perceive their ill child as more vulnerable and so pay close attention to the child and any emerging problems. The child responds by modelling the mother's behaviour and so sees himself as vulnerable and becomes more problem-focused. Fiese and Sameroff (1989) believe that a partial picture the child's environment at any one point in time can be gained by exploring the family belief system.

Family belief systems

Fiese and Sameroff (1989) divide the belief system into three levels – family paradigms, family stories and family rituals:

- *Family paradigms* consist of general beliefs held by each family member about how the world operates. Of relevance here would be family members' understanding of the patient's medical condition, of relationships with health professionals and, in cases where the ill member is a child, the understanding of child development.
- *Family stories* consist of family myths and legends passed down from generation to generation which contain within them the seeds of the family's tradition. Byng-Hall (1979) talks of the importance of family myths in giving families both an important sense of identity and models for behaviour. However, he also describes how myths can make it difficult for families to be flexible because they demand that family members respond in a predetermined way.
- *Family rituals* involve the prescription of a role and a set pattern of behaviour to each person for various family activities (e.g. Christmas dinner, where the head of the family is identified by sitting at the head of the table). These rituals provide a protection against stress; those families who can maintain clear routines and rituals are likely to have more success in coping with a chronic illness. Thus, Fiese and Sameroff argue that family belief systems are a major factor in determining a family's success or failure in coping with a chronic illness.

It is natural to assume that all family members will make efforts to rid the family of illness or reduce its harmful effects. But Minuchin *et al.*'s work questions this assumption. The work of Byng-Hall illustrates the way a transactional approach can account for such complex family pressures.

The function of illness

From clinical experience Byng-Hall identifies a pattern in some families in which the physical symptoms exhibited by a child appear to be related to the quality of the marital relationship. With these families, an increase in conflict between parents is followed by a resurgence of symptoms and then a drop in parental conflict. Byng-Hall explains his observations by suggesting that some couples find it so frightening to discuss emotionally charged subjects that they avoid them (cf. Minuchin *et al.*, 1978). This avoidance results in an increasing emotional distance between the couple. As they become more distant it becomes clear that they hold nothing in common and that they should separate. But this is also a frightening idea because they depend on each other for stability. Something is needed to stop the inexorable drift towards total separation.

Imagine that this couple has a child who suffers from a physiological disposition to a chronic illness such as asthma. At this point in time, whether coincidentally or because of the stress in the family, the child's asthma worsens. The parents understandably become concerned about the welfare of their child. In response to the asthma attack they begin to communicate and work together and the condition improves. The couple now feel closer and, with the asthma now in the background, they are free to consider their own relationship again. As they do so, they drift closer together, but areas of conflict that they have previously avoided by being distant with each other, become less easy to avoid. As a result, the tension rises again until it becomes unbearable. At this point the child's asthma worsens again. The couple become concerned once more and are quite distracted from their own difficulties. When the asthma again subsides the pattern continues. The child's symptoms are functioning as a homeostatic mechanism which ensures that the parents' emotional distance is kept at a tolerable level. When the parents become too close or too distant the asthma flares up.

In this section we have considered a transactional view of illness in which an individual with a chronic illness creates a particular family environment, which then further influences the development of the illness. At any one time, the environment is crystallized within the belief systems of family members.

An unspoken assumption about illness is that it is undesirable and that families will organize themselves in order to minimize its effect. The implications for nurses of work by Minuchin *et al.* and Byng-Hall is that, in a minority of cases, they will meet patients whose illness does not respond to treatment even though the patient and family have adequate knowledge of the illness and associated factors. In these cases, it is worth considering whether the illness fulfils a function for the families involved. Such families may be helped by a referral for family therapy.

Summary

The aim of this chapter has been to show how a different understanding of illness can be gained by viewing the whole family rather than just an individual. The issues raised in this chapter may be usefully summarized by a checklist:

- *The impact of illness.* Chronic illness is potentially stressful for all family members, but most families adapt to reduce the stress.
- *The family lifecycle.* If illness occurs at a developmentally abnormal time in the family lifecycle or at a time when the family is attempting to cope with other stressful changes, then the family will find it more difficult to cope.
- *The illness cycle.* There are three types of illness: (1) those in which improvement is probable, (2) those in which improvement is unlikely, and (3) those in which deterioration is likely. As improvement becomes unlikely and deterioration more likely the need for family support is likely to increase. The nature of the support may also need to change. At the acute phase of an illness, families need information and emotional support. During the chronic phase they will need concrete, practical help. In the terminal phase, the emphasis may return to emotional support.
- *Families in difficulties.* Families may be experiencing problems because of ignorance or lack of information. If this is the case, the solution is self-evident. If the reason for the family's difficulties is more complicated, a referral to a centre specializing in families may be useful so that the following factors can be considered (see the following Discussion Point). How is each family member coping with the illness? What strategies do they use? Are these strategies successful, or are they creating problems for themselves or anyone else in the family? What attempts are being made to solve the family's difficulties? Are these attempts serving to perpetuate those very difficulties? Alternatively, is the illness, or the difficulties arising from it, serving a useful function for part or all of the family?

DISCUSSION POINT

At what point do you decide that a family's difficulties are such that they would be better served by a referral to specialist family services rather than being helped by you?

Seminar questions

1. Do you agree with the definition of 'holistic' given in the Introduction to this chapter? What are the difficulties in providing holistic care?

2. How would you define the family? Are there problems with your definition or the one given in the chapter ? What is the role of the family in present-day society?

Further reading

A good, concise and detailed account of the relationship between psychology, families and health is given by the various contributors to: Akamatsu, T.J., Parris Stephens, M.A., Hobfoll, S.E. and Crowther, J.H. (eds) (1992) *Family Health Psychology*. Ohio: Hemisphere Publications. If this is read in conjunction with Beresford, B.A. (1994) 'Resources and strategies: How parents cope with the care of a disabled child', *Journal of Child Psychology and Psychiatry* **35** (1), 171–209, then a quite comprehensive account of the area will be achieved.

A less comprehensive but more readable account from a family therapy perspective is given by Lask, B. (1987) 'Physical illness, the family and the setting', in A. Bentovim, G. Gorell Barnes and A. Cooklin (eds.) *Family Therapy: Complementary frameworks of theory and practice*, 2nd edition, abridged. London: Academic Press.

A good introduction to the area of family therapy is given by Burnham, J. (1986) *Family Therapy*. London: Routledge.

References

Bateson, G., Jackson, D.D. Haley, J. and Weakland, J. (1956) 'Toward a theory of schizophrenia', *Behavioural Science* **1**, 251–64.

Beresford, B.A. (1994) 'Resources and strategies: How parents cope with the care of a disabled child', *Journal of Child Psychology and Psychiatry* **35** (1), 171–209.

Brown, G., Birley, J. and Wing, J. (1972) 'Influence of family life on the course of schizophrenic disorders: A replication', *British Journal of Psychiatry* **121**, 241–58.

Byng-Hall, J. (1979) 'Re-editing family mythology during family therapy', *Journal of Family Therapy* **1**, 103–16.

Campbell, T.L., McDaniel, S.H. and Seaburn, D.B. (1992) 'Families, systems, medicine: New opportunities for psychologists', in T.J. Akamatsu, M.A. Parris Stephens, S.E. Hobfoll and J.H. Crowther (eds.) *Family Health Psychology*. Ohio: Hemisphere Publications.

Carter, B. and McGoldrick, M. (1989) 'Overview: The changing family life cycle – a framework for family therapy', in B. Carter and M. McGoldrick. *The Changing Family Life Cycle*, 2nd edition. Boston: Allyn & Bacon.

Cheal, D. (1991) *Family and the State of Theory*. Hemel Hempstead: Harvester Wheatsheaf.

Coyne, J.C. and Anderson, B.J. (1988) 'The "psychosomatic family" reconsidered: Diabetes in context', *Journal of Marital and Family Therapy* **14**, 112–23.

Coyne, J.C. and Fiske, V. (1992) Couples coping with chronic and catastrophic illness', in T.J. Akamatsu, M.A. Parris Stephens, S.E. Hobfoll and J.H. Crowther (eds) *Family Health Psychology*. Ohio: Hemisphere Publications.

Doherty, W.J., McDaniel, S.H. and Hepworth, J. (1994) 'Medical family therapy: an emerging arena for family therapy', *Journal of Family Therapy* **16** (1), 31–47.

D'Zurilla, T.J. (1990) 'Problem solving training for effective stress management', *Journal of Cognitive Psychotherapy* **4** (4), 327–54.

Fiese, B. and Sameroff, A.J. (1989) 'Family context in pediatric psychology: A transactional perspective', *Journal of Pediatric Psychology* **14** (2), 293–314.

Fordyce, W.E. (1976) *Behavioral Methods for Chronic Pain and Illness.* St Louis: C.V. Mosby.

Hauser, S.T., Jacobson, A.M., Wertlieb, D., Weiss-Perry, B., Follansbee, D., Weolfsdorf, J.I., Herkowitz, R.D., Houlihan, J. and Rajapark, D.C. (1986) 'Children with recently diagnosed diabetes: Interactions within their families', *Health Psychology* **5**, 273–96.

Lask, B. (1994) 'Comment on W.J. Doherty, S.H. McDaniel and J. Hepworth (1994) "Medical family therapy: An emerging arena for family therapy"', *Journal of Family Therapy* **16**, 131–47.

Lazarus, R.S. (1966) *Psychological Stress and the Coping Process.* New York: McGraw-Hill.

Lebell, S.R., Marder, S.R., Mintz, J., Mintz, L.I., Tompson, W., Johnson, K. and McMenzie, J. (1993) 'Patients' perceptions of family emotional climate and outcome in schizophrenia', *British Journal of Psychiatry* **162**, 751–5.

McCubbin, H.I. and Figley, C.R. (1983) 'Bridging normative and catastrophic family stress', in H.I. McCubbin and C.R. Figley (eds) *Stress and the Family*, Vol. 1. *Coping with Normative Transition.* New York: Bruner Mazel.

McGoldrick, M. (1989) 'Ethnicity', in B. Carter and M. McGoldrick, *The Changing Family Life Cycle*, 2nd edition. Boston: Allyn & Bacon.

Minuchin, S., Rosman, B.L. and Baker, L. (1978) *Psychosomatic Families: Anorexia nervosa in context.* Cambridge, Mass.: Harvard University Press.

Mishler, E.G. and Waxler, N. (1968) *Interaction in Families: An experimental study of family process.* New York: John Wiley.

Moore, J. and Chaney, E. (1985) 'Outpatient group treatment of chronic pain: Effects of spouse involvement', *Journal of Consulting and Clinical Psychology* **53**, 326–34.

Norfleet, M.A., Hammett, B.C., Lichte, S.L., Lukensmeyer, W.W. and Payne, B.A. (1982) 'Helping families cope with chronic pain: An integral part of an interdisciplinary and multimodal treatment program', in L. Wolberg and M. Aronson (eds.) *Group and Family Therapy.* New York: Brunner Mazel.

Norfleet, M.A. and Payne, B.A. (1986) 'Chronic pain and the family: A review', *Pain* **26**, 1–22.

Owen, M.J. and Holmes, C.A. (1993) ' "Holism" in the discourse of nursing', *Journal of Advanced Nursing* **18**, 1688–95.

Parsons, T. (1955) 'The American family', in T. Parsons and R. Bales (eds.) *Socialization and Interaction Process.* Glencoe, Ill.: Free Press.

Peters, L.C. and Esses, L.M. (1985) 'Family environment as perceived by children with a chronically ill parent', *Journal of Chronic Disability* **38** (4), 301–8.

Reiss, D. and Kaplan De-Noir, A. (1989) 'The family and medical team in chronic illness: A transactional and developmental perspective', in C.N. Ramsey (ed.) *Family Systems in Medicine.* New York: Guilford Press.

Sameroff, A.J. and Chandler, M.J. (1975) 'Reproductive risk and the continuum of caretaking casuality', in F.D. Horowitz, M. Ketherington, Scarr-Salapatek and G. Sigel (eds.) *Review of Child Development Research*, Vol. 14. Chicago: University of Chicago Press.

Shovelar, G.P. and Perkel, R. (1990) 'Family systems interventions and physical illness', *General Hospital Psychiatry* **12**, 363–72.

Wood, B.L. (1994) 'One articulation of the structural family therapy model: A biobehavioural family model of chronic illness in children', *Journal of Family Therapy* **16** (1), 53–73.

Wood, B.L., Watkins, J., Boyle, J., Nogueira, J., Zimand, E. and Caroll, L. (1989) 'The "psychosomatic family": A theoretical and empirical analysis', *Family Process* **28**, 399–417.

CHAPTER 5

Attitudes and attitude change

LUCY JOHNSTON

Chapter outline

Introduction

'Abortion is murder'

'Scots are mean'

'BMW cars are classy'

The above are all statements of attitudes towards specific issues, persons or objects. Over half a century ago, Allport defined attitudes as 'the most distinctive and indispensable concept in American social psychology' (1935: p.298) and they still remain a dominant research topic today. Attitudes cannot be directly observed but are assumed to be good predictors of important behaviours. This intuitive link between attitudes and behaviour has been one of the focal points of research in social psychology. Understanding this link can assist in the prediction and interpretation of behaviour and it also opens a possible mechanism for behavioural change, through attitudinal change. The importance of behavioural prediction and change becomes evident when one considers not only traditional areas of social psychology (e.g. racism) but also, increasingly, issues such as health promotion. Influencing people's attitudes towards behaviours, such as using condoms, taking medication, eating healthily and attending for cervical smears, are of increasing social importance. This chapter will consider the psychological literature concerning the nature of attitudes, the link between attitudes and behaviour, together with the relation between attitude change and persuasion. This material will provide an overview of theoretical approaches to these areas, combined with practical examples of the application of such approaches to health issues.

Consider the following two examples:

- John, a young businessman, sleeps with many women on a casual basis. John has a negative attitude towards condom use. His negative attitude leads him to have unprotected sex and spread disease.
- Mary, a middle-aged housewife, receives a card inviting her to attend for a routine breast screening examination at a local clinic. With all the recent media attention on breast cancer on the importance of early detection, Mary has a positive attitude towards such screening. However, Mary failed to attend the clinic.

These are two examples of attitudes towards health-related topics. Such attitudes can have profound implications both for the individuals involved and for society. An understanding of how attitudes can predict behaviour may produce intervention programmes which result in Mary attending breast screening. An understanding of how attitudes can be changed may result in campaigns which encourage John to use condoms in casual sex.

Attitudes – definitions

DISCUSSION POINT

What attitudes do *you* hold towards trust hospitals, towards voluntary euthanasia, towards IVF? When did you adopt these attitudes and why do you hold them? What impact does your attitude have on your thinking about these issues?

The following section describes the nature of attitudes and how they affect thought processes. Read through this material and consider how it relates to the answers you have just given.

Attitudes and their impact on thinking

The basic tenet behind all definitions of attitudes is that they are relatively stable mental positions held towards specific issues, objects or persons. Petty and Cacioppo (1986: p. 127) define a person's attitudes as 'general evaluations about themselves, other persons, objects or issues'. Attitudes can develop through a variety of routes – through direct experience or through indirect experience (e.g. through media sources or from parents, teachers and peers).

Anything about which an attitude is held, be it an object, a person or an issue, is called an 'attitude object'. Attitudes are a combination of beliefs, feelings and evaluations about the attitude object. For example, people who differ in their attitudes towards safe sex will have different beliefs (e.g. safe sex does/does not offer protection from disease) and evaluations of safe sex (from extremely positive to extremely negative). These differences in turn are likely to lead to different behaviours (e.g. using condoms or not).

Attitudes can influence cognitive processes and may have an impact on a person's information processing. This is confirmed by research on selective perception. In general, research suggests that people show a preference for information consistent with their existing attitudes. Selective perception can be broken down into three processes:

1. *Selective exposure*: the seeking out of information consistent with a person's attitudes. Recent work has shown people to be biased in seeking information about particular social groups, preferring information consistent with their pre-existing attitudes about the group (Johnston and Macrae, 1994).
2. *Selective attention*: the focusing of attention on information consistent with attitudes. Studies suggest that, under some conditions, more time is spent attending to consistent than inconsistent information (e.g. Olson and Zanna, 1979).
3. *Selective interpretation*: the interpretation of ambiguous information in a way consistent with a prior attitude. Studies have shown, for example, that the attitudes people hold towards social groups influence their interpretation of behaviours performed by members of the group. Duncan (1976) showed the same 'gentle shove' to be interpreted as 'violent behaviour' when it was performed by a black actor, but as 'playing around' when it was performed by a white actor.

Attitudes may also influence memory for information, which may in turn influence subsequent judgements or behaviours. Memory for consistent information is especially dominant when adequate cognitive resources are not available to process fully and integrate the inconsistent information (e.g. Macrae, Hewstone and Griffiths, 1993).

Attitudes, then, are beliefs and evaluations held towards various objects or issues. Attitudes also influence the processing, interpretation and memory of attitude-relevant information and, in turn, influence attitude-related behaviours. Attitudes cannot be directly observed but must be inferred. The most commonly used method for measuring attitudes has been self-reported written responses to questionnaire items. In addition, combinations of both self-reports and behavioural measures have also been employed. For a clear account of the methods used to measure attitudes see Himmelfarb (1993).

Attitudes and behaviour

Predicting behaviour from attitudes

The link between attitudes and behaviour is an intuitively appealing one. It would seem logical that a person's behaviour should be affected by their attitudes. Heinnemann *et al.*'s (1980) measurement of attitudes suggested, however, that verbal attitudes and behaviour are not necessarily linked. In this section the relationship between attitudes and behaviour is examined (see also Chapter 2).

Early attempts to demonstrate the impact of attitudes on behaviour met with little success. Wicker (1969), in a review, suggested there is at best only a weak relationship between reported attitudes and observed behaviour. For example, a classic study by La Pière (1934) found little relationship between the recorded negative attitudes of restaurateurs towards the Chinese in a questionnaire and their positive behaviour towards a Chinese couple who came to their restaurant (the Chinese couple were actually part of the research team). Other studies have, however, demonstrated a strong relationship between attitudes and behaviour. Goodmonson and Glaudin (1971), for instance, showed there to be a high correlation between people's attitudes towards donation of body organs after death and the behaviour of carrying a donor card.

A number of *post hoc* explanations can be offered for why there is a strong attitude–behaviour relationship in some situations but not in others. In La Pière's study, it is possible that the people in the restaurants who completed the questionnaires might have been different from those who served the Chinese couple, or external factors, such as the reactions of other customers, may have prevented the owners behaving as negatively as they would have wished. Four main factors have been identified which help to explain a link between attitudes and behaviour. Each will be considered briefly.

Specificity

Attitudes can be very specific (e.g. attitudes towards kidney donation) or very general (e.g. racist, sexist or political attitudes). Most early research considered socially important general attitudes, which are very broad and encompass many features which may be expressed in a wide range of behaviours. Furthermore, these studies tended to consider only one or two specific behaviours relevant to the attitude (e.g. La Pière considered only whether or not the Chinese couple were refused service; other measures such as politeness or speed of service might have yielded stronger relationships between attitudes and behaviour). Since many different behaviours could be used to demonstrate general attitudes, it is hardly surprising that there are only weak relationships between these attitudes and each specific behaviour.

With specific attitudes there is a much more restricted range of relevant behaviours and hence there is likely to be a closer correspondence between these attitudes and behaviour. We see this in Davidson and Jaccard (1979), who considered the use of oral contraceptives over a two-year period. They found a negligible relationship between general attitudes to birth control (which could be manifest in a number of different behaviours) and use of oral contraceptives, but a strong relationship between specific attitudes towards birth control pills (involving only a few behaviours) and the use of oral contraceptives.

Direct experience

Attitudes formed through direct experience are more predictive of subsequent behaviour than the same attitudes formed through indirect experience, even if the attitudes are equal in strength. For example, attitude towards breastfeeding was found to be a better predictor of actual feeding for mothers who had attempted breastfeeding with previous children than for first-time mothers whose attitudes were formed through indirect experience, e.g. talking to other mothers (Manstead, Proffitt and Smart, 1983).

Outcome dependence

The greater the vested interest, the more highly related are attitudes and behaviour. For instance, Sivacek and Crano (1982) contacted students allegedly to elicit their support to oppose a proposed change in the law to raise the legal drinking age from 18 to 20. Virtually all the students expressed a negative attitude towards the change. However, only the younger students (aged between 18 and 20), who would be directly affected by the law, agreed to take part in the campaign. Those directly affected by the proposed change in the law did not hold stronger attitudes towards the issue, but there was a stronger relationship between their attitude and their behaviour.

We have seen that attitude–behaviour links are strengthened by direct experience and outcome dependence and that attitudes alone are not sufficient to predict behaviour. People with the same attitude can behave differently depending on other factors.

Separation of attitude components

In defining attitudes three separate components of the attitude – affective (feelings), cognitive (thoughts) and behavioural (actions) – have been identified. These components are not always in agreement. If this occurs, the attitude–behaviour link may be weakened. For example, a course of action (e.g. dieting) may be unpleasant but beneficial (giving a negative affective component but a positive cognitive component). Consequently, whether people diet or not, the relationship between the attitude as a whole and the dieting behaviour will be weak.

DISCUSSION POINT
The factors identified above show that, at least under certain circumstances, there is a strong relationship between attitudes and behaviour. Consider how knowledge of the factors which influence the link between attitudes and behaviour might influence the behaviour of a health educator. How important is it to be able to predict health-related behaviours? What strategies could be adopted to produce attitude-consistent behaviour? Is this necessarily a desirable strategy? (See later.)

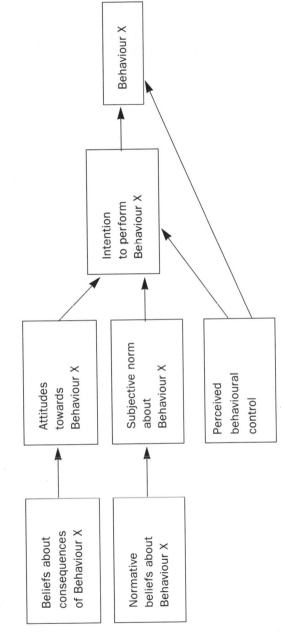

Figure 5.1 *The theory of planned action*

Source: After Ajzen (1985).

The relation of attitudes and behaviour: The theory of reasoned action and the theory of planned behaviour

The *theory of reasoned action* (Ajzen and Fishbein, 1980) and the *theory of planned behaviour* (Ajzen, 1985) were both proposed to predict social behaviour. These two theories assume that attitudes are not the best predictor of social behaviour. Rather, they treat attitudes as being only one influence on *intention to behave*. It is assumed that the intention to behave provides a better predictor of behaviour than does attitude towards that behaviour. Ajzen, Timko and White (1982), for example, found a stronger relationship between expressed *intention* to smoke marijuana and actual smoking behaviour over a specified four-week period than between *attitude* towards smoking marijuana and actual smoking behaviour.

In both theories, three main factors are believed to influence the intention to behave: (1) the attitude towards the behaviour; (2) the 'subjective norm' and (3) the degree of perceived behavioural control (this is included only in the theory of planned behaviour and is the major difference beween the theories). External influences (such as personality, age, gender, etc.), it is argued, affect behaviour only through their influence on these three factors (see Figure 5.1).

Attitudes are determined by a person's beliefs about the outcomes associated with the behaviour in question and their evaluations of those outcomes. The more strongly a person believes that certain outcomes are associated with a behaviour and the more favourably they value these outcomes, then the more favourable the attitude about the behaviour will be. For example, mothers who bottlefeed believe more strongly in the association between bottlefeeding (the behaviour) and the father's involvement with the baby (the outcome) than do mothers who breastfeed. In addition, the bottlefeeding mothers value this outcome of the behaviour, i.e. father's involvement, more than mothers who breastfeed (Manstead, Profitt and Smart, 1983).

The *subjective norm* is determined by the extent to which important people (e.g. spouse, parents, peers) would approve or disapprove of a person performing a specific behaviour and also the extent to which the person is motivated to comply with the wishes of these people. For mothers who bottlefed, in comparison to mothers who breastfed, it was found that important people (the baby's father and grandmother) more strongly approved of bottlefeeding. In addition, the mothers who bottlefed were more strongly motivated to comply with the wishes of these other people than were the mothers who breastfed (Manstead, Profitt and Smart, 1983).

A third factor, *perceived behavioural control*, was included in the theory of planned behaviour (Ajzen, 1985). Ajzen argued that the greater the perceived behavioural control over a behaviour, the greater should be the intention to be-have. The less a behaviour is seen to be under voluntary control, the weaker the impact of attitudes and subjective norm on intention to behave.

As Eiser (1983) has shown, those who consider themselves to be addicted have a low level of perceived behavioural control over the addictive behaviour (drinking,

| BOX 5.1 **THE THEORY OF PLANNED BEHAVIOUR** |

Prediction of Weight Loss*
Research on personality characteristics and general attitudes (locus of control, obesity, body image) had little success in predicting weight loss. Research based on the predictions of the theory of planned behaviour had much greater success in predicting actual weight loss in female college students over a six-week period.

Attitudes: Measured using the semantic differential, 'losing weight in the next six weeks' was rated on three bipolar scales: good/bad, harmful/beneficial, desirable/undesirable.

Subjective norm: Measured by two questions considering whether important others felt that they should lose or try to lose weight over the next six weeks (rated on a bipolar scale: should/should not) and two questions about whether those important others would support such an attempt (rated on a bipolar scale: support/oppose).

Perceived behavioural control: Measured by two questions assessing perceived likelihood of success if attempts were made to lose weight (rated on a scale 0–100).

Intention to behave: Measured by two ratings of 'intention to' and 'trying to' lose weight in the next six weeks (ratings made on a scale 1–7).

As predicted from the theory of planned behaviour, attitude, subjective norm and perceived behavioural control were all strongly related to the intention to behave. In addition, each of these three factors contributed to the prediction of intention to behave. As expected, intention to behave strongly predicted actual behaviour, measured in terms of weight loss over the six-week period. There was also a strong relationship between perceived behavioural control and actual weight loss, as predicted. A strong intention to lose weight resulted in increased weight loss only for those students who believed that they could attain the goal (i.e. high perceived behavioural control). If perceived control was low, the strength of the intention to behave had no effect on actual behaviour. A strong intention to behave, therefore, is not sufficient to produce the relevant behaviour. This behaviour must also be perceived to be under the control of the person.

What implications does this research have for intervention programmes? How might weight loss be improved? What sort of help and advice should be offered to those attempting to lose weight?

* After Schifter and Ajzen (1985).

smoking, etc.) and therefore show little behavioural change, despite strong attitudes and subjective norms towards a change in behaviour. Somebody may have a strong positive attitude towards giving up smoking, important others may also approve of their giving up smoking, but if smoking is perceived not to be under their own control, then behaviour will not change. Perceived behavioural control can also influence the relation between intention to behave and actual behaviour without there being a change in either attitudes or subjective norm. For instance, somebody may intend to donate blood, have a strong positive attitude towards giving blood and also significant others approve of their blood donation (high subjective norm). At the blood donating centre, however, there is a long queue so the intention to behave cannot be carried out. The attitude and subjective norm towards giving blood remain unchanged, but behavioural control was low.

Thus the stronger the attitude, the subjective norm and perceived behavioural control towards a particular behaviour, the greater is the intention to behave. Confirmation of this comes from a study concerning attendance for breast screening, which showed that the strongest predictors of attendance were attitudes towards attendance, subjective norms regarding attendance and also perceived behavioural control over attendance. These factors were much better predictors than individual variables such as age or social class (Rutter, Quine and Chesham, 1993).

The theories of reasoned action and planned behaviour have been applied to a number of situations with encouraging results. Attitudes, subjective norm and perceived behavioural control have all been shown to be good predictors of intention to behave. Similarly, intention to behave and behavioural control predict actual behaviour. There is much support for the theories from a wide range of behaviours, including a number from the health domain: weight loss (Schifter and Ajzen, 1985), family planning (Ajzen and Fishbein, 1980; Smetana and Adler, 1980; Vinokur-Kaplan, 1978), taking exercise after giving birth (Godin, Vezina and Lambert, 1989), limiting infants' sugar intake (Beale and Manstead, 1991), voluntary treatment programmes (Ajzen and Fishbein, 1980), condom use (Otis, Godin and Lambert, 1993) and blood donation (Pomazal and Jaccard, 1976). To illustrate the application of the theory of planned behaviour, the example of weight loss is considered in Box 5.1. The theory of planned behaviour is a general model of attitudes, which has been applied to various health-related behaviours. More specific models, especially developed to explain the dynamics of health behaviour (the *health belief model* and *protection motivation theory*), are discussed and evaluated in Chapter 6.

What happens when attitudes and behaviour are in conflict?

The previous section has considered the prediction of behaviour from attitudes. As has been shown, behaviour is not always well predicted by attitudes. Conflict between one's attitudes and behaviour results in an unpleasant state of inconsistency (e.g. Fazio and Cooper, 1983) called 'cognitive dissonance' (Festinger, 1957), which people are motivated to reduce. For example, people who eat high-fat foods, despite media campaigns and pleas from their family to change their dietary habits, may well suffer dissonance by feeling uncomfortable when eating such foods. As a result they are likely to seek to reduce this dissonance so that they can feel more comfortable with their diet.

Reduction of dissonance can be brought about through changes in any part of the attitude system. People eating high-fat food, therefore, can adopt a number of strategies; they can stop eating such foods; they can seek information which suggests that their diet is not bad for their health; or they can devalue the importance of diet (e.g. by highlighting all the other potential risks to health which are more dangerous than diet).

Consistent with the prevailing *cognitive miser* notion in social cognition (Fiske and Taylor, 1983), people are likely to choose the method of dissonance reduction that is the easiest, requiring least cognitive effort and resources. The easiest route to dissonance reduction is often through attitude change. Behaviour is often very resistant to change (see below) and acquiring new information or minimizing the importance of outcomes that really are important is quite difficult and effortful. Under such conditions, then, there is a situation of attitudes being predicted by behaviour rather than vice versa.

Supporting evidence for the changing of attitudes in line with behaviour comes from experimental situations of 'forced compliance', in which volunteers are required to perform counter-attitudinal behaviours (e.g. writing essays in support of the opposite attitude position to that which they hold, so that somebody who is in favour of abortion would have to write an essay opposing abortion) (Scher and Cooper, 1989). Performance of such attitude-inconsistent behaviour leads to a state of dissonance and a corresponding modification of existing attitudes to become consistent with the behaviour performed. This is especially likely when people believe they have freedom of choice over whether or not to perform the inconsistent behaviour and when they cannot attribute their behaviour to strong external pressures (e.g. Festinger and Carlsmith, 1959; Riess and Schlenker, 1977).

Being able to attribute the counter-attitudinal behaviour to a plausible external cause reduces the need for attitude modification. For example, somebody may voice agreement with their boss's proposal even though they think it is a bad one, because the last employee who voiced dissent was sacked. In this case dissonance is low since the behaviour is attributed to a strong external cause.

Just as in experimental situations of forced compliance, such attitude change can be seen in everyday situations. Consider the smoker who knows that smoking may be a health risk and hence suffers cognitive dissonance. Since addictive behaviours are difficult to change, it is likely that the smoker will reduce the cognitive dissonance through modification of his or her attitudes towards smoking. This could be done by believing that the negative aspects of smoking are less important than positive aspects (relaxing, peer approval) so that one's attitude towards smoking becomes overall more positive. As a result, the dissonance between attitudes and behaviour is reduced.

DISCUSSION POINT

Are you a smoker? If so, do you suffer from dissonance when you smoke? How do you resolve this dissonance and how do you cope with all the scientific evidence linking smoking with ill-health? If you are not a smoker, consider why people might smoke. How could smokers avoid the dissonance which results from their unhealthy behaviour?

Attitude change and persuasion

We are continually bombarded in everyday life with attempts to change our attitudes. Consider, for example, the number of advertisements we see which advocate
that we change anything from our brand of soap powder to our eating and sexual
habits. These attempts are usually aimed ultimately at changing a person's behaviour, expecting attitude change to produce a corresponding change in behaviour. Attitudes are defined as fairly stable entities and as such are resistant to
change. The utility of attitudes as organizing principles for incoming information
would be undermined if attitudes were continually changing in response to counter-
attitudinal information. In addition, attitudes are not always a good predictor of
behaviour and it is often more difficult to change behaviours that are more public
and involve more commitment than attitudes.

The nature of the persuasive message

Exposing people to persuasive messages does not, of course, guarantee a change in
attitudes or behaviours. There are a number of possible responses to a persuasive
message. The information contained in the message could be fully incorporated
into existing attitudes, which change in the direction of the persuasive message; the
persuasive message could be ignored; or the message could be interpreted in a
manner consistent with existing attitudes. The earlier discussion of selective perception of information showed evidence of selective exposure, selective attention and
selective interpretation in the processing of counter-attitudinal information. Such
biases in the processing of attitude-relevant information decrease the impact of that
information on the existing attitudes, making the attitudes more resistant to change.

   Fishbein (1984) identified three stages that are necessary for information to have
an effect on behaviour. The first is *awareness* – being aware that counter-attitudinal
information exists. The second stage is *general acceptance* – believing the counter-
attitudinal information at a general level (e.g. believing that there is a link between
smoking and cancer). Attitude change could conceivably be seen after these first
two stages. These two stages are necessary but not sufficient for behavioural
change, the third stage of *personalized acceptance* – accepting the counter-
attitudinal information at a personal level – also needs to occur.

   Examples of the separation of general and personal acceptance come from the
area of sexual behaviour. Kegeles, Adler and Irwin (1988) showed that in a
sample of 14–19-year-olds all believed condoms to be an efficient way of preventing sexually transmitted diseases (high *general* acceptance), while less than 10 per
cent of the sample reported using condoms in intercourse (low *personal* acceptance). Similarly, in a sample of gay men Valdiserri *et al.* (1987) found high levels
of knowledge about AIDS, its causes and consequences (high *general* acceptance)
but two-thirds of the sample still reported having had unprotected, risky sex with
more than one partner in the previous six months (low *personal* acceptance).

BOX 5.2 **CHANGING UNDERLYING BELIEFS**

Ajzen and Fishbein (1980) considered a group of alcoholics in hospital. These patients were asked to volunteer to participate in a special treatment programme. Ajzen and Fishbein developed a programme to persuade patients to volunteer for this treatment. Initial questionnaires identified the patients' beliefs regarding the treatment programme and showed that signing up for the programme was more under attitudinal than normative control. The persuasive message, aimed at encouraging patients to sign up for the treatment programme therefore focused on the beliefs underlying patients' attitudes towards signing up for the programme. Three versions of the persuasive message were constructed, each of which was given to a third of the patients:

Traditional message included ten arguments linking continued drinking to negative consequences. It then argued that the treatment programme offered a way of gaining control over their drinking and encouraged them to sign up.

Negative message included the same ten basic arguments as the traditional message but each argument linked 'not signing up for the programme' with a negative consequence. The message again ended by encouraging the patients to sign up for the programme.

Positive Message was the mirror image of the negative message. Again ten arguments were used and each linked 'signing up for the treatment programme' with a positive consequence. Again, patients were encouraged to volunteer for the programme.

The information contained in the three messages was virtually identical except for the focus of the message. In the traditional message focus was on 'continued drinking', in the negative message on 'not signing up for the treatment' and in the positive message on 'signing up for the treatment'. The negative and positive messages, therefore, attacked beliefs regarding the outcomes of the relevant behaviour (signing up for treatment) while the traditional message considered counter-attitudinal issues, but without actually attacking the beliefs underlying the patients' attitudes.

Results showed no overall difference in the patients' agreement with the three messages. However, the negative and positive messages were more influential than the traditional message in changing beliefs about the consequences of signing up for treatment. The positive and negative messages also actually increased the number of patients signing up for the treatment; the traditional message did not. Ajzen and Fishbein's research suggests that in order for a message to be successful in changing health-related behaviours, it must attack the beliefs underlying the attitudes and/or subjective norm of the behaviour in question. The traditional approach of linking the behaviour with negative consequences, they argue, is not sufficient.

This separation of general and personal acceptance may explain low attitude–behaviour correlations. Attitudes may change as a result of awareness and general acceptance of the counter-attitudinal information, but behavioural change will result only if there is also personal acceptance of the counter-attitudinal message.

Only a few investigations of attitude change have considered the content of the persuasive message itself and what is needed to make a message persuasive. However, research on stereotype change has provided some guidelines for the nature of any counter-attitudinal information. In order for the message to be effective in changing people's stereotypes it should be only mildly discrepant from the existing stereotype. This is because extremely discrepant information is not integrated into the existing stereotype (e.g. Johnston and Hewstone, 1992; Weber and Crocker, 1983).

Research based on the theory of reasoned action argues that counter-attitudinal information *per se* is insufficient to cause attitude or behaviour change (see Box 5.2). Instead, it is argued, the information should challenge the underlying beliefs regarding the behaviour in question. The theory of reasoned action proposes that this can be done in two ways: existing beliefs can be changed or new relevant beliefs can be introduced. Changing underlying beliefs will then lead to a change in the attitudes and normative beliefs about the behaviour (see Figure 5.1). For an example of the application of the theory of reasoned action to behaviour change of alcoholics, see Box 5.2.

The effects of a persuasive message will not be the same for all behaviour. Different people will hold different beliefs and the importance of these beliefs in predicting intentions to behave will vary. For instance, the subjective norm has been found to be a relatively better predictor of intention to attend for breast cancer screening than attitude towards attendance (Rutter, Quine and Chesham, 1993). In contrast, attitude towards losing weight was a better predictor of intention to lose weight than was the subjective norm regarding weight loss (Schifter and Ajzen, 1985). The strongest predictors may be different for different behaviours and hence require a different type of persuasive message. The persuasive message must, then, take into account what are the strongest influencing factors on the intention to behave and attempt to challenge those factors.

Not only may different behaviours require a different type of persuasive message, but also the effect of the message may change with the target audience. Fishbein (1984) showed that a single behaviour – intention to quit smoking – was most strongly influenced by different factors for two different groups. For teenagers the most influential factor in predicting intention to quit was attitudes towards stopping smoking, but for college-age women the strongest predictor of intention was the subjective norm. These two groups, then, needed a different emphasis in campaigns to try to make them stop smoking.

Traditional approaches to attitude change

The traditional, or Yale, approach to attitude change (developed largely by Hovland, Janis and Kelley, 1953) focused on identifying those external factors which influence the effectiveness of the persuasive message, either by enhancing or decreasing the persuasive impact of the message. Factors identified include the source of the message, the persuasive message itself and the audience for the message.

A message is more effective if presented by an attractive rather than an unattractive source, by an expert rather than a non-expert source, and by a likeable rather than a non-likeable source (e.g. Hovland and Weiss, 1951; Kiesler and Kiesler, 1969). These source effects can be seen in advertising campaigns today. Famous and popular sporting personalities are used to advertise products. Faster speakers are also more persuasive, fast speech conveying the impression that the source knows what they are talking about (Miller, Maruyama, Beaber and Valone, 1976).

Messages are more persuasive if they do not appear to be specifically designed to change our attitudes (Walster and Festinger, 1962). An obvious attempt at persuasion can actually lead to reactance, that is to say, a change in the opposite direction to that advanced in the persuasive message. Persuasive messages have more impact if they contain a two-sided rather than a one-sided argument. A two-sided approach gives an impression of fairness. It is easier to provide counter-arguments for a one-sided message and people look for information about the other side of the argument (e.g. Sears, 1965).

There are also *audience* effects on persuasion. Low self-esteem audiences are more susceptible to persuasive messages than high self-esteem audiences (Janis, 1954) and messages are more persuasive if the audience is distracted while listening to the message, paralleling everyday situations where people are rarely occupied on a single task (Allyn and Festinger, 1961).

This traditional approach to attitude change has provided much useful information about when attitude change is most likely to occur, which features enhance and which inhibit the impact of a message. This approach does not, however, provide much information about *why* people change their attitudes in response to persuasive messages. In the next section we shall consider in more detail the cognitive processes involved in attitude change.

Cognitive response analysis and attitude change

This approach considers attitude change to be a function of actively thinking about and elaborating the persuasive message. These elaborations can either support or oppose the message; the relative balance of such thoughts will influence the amount and direction of any attitude change. Attitude change is not, then, seen as a passive acceptance of the persuasive message but rather an active interaction with it. As well as providing a theoretical framework for attitude change, cognitive response analysis also provides a methodological tool – directly measuring the number of positive and negative thoughts in response to the persuasive message (see Cacioppo and Petty, 1981).

Two main models have developed from this perspective – the *heuristic systematic model* (HSM; Chaiken, 1980) and the *elaboration likelihood model* (ELM; Petty and Cacioppo, 1981). Although there are a number of differences between these two models, each is concerned with the processing of counter-attitudinal information and the impact of this on attitude change. Both models have proposed a dual

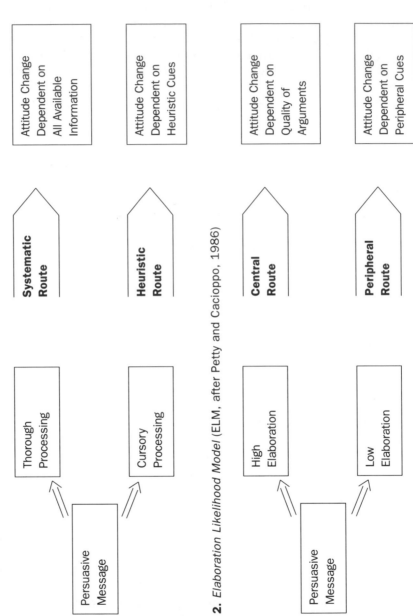

Figure 5.2 *Models of persuasion*

processing mechanism for persuasion (see Figure 5.2). Persuasion can occur as a result of processing counter-attitudinal information via either of the two routes. Each route is used under different conditions and different factors have more or less impact on persuasion depending on which route is being used (see below).

One of the processing routes in each model (the *systematic* route in the HSM and the *central* route in the ELM) involves thorough, effortful processing of all the available information before judgements and decisions are made. This mode of processing is characterized by a sensitivity to the quality of the persuasive message, by issue-relevant thoughts, by enhanced recall for the presented arguments and by relatively lasting change in attitudes. This mode of processing is capacity demanding, effortful and inevitably situations arise in which people do not have either sufficient processing resources or motivation to consider all the information. Under these conditions the second processing mode is used.

The *heuristic* (HSM) or *peripheral* (ELM) processing route is less effortful. Information processors do not fully evaluate all the available information before making judgements but, rather, base these judgements on shortcuts or heuristics. Cues in the persuasive situation are used to form a quick, easy judgement without fully analyzing all the information presented. Such heuristic cues can be rules of thumb such as 'experts can be trusted' or 'long arguments are strong arguments'. Many of the features identified in traditional research on attitude change as enhancing the persuasiveness of a message can be used as heuristic cues; for example, the source cues of credibility or expertise. Attitude change produced through heuristic/peripheral processing is characterized by insensitivity to message quality, by few issue-relevant thoughts, poor memory for the presented arguments and relatively short-lived change in attitudes.

Attitude change can, then, be brought about through two processing modes. Systematic/central route processing is capacity demanding and effortful and hence is likely to occur in situations of high involvement. Heuristic/peripheral processing, on the other hand, is likely under conditions of low involvement. Experiments have manipulated people's involvement with an issue; both message quality cues and a heuristic cue are then presented in the persuasive message.

In conditions of high involvement people were sensitive to message quality. People were not, however, sensitive to source cues of either credibility or likeability. That is, in high involvement conditions people agreed more with a high than a low quality message, and features of the message source had no impact on agreement with the message. This pattern of results is indicative of *systematic/central* route processing. More direct evidence for the mediation of cognitive processes on attitude change comes from people's thoughts about the presented message. Agreement with the persuasive message was predicted by the relative number of arguments for and against that a person generated. The higher the ratio of positive to negative thoughts that was evoked, the greater was the agreement with the message.

In conditions of low involvement people were insensitive to message quality but were sensitive to source cues. People showed more agreement with a message presented by either a highly credible or highly likeable source than the same message presented by a low credibility or unlikeable source. These effects are indicative of *heuristic/peripheral* route processing under conditions of low involvement (Chaiken, 1980; Petty, Cacioppo and Goldman, 1981).

In addition to high motivation, people must also have the available cognitive resources to undertake systematic/central processing. The introduction of a distraction task (which uses cognitive capacity) while people were reading a persuasive message was found to prevent thorough processing of the message and resulted in insensitivity to message quality, but also resulted in sensitivity to heuristic cues (Petty, Wells and Brock, 1976). This situation of distraction mimics the resource-usurping nature of everyday interaction when it is rare to be processing only one stimulus with no distraction. Under such everyday situations it is likely that counter-attitudinal information will be processed in a heuristic/peripheral manner and this may explain the relatively short-lived effects of persuasive arguments.

Before leaving the cognitive response analysis approach to attitude change it is worth highlighting a number of problems with this methodology. First, the HSM and ELM both assume that people are motivated to be accurate in their processing of attitude-relevant information. Although this may indeed be the case for some weak attitudes, this idea does not sit easily with findings of selective perception. In the case of strongly held attitudes and especially those with strong affective implications (Pyszczynski and Greenberg, 1987), people may be more motivated to maintain their own attitude than to process the available information accurately. This is likely to decrease the impact of counter-attitudinal information and decrease the likelihood of systematic or central processing of that information. Second, most of the work on attitude change in this framework has really been considering attitude formation since the persuasive messages employed are generally concerning issues about which the people will not have previously thought (often being fictitious issues). It is perhaps, therefore, somewhat premature to apply these findings to the area of change of strongly held attitudes. Current research on stereotype change is considering the applicability of such an approach to strongly held prior expectancies (Johnston and Coolen, in press).

DISCUSSION POINT

How could a health educator use the knowledge obtained from cognitive response analysis to encourage people to adopt a more healthy lifestyle (e.g. a low cholesterol diet)? Consider how a health professional could best induce a patient or client to adopt specific health-related behaviours. In doing this consider the importance of different factors, taking note of the conditions under which the persuasion takes place. Factors such as how keen the patient is to change his or her lifestyle or how busy the nurse is may be influential.

The role of fear and coping strategies in changing behaviour

Ajzen and Fishbein (1980) illustrate a common approach to attempts to change health-related behaviour. Health campaigns often try to evoke fears about an unhealthy behaviour by linking it with negative consequences (e.g. linking smoking with cancer, breathing difficulties and premature death). However, such fear-provoking messages are not always successful in promoting a switch to more healthy behaviours. Rogers (1983) suggested that both adaptive (giving up smoking) and maladaptive coping strategies (e.g. emphasizing positive aspects of smoking such as pleasure and peer approval; avoidance of the threatening information; fatalism – believing that behaviour will not influence health) are possible in response to the threatening message. Which strategy is adopted will depend on the relative costs and rewards associated with each. For a more detailed consideration of Rogers's *protection motivation theory*, see Chapter 6.

In a study concerning breast cancer, Rippetoe and Rogers (1987) considered factors which influenced whether women would use an adaptive (practising breast self-examination, BSE) or a maladaptive (religious faith, fatalism, wishful thinking, avoidance) coping strategy in response to a message describing the threat of breast cancer. They showed that a high fear-invoking message resulted in the adoption of more coping strategies (both adaptive and maladaptive) compared to a low fear-invoking message. However, fear evocation was not sufficient to ensure the adoption of an *adaptive* coping strategy. In order to encourage an adaptive strategy efficacy information was needed. An adaptive coping strategy was adopted in conditions where BSE was identified as a good coping strategy and information regarding the individual's ability to successfully perform BSE was provided. These findings, then, suggest that providing a persuasive message which emphasizes the negative consequences of current behaviour without offering a suitable replacement behaviour is unlikely to result in adaptive coping. This information regarding ability to perform the adaptive coping behaviour fits well with the idea of perceived behavioural control in the theory of planned behaviour.

We have seen, then, that the traditional persuasive message linking current behaviour with negative consequences is not sufficient to bring about adaptive behaviour change. Accordingly, Fishbein (1984) has argued that the effective persuasive message should include information linking current behaviour to negative consequences, but also information linking changed behaviour with positive consequences, along with information emphasizing the ability of the person to adopt the new, adaptive behaviour.

Summary

In this chapter the impact of attitudes on health-related behaviours and ways of changing those behaviours have been considered. The link between attitudes and behaviour is not a simple one. Attitudes can predict behaviours, but only under certain conditions. People may have a positive attitude towards condom use in terms of disease protection, but yet not use them themselves. Attitudes alone are not sufficient predictors of behaviour. Research on addictive behaviours, such as smoking, has shown that people may have a strong attitude towards not smoking but because they do not perceive the behaviour to be under their control, they continue to smoke. The theory of planned behaviour has indicated that attitudes, subjective norm and perceived behavioural control are all influential in predicting the intention to behave and, in turn, behaviour. Behaviours such as attendance at screening clinics depend on a strong positive attitude towards attendance, a strong subjective norm supporting attendance and a high level of perceived control over attendance. A change in any of these three components may result in a reduction in the intention to behave.

Many health campaigns aim to change people's attitudes and behaviours towards specific issues, such as condom use, healthy diets, and so on. In this chapter attitude change was shown to be difficult to achieve and also not necessarily to lead to a corresponding change in behaviour. The traditional approach of linking current behaviour with negative consequences is not sufficient to change behaviour. Many smokers are well aware of the health risks of their habit, yet do not change their smoking behaviour. More recent approaches, such as cognitive response analysis, have begun to identify under what conditions different factors are important in attitude change. Health campaigns need to be sensitive to the nature of their audience, to the factors which underlie the target behaviour (the underlying beliefs) and to the conditions under which the persuasive message is received.

Thus, although research on attitudes cannot specify exactly what should be done when attempting to change behaviour, the research does provide a set of issues to consider when making such attempts and is already suggesting which methods are more effective than others. It does need to be remembered that if attitude and behaviour change were easy then we, as people, would live in a very different social world with very different problems.

Seminar questions

1. How do attitudes influence information processing?
2. When do attitudes predict behaviour? Why is this useful?
3. How would you try to persuade people to change to a healthier lifestyle? What persuasion techniques would you use?

Further reading

Ajzen, I. (1988) *Attitudes, Personality and Behaviour.* Milton Keynes: Open University Press. This book provides a good overview of attitudes and their relation to behaviour, as well as considering additional factors such as the influence of personality factors.

Fiske, S.T. and Taylor, S.E. (1991) *Social Cognition*, 2nd edition. New York: McGraw-Hill. Chapter 11, pp.462–510, offers an excellent and easy to follow discussion of the cognitive analysis of attitudes and attitude change.

Rutter, D., Quine, L. and Chesham, D.J. (1993) *Social Psychological Approaches to Health.* Hemel Hempstead: Harvester Wheatsheaf. Provides in-depth examples of the application of attitude research to real-life settings (pregnancy, breast cancer and motorcycling).

Ajzen, I. and Fishbein, M. (1980) *Understanding Attitudes and Predicting Social Behaviour.* Englewood Cliffs, NJ: Prentice Hall. Provides a large number of examples of the application of the theory of reasoned action, in both health and other domains. Also contains a chapter on the application of the theory of reasoned action to attitude change.

Chaiken, S., Liberman, A. and Eagly, A.H. (1989) 'Heuristic and systematic information processing within and beyond the persuasion context', in J. Uleman and J. Bargh (eds.) *Unintended Thought*, Chapter 7. A detailed account of the heuristic systematic model and its predictions.

Petty, R.E. and Cacioppo, J.T. (1986). 'The elaboration likelihood model of persuasion', in L. Berkowitz (ed.) *Advances in Experimental Social Psychology*, Vol. 19. New York: Academic Press. A detailed account of the elaboration likelihood model and its predictions.

Rogers, R.W. (1975) 'A protection motivation theory of fear appeals and attitude change', *The Journal of Psychology* **91**, 93–114. A theoretical account of the impact of fear on attitude change.

Rippctoc, P.A. and Rogers, R.W. (1987). 'Effects of components of protection-motivation theory on adaptive and maladaptive coping with a health threat', *Journal of Personality and Social Psychology* **52**, 596–604. An application of Rogers's theoretical model to a situation of real health threat (breast cancer).

References

Ajzen, I. (1985) 'From intentions to actions: A theory of planned behaviour', in J. Kuhl and J. Beckmann (eds.) *Action-Control: From cognition to behaviour.* Heidelberg: Springer.

Ajzen, I. and Fishbein, M. (1980) *Understanding Attitudes and Predicting Social Behaviour.* Englewood Cliffs, NJ: Prentice Hall.

Ajzen, I., Timko, C. and White, J.B. (1982) 'Self-monitoring and the attitude–behaviour relation. *Journal of Personality and Social Psychology* **42**, 426–35.

Allport, G.W. (1935) 'Attitudes', in C. Murchinson (ed.) *A Handbook of Social Psychology.* Worcester, Mass.: Clark University Press.

Allyn, J. and Festinger, L. (1961) 'The effectiveness of unanticipated persuasive communications', *Journal of Abnormal and Social Psychology* **62**, 35–40.

Beale, D.A. and Manstead, A.S.R. (1991) 'Predicting mothers' intentions to limit frequency of infants' sugar intake: Testing the theory of planned behaviour', *Journal of Applied Social Psychology* **21**, 409–31.

Cacioppo, J.T. and Petty, R.E. (1979) 'The effects of message repetition and position in cognitive response, recall and persuasion', *Journal of Personality and Social Psychology* **37**, 97–109.

Cacioppo, J.T. and Petty, R.E. (1981) 'Social psychological procedures for cognitive response assessment: The thought-listing technique', in T. Merluzzi, C. Glass and M. Genest (eds.) *Cognitive Assessment*. New York: Guilford Press.

Chaiken, S. (1980) 'Heuristic versus systematic information processing and the use of source versus message cues in persuasion', *Journal of Personality and Social Psychology* **39**, 752–66.

Davidson, A.R. and Jaccard, J.J. (1979) 'Variables that moderate the attitude–behaviour relation: Results of a longitudinal survey', *Journal of Personality and Social Psychology* **37**, 1364–76.

Duncan, B.L. (1976) 'Differential social perception and attribution of intergroup violence: Testing the lower limits of stereotyping of blacks', *Journal of Personality and Social Psychology* **34**, 590–8.

Eiser, R. (1983) 'Smoking, addiction and decision-making', *Journal of Applied Social Psychology* **32**, 11–28.

Fazio, R.H. and Cooper, J. (1983) 'Arousal in the dissonance process', in J.T. Cacioppo and R.E. Petty (eds.) *Social Psychophysiology*. New York: Guilford Press.

Festinger, L. (1957) *A Theory of Cognitive Dissonance*. Evanston, Ill.: Row, Peterson.

Festinger, L. and Carlsmith, J.M. (1959) 'Cognitive consequences of forced compliance', *Journal of Abnormal and Social Psychology* **58**, 203–10.

Fishbein, M. (1984) 'Consumer beliefs and behaviour with respect to cigarette smoking: A critical analysis of the public literature', in J. Murphy, M. John, and H. Brown (eds.) *Dialogues and Debates in Social Psychology*. London: Open University.

Fiske, S.T. and Taylor, S.E. (1983) *Social Cognition*. New York: Random House.

Godin, G., Vezina, L. and Lambert, O. (1989) 'Factors influencing intentions of pregnant women to exercise after giving birth', *Public Health Reports* **104**, 188–95.

Goodmonson, C. and Glaudin, V. (1971) 'The relationship of commitment-free behaviour and commitment behaviour: A study of attitudes toward organ transplantation', *Journal of Social Issues* **27**, 171–83.

Heinnemann, W., Pellander, F., Vogelbusch, A. and Wojtek, B. (1980) 'Meeting a deviant person: Subjective norms and affective reactions', *European Journal of Social Psychology* **11**, 1–25.

Himmelfarb, S. (1993) in Eagly, A.H. and Chaiken, S. (eds.) *The Psychology of Attitudes*, Orlando: Harcourt, Brace Jovanovich.

Hovland, C.I., Janis, I.L. and Kelley, H.H. (1953) *Communication and Persuasion: Psychological studies of opinion change*. New Haven, Conn.: Yale University Press.

Hovland, C.B.I. and Weiss, W. (1951) 'The influence of source credibility on communication effectiveness', *Public Opinion Quarterly* **15**, 635–50.

Janis, I.L. (1954) 'Personality correlates of susceptibility to persuasion', *Journal of Personality* **22**, 504–18.

Johnston, L. and Coolen, P. (in press) 'A dual process approach to stereotype change', *Personality and Social Psychology Bulletin*.

Johnston, L. and Hewstone, M. (1992) 'Cognitive models of stereotype change (3): Subtyping and perceived typicality of disconfirming group members', *Journal of Experimental Social Psychology* **28**, 360–86.

Johnston, L. and Macrae, C.N. (1994) 'Stereotype change: The case of the information seeker', *European Journal of Social Psychology* **24**, 581–92.

Kegeles, S.M., Adler, N.E. and Irwin, C.E. (1988) 'Sexually active adolescents and condoms: Change over one year in knowledge, attitudes and use', *American Journal of Public Health* **78**, 460–1.

Kiesler, C.A. and Kiesler, S.B. (1969) *Conformity.* Reading, Mass.: Addison-Wesley.

La Piére, R.T. (1934) 'Attitudes and actions', *Social Forces* **13**, 230–7.

Macrae, C.N., Hewstone, M. and Griffiths, R.J. (1993) 'Processing load and memory for stereotype-based information', *European Journal of Social Psychology* **23**, 77–87.

Manstead, A.S.R., Profitt, C. and Smart, J.L. (1983) 'Predicting and understanding mothers' infant-feeding intentions and behaviour: Testing the theory of reasoned action', *Journal of Personality and Social Psychology* **44**, 657–71.

Miller, N., Maruyama, G., Beaber, R.J. and Valone, K. (1976) 'Speed of speech and persuasion', *Journal of Personality and Social Psychology* **34**, 615–24.

Olson, J.M. and Zanna, M.P. (1979) 'A new look at selective exposure', *Journal of Experimental Social Psychology* **15**, 1–15.

Osgood, C.E., Suci, G.J. and Tannenbaum, P.H. (1957) *The Measurement of Meaning.* Urbana: University of Illinois Press.

Otis, J., Godin, G. and Lambert, J. (1993) 'AIDS prevention: Intentions of high school students to use condoms', *Advances in Health Education*, in press.

Petty, R.E. and Cacioppo, J.T. (1981) *Attitudes and Persuasion: Classic and contemporary approaches.* Dubuque, Ind.: Wm. C. Brown.

Petty, R.E. and Cacioppo, J.T. (1986) 'The elaboration likelihood model of persuasion', in L. Berkowitz (ed.) *Advances in Experimental Social Psychology* **19**. New York: Academic Press.

Petty, R.E., Cacioppo, J.T. and Goldman, R. (1981) 'Personal involvement as a determinant of argument-based persuasion', *Journal of Personality and Social Psychology* **41**, 847–55.

Petty, R.E., Wells, G.L. and Brock, T.C. (1976) 'Distraction can enhance or reduce yielding to propaganda: Thought disruption versus effort justification', *Journal of Personality and Social Psychology* **34**, 874–84.

Pomozal, R.J. and Jaccard, J.J. (1976) 'An informational approach to altruistic behaviour', *Journal of Personality and Social Psychology* **33**, 317–26.

Pyszczynski, T. and Greenberg, J. (1987) 'Toward an integration of cognitive and motivational perspectives on social inference: A biased hypothesis-testing model', in L. Berkowitz (ed.) *Advances in Experimental Social Psychology*, Vol. 20. New York: Academic Press.

Riess, M. and Schlenker, B.R. (1977) 'Attitude change and responsibility avoidance as modes of dilemma resolution in forced-compliance situations', *Journal of Personality and Social Psychology* **35**, 21–30.

Rippetoe, P.A. and Rogers, R.W. (1987) 'Effects of components of protection-motivation theory on adaptive and maladaptive coping with a health threat', *Journal of Personality and Social Psychology* **52**, 596–604.

Rogers, R.W. (1983) 'Cognitive and physiological processes in attitude change: A revised theory of protection motivation', in J.T. Cacioppo and R.E. Petty (eds.) *Social Psychophysiology.* New York: Guilford Press.

Rutter, D.R., Quine, L. and Chesham, D.J. (1993) *Social Psychological Approaches to Health.* Hemel Hempstead: Harvester Wheatsheaf.

Scher, S.J. and Cooper, J. (1989) 'Motivational basis of dissonance: The singular role of behavioural consequences', *Journal of Personality and Social Psychology* **56**, 899–906.

Schifter, D.B. and Ajzen, I. (1985) 'Intention, perceived control and weight loss: An application of the theory of planned behaviour', *Journal of Personality and Social Psychology* **49**, 843–51.

Sears, D.O. (1965) 'Biased indoctrination and selectivity of exposure to new information', *Sociometry* **28**, 363–76.

Sivacek, J. and Crano, W.D. (1982) 'Vested interest as a moderator of attitude–behaviour consistency', *Journal of Personality and Social Psychology* **43**, 210–21.

Smetana, J.G. and Adler, N.E. (1980) 'Fishbein's value x expectancy model: An examination of some assumptions', *Personality and Social Psychology Bulletin* **6**, 89–96.

Valdiserri, R., Lyter, D., Kingsley, L., Leviton, L., Schofield, J., Hoggins, J., Ho, M. and Rinaldo, C. (1987) 'The effect of group education on improving attitudes about AIDS risk reduction', *New York State Journal of Medicine* **87**, 272–8.

Vinokur-Kaplan, D. (1978) 'To have – or not to have – another child: Family planning attitudes, intentions and behaviour', *Journal of Applied Social Psychology* **8**, 29–46.

Walster, E. and Festinger, L. (1962) 'The effectiveness of "overheard" persuasive communication', *Journal of Abnormal and Social Psychology* **65**, 395–402.

Weber, R. and Crocker, J. (1983). 'Cognitive processes in the revision of stereotypic beliefs', *Journal of Personality and Social Psychology* **45**, 961–77.

Wicker, A.W. (1969) 'Attitudes versus actions: The relationship of verbal and overt behavioural responses to attitude objects', *Journal of Social Issues* **25**, 41–78.

CHAPTER 6

Social cognition and health behaviour

PETER HARRIS AND WENDY MIDDLETON

Chapter outline

Introduction

Social cognition involves the extension of the concepts, theories and methods of cognitive psychology to the understanding of social phenomena. The aim of this branch of social psychology is to specify the cognitive processes that underpin social behaviour. The focus is on the cognitive elements and processes that are involved when people think about themselves and others (Fiske and Taylor, 1991).

In this chapter we shall explore some of the ways in which social cognition research has contributed to our understanding of health behaviour. Why do some people give up smoking, change their diets and exercise regimes or attend health screening appointments while others do not? Attempts to answer questions such as these have led to the creation of models in which the key components are the social and especially the cognitive processes postulated to be involved in the take-up and implementation of health precautions – the *social cognition models of health behaviour.*

There is, of course, much more to social cognition than just these models. We have chosen to focus on these models here because they constitute one of the major ways in which this field of research has contributed to what has become known as health psychology. If you wish to find out more about social cognition generally, you will find a reference at the end of this chapter to Fiske and Taylor (1991) who provide a comprehensive overview of the area.

The social cognition models of health behaviour

There are two basic types of social cognition models of health behaviour: models that have been developed to account for social behaviour in general and models that have been developed to account for some aspect of health behaviour in particular. For clarity, we shall call the first type 'general' models and the latter 'health' models.

The general models are more encompassing than the health ones – they attempt to explain other forms of social behaviour as well. Two such models – Ajzen and Fishbein's (1977, 1980) theory of reasoned action (TRA) and its subsequent extension, the theory of planned behaviour (TPB; Ajzen, 1985, 1988) – are described and evaluated in Chapter 5. In this chapter, we shall focus primarily on the health models. We shall look at two of the most widely employed examples of this type of model here, the health belief model and protection motivation theory, together with a recent attempt by Schwarzer to enhance their explanatory power in his health action process approach (Schwarzer, 1992a). Nevertheless, the TRA/TPB are also relevant to the issues raised in this chapter and, where appropriate, we shall discuss them here as well.

Both classes of model have their strengths and weaknesses. The pivotal question is whether health behaviour can be explained in the same way as other forms of social behaviour or whether there is something distinctive about the factors that prompt and sustain it. This issue will surface in the discussion that follows. In part, the answer may depend on what type of health behaviour we consider.

Health behaviour is a general label for behaviours that have implications for one's health. Such behaviours fall into two broad classes – those that are *health-promoting* and those that are *health-damaging* (Adler, Kegeles and Genevro, 1992). Within each class, however, there may be important distinctions to be made between different types of behaviour. They might differ, for instance, in terms of knowledge of the consequences for health or in terms of the primacy of the health consequences in motivating and sustaining the behaviour. Thus we may sunbathe in ignorance of the consequences for our health or in spite of them (see Box 6.1). Likewise, we may attempt to lose weight on medical grounds, to make ourselves feel more attractive, or both. In the end, going for a run might be stimulated more by the highs that accompany it and the routine involved than by concerns over fitness, and so on.

Differences such as these may have implications for the models we devise to explain behaviour, as well as for appropriate methods of health promotion and treatment (see Box 6.1). While useful to us as a general term, therefore, you should bear in mind the fact that health behaviour covers a range of potentially different activities.

The health models

One of the most significant changes in health and disease during the twentieth century has been the shift in Western societies from the primacy of acute infectious diseases as causes of death to chronic, non-infectious ones (Crawford, 1987). Consequently, many of the people you will treat will be victims of their own behaviour. If they had cut down on alcohol, given up smoking sooner, changed their diet, taken more exercise, learnt how to relax more effectively, avoided unprotected sexual intercourse or spent less time in the sun, they might not have been ill today (Box 6.1).

BOX 6.1 SHOULD WE WITHHOLD TREATMENT FROM PEOPLE WHO KNOWINGLY DAMAGE THEIR OWN HEALTH?

Knowledge of the links between behaviour and health has grown massively in recent years as scientific evidence has accumulated. Consequently, many of your current patients/clients may well have been ignorant of the risks that they were running with their long-term health. Equally, as with all scientific progress, there is often dispute among 'experts' about the evidence. It is not hard to get confused over the conflicting advice and it may be easy to persuade yourself that expert opinion lacks credibility and can be ignored. In the area of diet, for instance, expert advice about what constitutes a healthy diet has changed remarkably in the post-war period. Other people, therefore, may simply not have believed the advice they were given. However, there is clear evidence that some people persist in unhealthy behaviour even when the risks are known and accepted.

DISCUSSION POINT
Given the limits on health budgets, should treatment be withheld from those who wilfully persist in unhealthy behaviour?

The issue of treatment for such people was brought to the fore by a recent case in which a smoker died shortly after he had been refused treatment for his heart condition at a Manchester hospital. The consultant refused to consider the patient for a coronary bypass operation until he gave up smoking. The patient, who smoked 25 cigarettes a day, eventually gave up, but died shortly before he was due to go into hospital for tests. The case brought a public outcry in which the decision was widely condemned as discriminatory and unethical.

In fact, treatment was not withheld simply to punish the patient for continuing to smoke when it had already predisposed him to disease, but because post-operative recovery from this expensive procedure is compromised by continuing to smoke. Nevertheless, the case raises important ethical issues which you might like to address in group discussions. It also raises a related psychological question:

■ Would it help to encourage healthier behaviour if people were made aware that they would not be treated for diseases that could be traced to their risk-taking?

In your discussions, you might like to ponder the kinds of risk-taking involved and to think about any relevant cases that you have encountered. Below are some additional questions you might like to consider:

- How might the health care given by health professionals be affected by knowing that a patient/client is, in part or wholly, responsible for the condition requiring treatment? (See Chapter 2 for discussion of how nurses' attributions about patients affect the care given.)
- As well as behaviour that contributes to chronic disease, what about activities that drain resources by requiring treatment for acute conditions, such as sports injuries? Should treatment be withheld from people who persist in playing rugby or climbing mountains when they are aware of the risks they run? How does this differ from the case of the smoker?
- What about cases in which people actually intend to damage themselves, such as when they attempt suicide?

Why do people take risks with that most precious of their assets, their health? The various social cognition models attempt to describe and predict the adoption of *precautionary* or *self-protective behaviour* once the risks become known. The key assumption that unites these models is the *expectancy-value assumption*. This is the assumption that people weigh up the relative costs and benefits of various courses of action and choose the course that provides the best return. The expectancy refers to a person's estimates of the likely consequences of a given course of action, such as smoking or taking regular exercise; the value concerns how important these outcomes are to the person concerned. Thus, if you value many of the consequences of smoking and perceive the associated risks to be low, the assumption is that you will persist in smoking; if, however, you perceive the risks to outweigh the benefits, then you are likelier to give up. The assumption is, therefore, essentially 'rational' – it assumes that risks are taken in the pursuit of valued outcomes, rather than for trivial returns.

At first glance, however, the data appear to be quite at odds with this assumption. Looked at individually, campaigns to encourage various forms of self-protective behaviour are often strikingly unsuccessful, even when the precautionary behaviour seems to be comparatively straightforward, involves little apparent cost and can result in a sizeable reduction in objective risk (e.g. installing a smoke alarm, wearing a car seat-belt, using a condom; see Weinstein, 1987). However, the key words in the above sentence are 'seems' and 'apparent'. The expectancy-value assumption, together with the models based on it, deal with the world as seen by the people concerned. In order to deem the failure to wear a car seat-belt or use a condom irrational, we have to understand the expectancies and values of the people who are failing to take these precautions.

Moreover, whereas the results of individual campaigns are often disappointing, the cumulative effects of health education programmes over the years are much more encouraging (Gatchel, Baum and Krantz, 1989). For example, whereas 52 per cent of British men and 41 per cent of British women over 16 years of age could be classified as regular smokers twenty years ago, the respective figures are now down to 31 per cent and 29 per cent (Rutter, Quine and Chesham, 1993). What is certainly clear, however, is that there are considerable differences between people both in their readiness to listen to and to act on health-related advice (inter-individual differences) and in their readiness to respond in this way to advice in particular domains of health (intra-individual differences). The social cognition models are attempts to alert us to general principles that help to explain such different responses. As such, they attempt the dual task of promoting theoretical understanding and offering practical solutions to the problems of promoting healthier behaviour.

DISCUSSION POINT

Think of an example of your own health-damaging behaviour (e.g. smoking, eating food high in saturated fat, not taking enough exercise) and an example of something you have done or do regularly that is health-promoting (e.g. cutting down or giving up alcohol or cigarettes, changing some aspect of your diet for reasons of health, taking up some form of regular exercise). Bear these separate examples in mind as you work through each of the models that follow. Below are some questions that you might think about when doing so:

■ To what extent do these models capture the processes by which you maintain your unhealthy behaviour or changed to a healthier regime?
■ What does thinking about your own behaviour in this way tell you about the expectancy-value assumption? Is it a sensible assumption? Can you think of something you do that does not appear to satisfy this assumption?
■ Are there any important differences among your health behaviours? Do you do some things in spite of their implications for your health? If so, why? How much of your health-promoting behaviour is prompted primarily by health concerns? Can you identify any aspects of your own behaviour that you carry out solely or at least principally for reasons of health?

The health belief model (HBM)

The first model we shall discuss is the health belief model (HBM; see Figure 6.1). This was originally formulated as an attempt to account for people's failure to take advantage of preventive health services, such as screenings and inoculation (Becker, 1974; Rosenstock, 1966, 1974). It has subsequently been extended to more general aspects of precautionary health behaviour and has become one of the most influential frameworks in the area (Adler, Kegeles and Genevro, 1992; Schwarzer, 1992a). In the process it has, of course, been both extended and refined (Becker and Maiman, 1975; Rosenstock, Strecher and Becker, 1988; Schwarzer, 1992a). We shall first describe the basic model.

According to the HBM, precautionary behaviour is prompted by appropriate *cues to action*. These can be external (e.g. receiving an appointment card, reading a health promotion leaflet) or internal (e.g. pains in the chest, repeated breathlessness).

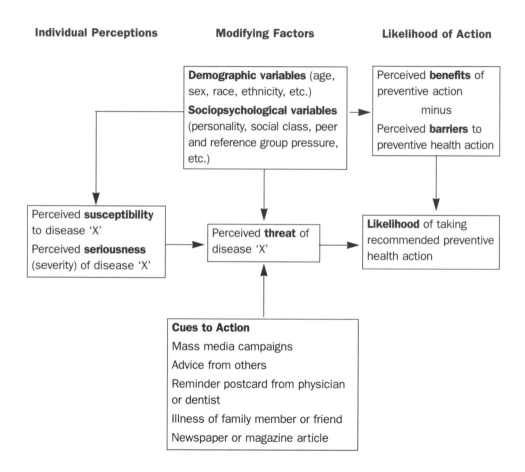

Figure 6.1 *The health belief model*

Source: Adler *et al.* (1992), in J. F. Yates (ed.) *Risk-taking Behaviour*. Chichester: John Wiley; from Becker and Maiman (1975).

The assumption is that precautionary behaviour is less likely to occur in the absence of relevant cues. This is an important assumption, as it suggests that we generally have to be prompted or provoked into such behaviour. However, the presence of the cue alone is not sufficient to prompt the behaviour. Thus, sending out appointments to attend for a screening test will be sufficient to prompt some people into attending, but not others. What differentiates the attenders from the non-attenders? According to the HBM there are several critical conditions that have to be met in order for such attendance to become likely.

One factor is that the person has to see her or himself as threatened by the disease. There are two components to this perceived *threat*: in order to feel threatened, the person must perceive her or himself to be at risk of the disease (perceived *susceptibility*) and believe that the disease is sufficiently serious to warrant action (perceived *seriousness*). Figure 6.1, however, shows that although perceiving oneself to be threatened by a given disease increases the likelihood of taking a recommended preventive health action, it is not the only factor that contributes to this likelihood. The likelihood of taking action is further increased if the person concerned considers that the preventive action has *benefits* that outweigh the perceived *barriers* in the way of taking the preventive action. Thus, according to the HBM, a woman is more likely to attend for breast cancer screening if she sees herself as potentially at risk for this cancer, acknowledges that breast cancer is dangerous, accepts that screening will be of benefit in detecting a cancer early and feels that the barriers to attending – such as finding the time and being able to get to the screening site – are worth overcoming for these benefits. In the terms of the theory, these perceptions make her 'psychologically ready' to act if prompted. She might be prompted to attend by, for example, receiving an invitation to a screening, by discovering a lump in her breast, by being offered a lift to the clinic by a friend who had decided to attend or by reading an article in a magazine that reminded her of her vulnerability to breast cancer.

Note that the model is clearly cognitive. The central factors are the person's perceptions of things such as their susceptibility to the disease and the likely benefits of the preventive action, rather than any 'objective' assessment of these factors. Thus, even though to an outsider the barriers to action might appear minimal and the threat great, it matters more that the person concerned believes the reverse.

The model also provides a role for variables such as a person's age, sex, social class, personality and perceptions of the attitudes of family and friends towards the behaviour (summarized in the model as *demographic* and *sociopsychological* variables). These are factors that potentially influence the central perceptions and beliefs. Thus, females will be more alert than males to the possibility of contracting cystitis, for instance, while a husband's hostility to his wife's attendance for breast cancer screening may be more of a barrier among certain social classes or in certain ethnic groups than in others. The direction of the arrows in Figure 6.1 indicates that these factors can influence all the perceptions central to the model.

From its origins as an attempt to understand non-attendance for precautionary health checks, the HBM has grown to be one of the dominant frameworks for predicting health behaviour. It has provided the impetus for a wide range of studies and has received widespread empirical support (for reviews see Adler, Kegeles and Genevro, 1992; Conner and Norman, in press; Janz and Becker, 1984; Rutter, Quine and Chesham, 1993). Research on preventive health behaviours has shown that perceived barriers tend to be the strongest predictor of behaviour in the model and that perceived seriousness tends to be the weakest (Rutter, Quine and Chesham, 1993).

The HBM currently comprises one of the principal contributions of social cognition to the understanding of health behaviour. It is not, however, without its problems or its critics and we shall consider some of the more central of these next.

Problems with the health belief model

Theories and models in science serve not only to summarize and integrate knowledge but also to focus attention on areas where understanding is inadequate. In this respect the HBM is no exception. Among the problems with it are:

- There is no consensus over how key components of the model should be operationalised (i.e. how they should be measured), with the result that there is great variation in practice. Indeed, some of the critical variables – such as 'cues to action' – have been omitted from studies altogether because of difficulties in their operationalisation (Adler, Kegeles and Genevro, 1992).
- The relationships between the variables in the model have been found to vary greatly from study to study and even within the same study itself. Adler, Kegeles and Genevro (1992) suggest that this might be related in part to the lack of consensus over operationalising key components of the model.
- The HBM often explains less of the variance in health behaviour than we would expect if it were adequately capturing what goes on (Rosenstock, Strecher and Becker, 1988). This raises the possibility that factors other than those specified in the model are having an influence on the behaviours of interest.
- Although the model specifies key perceptions thought to contribute to health behaviour, it does not explicitly tie these together into a coherent theoretical framework. It does not specify, for instance, what *psychological* processes are involved in comparing the benefits of action with the barriers to action or by what *psychological* principles demographic and sociopsychological factors exert their influence on the central beliefs and perceptions. The model, therefore, tells us about where we might look if we want to understand something about the adoption of precautionary health behaviour, but it does not tell us much about the psychological principles and processes that make these variables hang together.

One response to such problems has been to use the alternative models of health behaviour, such as the TRA, TPB and protection motivation theory (see below). However, several authors have suggested refinements to the HBM that have served to improve its capacity to predict health behaviour.

Refinements to the HBM

Two subsequent refinements to the HBM have been (1) the introduction of a role for the person's *general motivation for health* (Becker and Maiman, 1975), and (2) the incorporation of the concept of *self-efficacy* (Rosenstock, Strecher and Becker, 1988). The former refers to a general tendency to be interested in health and to feel in control of one's health, which is postulated to be stable over time for any given person and to vary between people. Thus, some people will be motivated by concerns about their health, while others will not, and this will clearly influence their perceptions and their respective responses to health threats.

However, if people feel that they simply cannot do what is required by way of preventive behaviour, they will fail to take preventive action, even though they accept that they are at risk and acknowledge that the preventive action will significantly reduce that risk. Such people are said to have low self-efficacy for the behaviour in question. Thus, a cigarette smoker may acknowledge the risk to his health posed by his smoking, accept that he ought to give up and that there are, in principle, no insurmountable external barriers to him so doing, but fail to do so simply because he sees giving up as beyond him (i.e. his self-efficacy for this behaviour is low). Although it might be argued that this is captured in the model as an internal barrier to action, Rosenstock, Strecher and Becker (1988) have argued that the addition of the concept of self-efficacy to the HBM adds to the model's explanatory power. The concept of self-efficacy has been widely researched in its own right (e.g. Schwarzer, 1992b) and features in both of the models we will discuss next.

Interestingly, the HBM summarized in Figure 6.1 does not include an element that is central to general models like the TRA and TPB. This is the *intention* to perform the behaviour in question. Ajzen and Fishbein (1977) introduced this concept in order to improve our understanding of the relationship between attitudes and behaviour and it has been shown to be a stronger predictor of eventual behaviour than attitude alone (see Chapter 5). In the HBM, however, the central beliefs and perceptions act directly on the likelihood of behaviour, without being explicitly mediated by the formation of any intention to perform the act. Adding intention to the HBM has been shown to increase the level of prediction obtained and this component is now typically added to the model in studies testing it (Conner and Norman, in press). One of the consequences of such refinements to the HBM has been to erode the distinctions between it and models like the TRA/TPB and protection motivation theory (PMT). Indeed, the trend seems to be towards the development of a generic model of health behaviour that incorporates the best predictors from various models. We shall discuss one such recent example, Schwarzer's health action process approach (HAPA). This incorporates elements from the HBM, the TRA/TPB and PMT. Before considering the HAPA, therefore, we will briefly describe protection motivation theory.

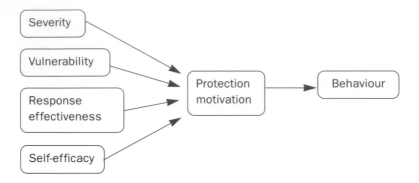

Source: adapted from R. Schwarzer (1992) 'Self-efficacy in the adoption and maintenance of health behaviours'. In R. Schwarzer (ed.) *Self-efficacy: Thought control of action.* Washington; Hemisphere.

Figure 6.2 *Protection motivation theory*

Protection motivation theory (PMT)

Like the HBM, PMT is based on the expectancy-value assumption. The focus of PMT, however, is on the way in which fear acts as a motivating factor for health behaviour. Like the HBM, it is a cognitive model. However, unlike the HBM, PMT posits the existence of a motivation to protect oneself from danger – *protection motivation.* Once aroused, protection motivation acts to promote, sustain and direct self-protective activity.

PMT (Rogers, 1975, 1983, 1985) was devised to explain the impact of 'fear appeals' on the adoption, or otherwise, of precautions. Fear appeals are attempts to provoke the adoption of appropriate methods of protection among the target audience by making them fearful of the consequences if they do not. Some versions of the model are quite complicated (see, for example, Rippetoe and Rogers, 1987), but a simplified version that captures the essentials is depicted in Figure 6.2.

Protection motivation is hypothesized to be determined by four factors (Figure 6.2). These are the person's perceptions of (1) the *severity* of the disease, (2) her susceptibility or *vulnerability* to the disease, (3) the *effectiveness* of the health precaution, and (4) her *self-efficacy* regarding the action. Thus someone might decide to take up running for health reasons to the extent that he perceived himself to be at risk for heart disease, acknowledged that heart disease was life-threatening, accepted that running regularly would help to reduce the threat of heart disease and believed that he would be able to sustain his running programme.

In support of PMT, Rippetoe and Rogers (1987) found that motivation to perform breast self-examination was highest under conditions of high severity, high vulnerability, high self-efficacy for the behaviour in question and with higher levels of belief in the health benefits of breast self-examination.

Similarities and differences among the models

Although there is no equivalent of protection motivation in the HBM, in other respects the elements of PMT resemble those of the HBM. However, one central feature of both models – their respective emphases on threat and fear – marks a key distinction between them and the TRA/TPB.

Neither threat nor fear plays any role in the TRA/TPB. This is interesting, as it tells us something about theorists' perceptions of the factors that prompt self-protective behaviours in the domain of health and how these differ from the assumptions they hold about behaviour in general. It seems that self-protective behaviours are presumed to be things we need to be triggered or prodded into doing, not things we typically do naturally. Left to our own devices, it seems, the assumption is that we do things that place us at risk. This, of course, is the crux of the problem for health promotion – if self-protective actions came as naturally as risky ones, there would be no problem. On the other hand, it has been argued (e.g. Schwarzer, 1992a) that protection motivation is synonymous with the intention to behave. Thus PMT incorporates features to be found in both the HBM and the TRA/TPB. Recently, Schwarzer (1992a) has taken this a stage further and has proposed a model that explicitly synthesizes elements from all three into a generic model he calls the health action process approach.

The health action process approach (HAPA)

The health action process approach (HAPA; Figure 6.3) has two distinct stages. The left-hand side of Figure 6.3 represents what Schwarzer calls the *decision-making/motivational stage* of the process. The right-hand side of this figure represents what he calls the *action/maintenance stage*. The inclusion of this second stage is one of the principal innovations of the HAPA. First, however, we will consider the decision-making/motivational stage.

The decision-making/motivational stage

The models discussed so far – including the TRA/TPB – confine themselves to the first stage of the process and, as you can see from Figure 6.3, in many respects this stage of the HAPA employs concepts that are by now familiar to you. *Threat* we met in the HBM; *self-efficacy expectancies* featured in both the HBM and PMT; *intention* is an import from the TRA/TPB and is synonymous with 'protection motivation' from PMT. Although *outcome expectancies* may seem unfamiliar, it is, in effect, the variable labelled 'response effectiveness' in PMT.

The HAPA does, however, introduce some new relationships between these variables. Whereas in PMT *severity* and *vulnerability* made independent contributions to intention (Figure 6.2), here their impact is mediated by threat (as in the

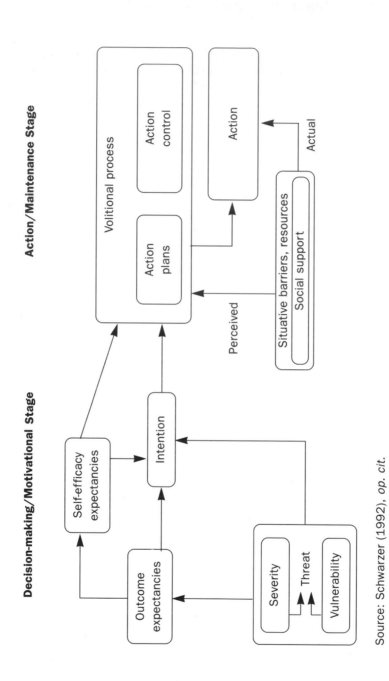

Source: Schwarzer (1992), op. cit.

Figure 6.3 The health action process approach

HBM). However, as well as contributing to intention, threat is also linked now to outcome expectancies. Likewise, in PMT outcome expectancies and self-efficacy expectancies simply made independent contributions to intention. However, Bandura, the originator of the notion of self-efficacy, has repeatedly argued that the impact of outcome expectancies on intention is partly governed by the person's self-beliefs about efficacy (e.g. Bandura, 1989) and this is incorporated in Schwarzer's model. Thus a smoker's intention to give up smoking will not be governed simply by his belief that giving up will reduce his likelihood of contracting lung cancer, but will be mediated by his assessments of his capacity to give up. If he feels that giving up will be hard for him to do, he will not form the intention to do so, however convinced he is that giving up will significantly reduce his risk (according to this model). In the HAPA, therefore, there is a link between outcome expectancies and self-efficacy expectancies (Figure 6.3).

After reviewing the available evidence, Schwarzer (1992a) posits the following order of importance for the three direct paths to intention: (1) self-efficacy, (2) outcome expectancy and (3) threat. Indeed, consistent with the above argument, he suggests that the latter variables (especially threat) may exert most of their impact on intention via the indirect rather than the direct paths. Thus, perceiving yourself to be at risk of lung cancer may be more influential in creating the intention to give up smoking if it prompts you to think about ways in which you might enhance your self-efficacy for stopping smoking. It will be less influential if it contributes only to an intention to give up that you feel it will be difficult for you to fulfil.

The decision-making/motivation stage is an attempt to delineate the key general processes involved when people make up their minds about whether or not to adopt health precautions. The action/maintenance stage attempts to model the factors that determine how hard they try and how long they persist.

The action/maintenance stage

One of the major frustrations of life is the cavernous gap that often seems to appear between good intentions and behaviour. Psychological data (e.g. Prochaska, DiClemente and Norcross, 1992), as well as everyday experience, testify to the fact that having the motivation or the intention to become healthier is sadly no guarantee that this intention will be translated into action or that one will do much more than dabble with the new behaviour before reverting to old habits. The HBM, PMT and TRA/TPB have nothing to say about the factors that promote effective and sustained action once action becomes likely. The action/maintenance stage of the HAPA is Schwarzer's attempt to fill this gap. In it, he addresses the factors that contribute to or undermine the adoption and maintenance of effective health behaviour, once the good intention has been established.

The first step, according to the model, is to translate the intention into more precise *action plans*. It is all very well forming an intention to reduce saturated fat consumption, to start exercising or to give up cigarettes, but these intentions need to be translated into action in order to be realized. According to Schwarzer, a high sense of self-efficacy for the task ahead will facilitate this process, both by helping the person to generate different ways in which the goal can be realized and by enhancing his or her capacity to evaluate the different options. Thus a woman who really believes she can cut down on her alcohol consumption will not only tend to think up more ways of achieving this goal (e.g. not having alcohol in the house, leaving for the pub later than usual, drinking with friends less often) but will also tend to be more realistic about what will work (e.g. trying to cut down rather than to give up immediately, avoiding situations in which drink is available rather than assuming that she will simply be able to refuse alcohol when it is offered).

Once a course of action has been initiated, it has to be maintained. Schwarzer (1992a) again sees self-efficacy as one of the critical variables influencing the outcome of this *action control* phase of the process. He argues that self-efficacy determines the amount of effort invested in the task and the degree to which people will persevere in the face of obstacles.

Indeed, one of the central difficulties people face when adopting healthier behavioural regimes is precisely the fact that the regime typically represents a change. Not only does changing behaviour tend to have all manner of psychological and social consequences, but there are invariably powerful psychological and social factors remaining to encourage a return to old habits. Lapses are common, even when the commitment to change is strong (Prochaska, DiClemente and Norcross, 1992). For this reason, health educators are placing increasing emphasis on catching youngsters early, before they have developed bad habits, as it may well be easier to encourage the formation of good habits than to encourage people to change long-standing bad ones (Weinstein, 1987).

Schwarzer suggests that a key capacity for successful action control is self-reinforcement – the capacity to reward oneself for 'being good'. One of the problems we face in adopting healthier behaviour is that, while we immediately lose the rewards that come with the old bad habits, the rewards that come with the new good ones tend to be more remote, less tangible and, at least in the short term, less powerful. Thus, giving up smoking involves trading the tangible and powerful rewards you know and love for the long-term possibility that you might not now die of a smoking-related disease. Not only is this rather a distant and remote reward, but there was, of course, no guarantee that you would have died of such a disease had you continued smoking; nor, sadly, is giving up itself a guarantee that you will not die in the meantime in some equally unpleasant way. As a consequence, some people are ready to take risks with their health precisely because they construe this in terms of a gamble – they hope that they will be among the lucky few who will not get ill or believe that there are many other risks out of their control and that they might as well reap the benefits of their unhealthy habits in the meantime (Davison, Smith and Frankel, 1991; Regis, 1988). Thus in one study 85 per cent of smokers accepted that, if they did get ill, smoking would be at least partly to blame (Marsh and Matheson, 1983), while McKenna, Warburton and Winwood (1993) found that smokers rated their risk of smoking-related diseases to be higher than that of non-smokers, but lower than that of the average smoker.

Change is probably more likely to be permanent, therefore, if people focus on the short-term rewards of the change itself (e.g. feeling fitter, feeling better about oneself). It is interesting to note, for instance, that as smokers give up, they form increasingly negative impressions of the 'typical smoker' and come to see this figure as less similar to themselves (Gibbons *et al.*, 1991). This cognitive process has the dual effect of discouraging smoking (in order to avoid associating the self with this negative figure) and rewarding non-smoking (via the positive self-regard that comes from the gap between the self and this increasingly negative figure).

The rewards that you lose when giving up certain types of unhealthy habit are not only intrinsic, however, but often also social. Many kinds of drug-taking, for example, whether socially acceptable or not, are often shared experiences. Not only does this mean that changing such habits involves the loss of these additional rewards (e.g. drinking with your friends, sharing a cigarette or a chocolate cake after a trying day), but it may also mean that there are important social obstacles to face when negotiating the process of change. Your friends and even your family, for example, might well find the changes in your habits and routines inconvenient or even threatening and may mobilize the resources available to them to resist your attempts to change. On the other hand, they might very much welcome the new you and offer all kinds of support and reassurance in the process. These kinds of factor appear in the HAPA as *situative barriers*, *situative resources* and *social support*. However, Schwarzer makes a key distinction between one's perceptions of these factors and their actual status. The arrows in Figure 6.3 indicate that while perceptions are thought to influence the volitional process, the actual status of these factors has a direct impact on action. Although Schwarzer does not comment on this, it is not unreasonable to assume that perceptions of the reactions of your family and friends may well influence how you construct your plans and act to maintain your new habits (the volitional process), but that their actual reactions (social support) will have some bearing on the eventual outcome. (See Box 2.4, p. 43, for strategies used to enhance adherence to medical treatments and life-style changes.)

At the time of writing it is too early to tell what impact the HAPA will have on research into health behaviour. The decision-making/motivational phase is an interesting and potentially important synthesis of the existing models. The action/maintenance stage is rather more speculative, but nevertheless represents a welcome broadening of concerns to embrace the factors that may contribute to sustained and effective health behaviour. However, this stage is vague in places and it has yet to be integrated with alternative approaches to the initiation and maintenance of action, such as Carver and Scheier's (1981, 1982) control theory of self-regulation, models of the adoption of self-protective action such as Prochaska's trans-theoretical model (Prochaska, 1994) and Weinstein's precaution adoption process model (Weinstein and Sandman, 1992), and Gollwitzer's work on goal achievement (Gollwitzer, 1993; Gollwitzer and Kinney, 1989).

In many respects the HAPA represents the culmination of this tradition of research and, as such, it embodies both its strengths and its weaknesses. Before turning to these, however, we want to consider another aspect of social cognition that has implications for health behaviour – unrealistic optimism.

Unrealistic optimism

Consider the illnesses in Box 6.2. If you attempt the exercise in that box the chances are that you will see yourself as at or below average risk for most of the diseases. Indeed, the odds are that you will see yourself as less at risk for the more serious disorders, the rarer disorders, those with which you have had no direct personal experience (for example, no one close to you has suffered it) and, especially, those you perceive to be preventable by your own actions (Weinstein, 1989). This effect has been demonstrated across a wide range of samples and a variety of risks, not simply risks to health (Hoorens, 1993, in press; Weinstein, 1989). It has been called

---

BOX 6.2   PERCEIVED VULNERABILITY TO DISEASE

Look at each of the diseases below:

- Heart disease
- Stomach ulcers
- Tuberculosis
- Parkinson's disease
- Liver trouble
- Stroke
- Lung cancer
- Obesity
- AIDS
- Clinical depression

What do you think are the approximate chances that you will get each of these diseases or disorders at some stage in your life? In particular, how do your chances of getting each disease compare with the chances that *an average person of the same age, sex, background and occupation as yourself* will get it? Of course, you can only guess, but what's your best guess of your relative chances at the moment? Use the following scale to make your judgements:

1	2	3	4	5	6	7
Much less than average	Less than average	Slightly less than average	Average	Slightly more than average	More than average	Much more than average

Your Chances of Getting the Disease

unrealistic optimism (Weinstein, 1980). Unrealistic optimism is one of a range of ways in which we appear to operate on the assumption that we are superior to those around us (Hoorens, 1993, in press). Social cognition research has been instrumental in uncovering these biases in our self-perceptions (Fiske and Taylor, 1991; Taylor and Brown, 1988).

Weinstein chose to call this phenomenon 'unrealistic' optimism because the average judgement made by groups of respondents asked to estimate the likelihood of future events in their lives is typically below 'average chance' for negative events (and often above 'average chance' for positive events as well, e.g. Weinstein, 1980). This suggests that some of them see themselves as below average risk when they should not (as, in most circumstances, we cannot all be below average risk). Those who fail to recognize that they are at or above average risk, therefore, are being unrealistically optimistic.

As we have seen, perceived susceptibility or vulnerability to disease is a central element of all the health models we have considered. The implication of unrealistic optimism, however, is that we may see ourselves as less vulnerable than we should. According to the models, this will undermine the extent to which we adopt health precautions. However, it can be very hard to shake off a compelling sense that we are somehow less vulnerable to the kinds of problem and difficulty others face. For most of us, most of the time, serious illnesses, accidents and other problems happen to other people, not to us. Indeed, there is evidence that we typically come to acknowledge our own susceptibility to risk only after first believing that others are more at risk than we are (Weinstein, 1988).

AIDS is an important contemporary case in point. (See Chapter 16 for a discussion of the psychological implications of HIV infection.) In a recent study we conducted at the University of Hertfordshire, the students saw themselves as much less likely than average to contract AIDS and saw AIDS as one of the least likely diseases they would suffer from (it ranked 14th out of the 15 illnesses they were asked to rate; Harris and Middleton, 1994). One of the problems health educators face is that, for most people, AIDS fits perfectly the profile of a risk for which people tend to manifest unrealistic optimism, being serious, still comparatively rare, one for which most people still typically lack personal experience and highly preventable by their own actions. Thinking back to the exercise in Box 6.2, the likelihood is that most of you also saw your chances of contracting AIDS as below average and felt you had good grounds for doing so.

Strengths and weaknesses of the social cognition models of health behaviour

In this chapter we have outlined several social cognition models. What are their strengths and weaknesses?

The principal strength of the social cognition models is their capacity to explain and predict health behaviour. Although the level of understanding is currently far from perfect, it seems likely that the models identify and describe some of the key factors underlying and influencing decisions about health behaviour. Such information should be of help to practitioners and health educators. Models such as the HAPA hold out the prospect that in the future we will be able to explain even more.

Conner (1992) suggests that the models also provide a clear theoretical background that serves to guide research, that they give the area some coherence and that they help us to identify the critical variables underlying unhealthy behaviour. In so doing, he argues, they suggest both where interventions to alter cognitions underlying unhealthy behaviour should be targeted and what form such interventions might take. Nevertheless, the models are still some way from telling the complete story and it may even be that they never will. Some of the problems are potentially surmountable. Others, if the critics are right, are more fundamental.

The models may not be applicable to all health behaviour. Conner (1992) suggests that the kinds of cost–benefit analysis underlying the models may be applicable only to certain types of health behaviour (e.g. where the outcomes are important). We may not always be as thoughtful or even as rational about our health as the models assume (see Box 6.3). There may be limits on the applicability of the expectancy-value assumption.

The models may place too much emphasis on people's capacity to decide for themselves about their behaviour. Although they are called social cognition models, in terms of their emphasis they are rather more cognitive than social. Thus, while social and economic factors may well be vital to the process of change, these factors tend to be confined to such notions as the sociopsychological variables that 'moderate' beliefs or that constitute one class of 'barrier' to action (HBM), or to the 'normative beliefs' about the behaviour that contribute to the intention to do it via the subjective norm (TRA). In particular, a sense of the social network as an *active* resistor of change, rather than a passive 'barrier' to be overcome, is frequently missing from these models. It may well be no exaggeration to say, for instance, that for some people and for some habits the prospect of change may well amount to a decision whether or not to lose their friends. As a consequence, some models that pay less lip service to social factors have appeared very recently (Breakwell, Fife-Schaw and Clayden, 1991; Rutter, Quine and Chesham, 1993).

The models are very general. They are designed to cover everything from taking medicines for trivial illnesses to major changes of lifestyle, and in the case of the models such as the TRA/TPB, even non health-related behaviour. Not only is this a daunting task – at its most general it seems to be little short of the task of the discipline of psychology itself – but it might be that the assumption that we can model behaviour in such general terms is invalid. Either way, it seems a tall order to expect to model such an apparently complex phenomenon as human behaviour adequately with a sketch that can fit on the back of a medium-sized envelope. Indeed, there have been appeals (e.g. Cleary, 1987) for researchers to be less ambitious, to explore the factors that determine specific acts rather than behaviour in general. Recently, there have been more specific attempts to model behaviour in

BOX 6.3 **THE PSYCHOLOGY OF HEALTH SCREENING**

One area of certain growth in modern health care provision is in providing screening for an increasing range of conditions. Yet surprisingly little is known about the psychology of health screening.

In and of itself, of course, screening does not reduce your risk of disease; rather, it provides you with clearer evidence of your potential risk of a disease. The effectiveness of screening in prevention depends on how we respond subsequently – whether, for example, we attend for further tests, have lumps and other growths removed, act to reduce our cholesterol levels, agree to follow a healthier diet.

All these things entail changes in current behaviours and, perhaps even more importantly, facing up to threatening information about ourselves. We may even be reluctant to make a check-up or screening appointment precisely because we are afraid of what we may find out. What would happen, however, if the opportunity arose to cheat on a screening test? Would we do so? On the face of it, this would be an extremely irrational response, for it would mean that we would then fail to take necessary preventive or precautionary measures and risk illness and even premature death. Quattrone and Tversky (1986) tested this very notion.

People attending an experiment on the 'psychological and medical aspects of athletics' were required to undertake the cold-pressor pain task, which involves submerging the forearm in circulating cold water for as long as it is tolerable. Once their baseline tolerance had been established, participants then pedalled an exercise bike for 1 minute. They were then introduced to the experimental manipulation: as part of a mini-lecture the participants were told that there were two types of heart, Type 1 and Type 2. People with Type 1 hearts were frequently ill, prone to heart disease and had a shorter than average life expectancy; those with Type 2 hearts enjoyed good health and had a longer than average life expectancy. Participants were also told that heart type determines how exercise changes the person's ability to tolerate cold water: half of them were told that Type 1 hearts increase tolerance to cold water after exercise while Type 2 hearts decrease this tolerance, while half were told that Type 2 hearts increase tolerance and Type 1 hearts decrease it. They then repeated the cold-pressor pain task, again to their tolerance threshold.

Given that this is a diagnostic test, cheating serves no rational purpose. Yet over 70 per cent of the subjects shifted their performance on the cold-pressor task in the direction favouring having the Type 2 heart. Indeed, where this involved keeping the forearm in the cold water longer than during the first phase of the experiment, there was a mean (average) increase in immersion of almost 12 seconds. Yet, only 24 per cent of the participants indicated that they had shifted their performance intentionally.

Clearly, we need to know more about the psychology of screening – especially as we move away from reactive medicine to preventive programmes.

- In your experience, what reasons have people given for (a) attending or (b) not attending a voluntary screening programme? How do these reasons relate to the models you have read about?

response to the threat of AIDS, such as the AIDS risk reduction model (Catania, Kegeles and Coates, 1990) and the information motivation behavioral skills model (Fisher and Fisher, 1992, 1993; Fisher *et al.*, 1994).

Summary

In this chapter we have introduced three health models of health behaviour – the HBM, PMT and a very recent model, the HAPA, based in part on the first two. All three models have a common basis in the assumption that our behaviour is rational. They share this assumption with some of the general models that have also been used to explain and predict health behaviour, such as the TRA/TPB.

The HBM is currently the most influential of the health models. However, modifications to the models have served to render them increasingly similar to one another and the trend seems to be towards developing a generic model of health behaviour that employs the best predictors from the other models. The HAPA is a recent example of such a model. As well as being a synthesis of elements from the HBM, PMT and the TRA/TPB, the HAPA is novel in that it attempts to delineate the processes involved in initiating and maintaining health behaviour. It is too early to say what the prospects are for the HAPA, but it offers the potential of a more complete understanding of health behaviour than the earlier models.

One of the elements of the health models that sets them apart from the general ones is the place they afford threat and fear in health behaviour. Social cognition research on unrealistic optimism, however, suggests that we may have a basic tendency to underestimate our susceptibility to disease relative to others. Unrealistic optimism, therefore, potentially lessens the extent to which we feel threatened and undermines the prospect of health-promoting activity.

We ended by considering some of the principal strengths and weaknesses of the social cognition models of health behaviour. Though currently far from offering a complete understanding of the processes involved, they provide a framework for research and work on health promotion. As they become refined and improved by further empirical and theoretical work, they offer the hope of a fuller understanding of those aspects of our health behaviour that are rational.

Acknowledgement

We would like to thank Dr Paul Sparks of the BBSRC Institute for Food Research, Reading, for his helpful comments on an earlier draft of this chapter

Seminar questions

1. Provide a case study based on one of your patients. Use this study to examine the strengths and weaknesses of one or more of the models discussed in this chapter.

2. Complete the exercise in Box 6.2 or get a group of people to do it. What are the average responses to each disease? Do you have evidence of unrealistic optimism? What are the implications of such optimism for the threat component of the various models? What are the implications for the likelihood of health behaviour?
3. What implications do the models hold for (a) health promotion; and (b) patient/client care?

Further reading

Adler, N.E., Kegeles, S.M. and Genevro, J.L. (1992) 'Risk taking and health', in J.F. Yates (ed.) *Risk-taking Behavior*. Chichester: John Wiley. Includes coverage of the HBM, PMT and unrealistic optimism, together with a discussion of the AIDS risk reduction model.

Rutter, D.R. (ed.) (in press) *The Social Psychology of Health and Safety: European perspectives*. Aldershot: Avebury. An up-to-date, edited collection of advanced chapters of relevance to the topics covered in this chapter written by European researchers. See especially Conner and Norman's chapter comparing the HBM and the TPB in health screening, Hoorens on unrealistic optimism and Sparks on issues surrounding the use of the TPB in the area of food choice.

Rutter, D.R., Quine, L. and Chesham, D.J. (1993) *Social Psychological Approaches to Health*. Hemel Hempstead: Harvester Wheatsheaf. Reasonably up-to-date and affordable. Includes discussion of the TRA/TPB and the HBM as well as Rutter *et al.*,'s own model and a consideration of some of the broader issues.

Stainton Rogers, W. (1991) *Explaining Health and Illness*. Hemel Hempstead: Harvester Wheatsheaf. The social cognition approach represents the dominant 'mainstream' tradition of research in this area. Some researchers question the utility of this approach. This book provides an interesting and accessible introduction to the arguments against the social cognition approach and to some of the alternatives that are being pursued.

Taylor, S.E. (1989) *Positive Illusions*. New York: Basic Books. Unlike Weinstein, Taylor emphasizes the positive consequences of optimism and argues that creative self-deception is healthy.

References

Adler, N.E., Kegeles, S.M. and Genevro, J.L. (1992) 'Risk taking and health', in J.F. Yates (ed.) *Risk-taking Behavior*. Chichester: John Wiley.

Ajzen, I. (1985) 'From intentions to actions: a theory of planned behavior', in J. Kuhl and J. Beckman (eds.) *Action Control: From Cognition to Behavior*. Heidelberg: Springer.

Ajzen, I. (1988) *Attitudes, Personality and Behaviour*. Milton Keynes: Open University Press.

Ajzen, I. and Fishbein, M. (1977) 'Attitude–behavior relations: A theoretical analysis and review of empirical research', *Psychological Bulletin* **84**, 888–918.

Ajzen, I. and Fishbein, M. (1980) *Understanding Attitudes and Predicting Social Behavior.* Englewood Cliffs, NJ: Prentice Hall.

Bandura, A. (1989) 'Human agency in social cognitive theory', *American Psychologist* **44**, 1175–84.

Becker, H.M. (1974) *The Health Belief Model and Personal Health Behavior.* Thorofare, NJ: Slack.

Becker, M.H. and Maiman, L.A. (1975) 'Sociobehavioral determinants of compliance with health and medical care recommendations', *Medical Care* **13**, 10–24.

Breakwell, G.M., Fife-Schaw, C.R. and Clayden, K. (1991) 'Risk-taking, control over partner choice and intended use of condoms by virgins', *Journal of Community and Applied Social Psychology* **1**, 173–87.

Carver, C.S. and Scheier, M.F. (1981) *Attention and Self-regulation: A control-theory approach to human behavior.* New York: Springer.

Carver, C.S. and Scheier, M.F. (1982) 'Control theory: A useful conceptual framework for personality-social, clinical and health psychology', *Psychological Bulletin* **92**, 111–35.

Catania, J.A., Kegeles, S.M. and Coates, T.J. (1990) 'Towards an understanding of risk behavior: An AIDS risk reduction model (ARRM)', *Health Education Quarterly* **17**, 53–72.

Cleary, P.D. (1987) 'Why people take precautions against health risks', in N.D. Weinstein (ed.) *Taking Care: Understanding and encouraging self-protective behaviour.* Cambridge: Cambridge University Press.

Conner, M. (1992) 'Pros and cons of social cognition models in health psychology'. Paper given to the British Psychological Society, Health Psychology Section Conference, University of St Andrews, September.

Conner, M. and Norman, P. (in press) 'Comparing the health belief model and the theory of planned behaviour in health screening', in D.R. Rutter (ed.) *The Social Psychology of Health and Safety: European perspectives.* Aldershot: Avebury.

Crawford, R. (1987) 'Cultural influences on prevention and the emergence of a new health consciousness', in N.D. Weinstein (ed.) *Taking Care: Understanding and encouraging self-protective behaviour.* Cambridge: Cambridge University Press.

Davison, C., Smith, G.D. and Frankel, S. (1991) 'Lay epidemiology and the prevention paradox: The implications of coronary candidacy for health education', *Sociology of Health and Illness* **13**, 1–19.

Fisher, J.D. and Fisher, W.A. (1992) 'Changing AIDS risk behavior', *Psychological Bulletin* **111**, 454–74.

Fisher, J.D. and Fisher, W.A. (1993) 'A general social psychological model for changing AIDS risk behaviour', in J.B. Pryor and G.D. Reeder (eds.) *The Social Psychology of HIV Infection.* Hove: Lawrence Erlbaum.

Fiske, S.T. and Taylor, S.E. (1991) *Social Cognition.* New York: McGraw-Hill.

Gatchel, R.J., Baum, A. and Krantz, D.S. (1989) *An Introduction to Health Psychology*, 2nd edition. New York: Random House.

Gibbons, F.X., Gerrard, M., Lando, H.A. and McGovern, P.G. (1991) 'Social comparison and smoking cessation: The role of the "typical smoker" ', *Journal of Experimental Social Psychology* **27**, 239–58.

Gollwitzer, P.M. (1993) 'Goal achievement: The role of intentions', in W. Stroebe and M. Hewstone (eds.) *European Review of Social Psychology*, Vol. 4. Chichester: John Wiley.

Gollwitzer, P.M. and Kinney, R.F. (1989) 'Effects of deliberative and implemental mind-sets on illusion of control', *Journal of Personality and Social Psychology* **56**, 531–42.

Harris, P. and Middleton, W. (1994) 'The illusion of control and optimism about health: On being less at risk but no more in control than others', *British Journal of Social Psychology*, **33**, 319–86.

Hoorens, V. (1993) 'Self-enhancement and superiority biases in social comparison', in W. Stroebe and M. Hewstone (eds.) *European Review of Social Psychology*, Vol. 4. Chichester: John Wiley.

Hoorens, V. (in press) 'Unrealistic optimism in social comparison of health and safety risks', in D. Rutter (ed.) *The Social Psychology of Health and Safety*. Aldershot: Avebury.

Janz, N.K. and Becker, M.H. (1984) 'The Health Belief Model: A decade later', *Health Education Quarterly* **11**, 1–46.

Marsh, A. and Matheson, J. (1983) *Smoking Attitudes and Behaviour: An enquiry carried out on behalf of the Department of Health and Social Security*. London: HMSO.

McKenna, F.P., Warburton, D.M. and Winwood, M. (1993) 'Exploring the limits of optimism: The case of smokers' decision-making', *British Journal of Psychology* **84**, 389–94.

Prochaska, J.O. (1994) 'Strong and weak principles for progressing from precontemplation to action on the basis of twelve problem behaviors', *Health Psychology* **13**, 47–51.

Prochaska, J.O., DiClemente, C.C. and Norcross, J.C. (1992) 'In search of how people change: Applications to addictive behaviors', *American Psychologist* **47**, 1102–14.

Quattrone, G.A. and Tversky, A. (1986) 'Self-deception and the voter's illusion', in J. Elster (ed.) *The Multiple Self*. Cambridge: Cambridge University Press.

Regis, D. (1988) 'Conformity, consistency and control', *Education and Health*, March, 4–9.

Rippetoe, P.A. and Rogers, R.W. (1987) 'Effects of components of protection motivation theory on adaptive and maladaptive coping with a health threat', *Journal of Personality and Social Psychology* **52**, 596–604.

Rogers, R.W. (1975) 'A protection motivation theory of fear appeals and attitude change', *Journal of Psychology* **91**, 93–114.

Rogers, R.W. (1983) 'Cognitive and physiological processes in fear appeals and attitude change: A revised theory of protection motivation', in J.R. Cacioppo and R.E. Petty (eds.) *Social Psychophysiology: A sourcebook*. New York: Guilford Press.

Rogers, R.W. (1985) 'Attitude change and information integration in fear appeals', *Psychological Reports* **56**, 179–82.

Rosenstock, I.M. (1966) 'Why people use health services', *Milbank Memorial Fund Quarterly* **44**, 94.

Rosenstock, I.M. (1974) 'Historical origins of the health belief model', *Health Education Monographs* **2**, 328.

Rosenstock, I.M., Strecher, V.J. and Becker, M.H. (1988) 'Social learning theory and the health belief model', *Health Education Quarterly* **15**, 175–83.

Rutter, D.R., Quine, L. and Chesham, D.J. (1993) *Social Psychological Approaches to Health*. Hemel Hempstead: Harvester Wheatsheaf.

Schwarzer, R. (1992a) 'Self-efficacy in the adoption and maintenance of health behaviors: Theoretical approaches and a new model', in R. Schwarzer (ed.) *Self-efficacy: Thought control of action*. Washington: Hemisphere.

Schwarzer, R. (ed.) (1992b) *Self-efficacy: Thought control of action*. Washington: Hemisphere.

Taylor, S.E. and Brown, J. (1988) 'Illusion and well-being: Some social psychological contributions to a theory of mental health', *Psychological Bulletin* **103**, 193–210.

Taylor, S.E. (1989) *Positive Illusions*. New York: Basic Books.

van der Pligt, J., Otten, W., Richard, R. and van der Velde, F. (1992) 'Perceived risk of AIDS: Unrealistic optimism and self-protective action', in J.B. Pryor and G. Reeder (eds.) *The Social Psychology of HIV Infection*. Hillsdale, NJ: Lawrence Erlbaum.

Weinstein, N.D. (1980) 'Unrealistic optimism about future life events', *Journal of Personality and Social Psychology* **39**, 806–20.

Weinstein, N.D. (1987) 'Introduction: studying self-protective behaviour', in N.D. Weinstein (ed.) *Taking Care: Understanding and encouraging self-protective behaviour*. Cambridge: Cambridge University Press.

Weinstein, N.D. (1988) 'The precaution adoption process', *Health Psychology* **7**, 355–86.

Weinstein, N.D. (1989) 'Optimistic biases about personal risks', *Science* **246**, 1232–3.

Weinstein, N.D. and Sandman, P.M. (1992) 'A model of the precaution adoption process: Evidence from home radon testing', *Health Psychology* **11**, 170–80.

Psychological concepts applied to health care professionals

Psychological concepts that have particular relevance to today's health care professionals are considered in Part II. Some of these topics are part of mainstream psychology (e.g. personality and memory); some do not yet have this status but are included because of their relevance and because they exhibit important aspects of the work of psychologists (e.g. error, psychopharmacology and brain damage).

We start with a consideration of personality, a topic that non-psychologists often consider to be central to psychology. Chapter 7 first describes the methods used to identify and assess personality. Such knowledge is extremely useful in understanding the limitations and benefits of using personality tests. The chapter then considers the issue of personality in relation to three important domains for health professionals: patients and clients; health professionals themselves; and managers of health professionals.

Some of the earliest studies in psychology were concerned with memory. Chapter 8 provides an up-to-date examination of this topic by identifying the processes involved in remembering different types of material. A central finding is that memory processes should no longer be seen as separate cognitive operations isolated from the rest of a person's experience, thoughts and knowledge; rather, a person's memory is influenced by and in turn influences these other processes. Because memory is central to so many aspects of everyday living, it is clearly important for an understanding of the way that people function.

We all make errors, but errors made by health professionals can have fatal consequences. Chapter 9 examines those issues that should be considered in relation to such problems. We all fall into the habit of blaming an individual when something goes wrong. But the key point made in this chapter is the need to examine error from a wider perspective. Systems theory points to the benefits of taking a broader perspective to the understanding and prevention of error.

In a number of areas psychology has ill-defined boundaries with other disciplines. One of these is psychopharmacology; Chapter 10 considers the effects of drugs. Because some nurses are now assuming responsibility for prescribing drugs, this chapter is particularly timely. The chapter also provides a useful perspective on the biological basis of behaviour and the way that some drugs are responsible for health problems, while others are a vital tool in the treatment of psychological conditions. Understanding the way that drugs can affect psychological processes is fundamental to many aspects of health care.

The brain is the centre of psychological processes. However, much still remains to be discovered about its operation and the mechanisms that cause impairments. The final chapter in Part II provides an introduction to the structure and function of the brain. This leads on to a consideration of the causes, consequences and treatment of brain damage. The chapter shows the way that physiological damage can result in a number of disabilities affecting psychological functioning.

The chapters in Part II cover a diverse range of topics. The connecting thread running through all of them is that the understanding of a particular area of psychology has relevance to the issues facing health professionals. It also emerges that the study of health-related issues feeds back into psychology so that a better understanding of the psychological process under consideration is achieved.

CHAPTER 7

Personality

JOHN GOSLING

Chapter outline

Introduction

The purpose of this chapter is to examine the ways in which the study of personality can be relevant to nursing. It is assumed that an understanding of personality can provide the nurse with important guidelines regarding how best to understand an individual patient's illness and how best to care for each patient as an individual. Furthermore, the study of personality can provide insight into how each individual nurse approaches his or her role in caring for the patient.

We begin with an example of why personality is relevant to nursing and then discuss the meaning of the term personality. This is followed by a brief discussion of theories of personality and of the means by which psychologists have attempted to assess the personality of individuals. The next section examines in detail ways in which research has demonstrated links between the personality of the patient and the origin and course of his or her illness. It is argued that certain personality attributes have been linked to specific kinds of illness. The chapter ends by considering the personality of the nurse, first, in terms of how particular attributes may be of relevance to patient care; and second, in terms of how personality is important to the management skills of senior nurses.

| BOX 7.1   **THE RELEVANCE OF PERSONALITY TO NURSING** |

David Jones and Gary Smith were both admitted on the same day to Lister Ward at St Miriam's Hospital for a period of observation following complaints of irregular heart beats. Staff Nurse Sue Peters was on duty during the morning of their admission and Staff Nurse Jane Thompson took over later that afternoon. David was very worried about what might be wrong with him and asked his wife to stay with him for as long as she could. Gary, on the other hand, seemed quite calm. His view was that it was probably nothing serious, and even if it were, he knew he was in good hands at St Miriam's. Sue had noticed immediately that David was rather anxious. As soon as he was settled in, she spent a little time with him explaining about the tests he was to have and doing her best to reassure him. She could see that Gary was fine and so did not feel that he needed any special attention. Throughout the shift, she kept an eye on David to make sure he was all right and, when handing over to Jane in the afternoon, pointed out that she might need to have a word with him from time to time. Jane, however, took the view that her job, and that of the hospital, was to tend for the patients' physical needs rather than their emotional needs and so did not follow Sue's recommendation.

Sue was glad to get off shift. The pressures of work had been mounting over the previous six months. She had felt an increasing sense of being emotionally exhausted and was beginning to find it difficult to maintain her feelings of commitment to the job, despite her real love of nursing. But because of her caring nature, she still gave her utmost to each of her patients and her concern about David was a good illustration of this. In contrast, Jane was coping very well with the job. She had always been tough by nature, able to brush problems aside and always able to get through on her own resources. Despite the fact that she had experienced the same pressures as Sue over the past few months, she was coping far better.

By 11.00 pm David was obviously in a state of distress. His pulse was 115 and his blood pressure had risen significantly from the reading taken at admission to hospital and had remained high. After consulting her nursing colleagues Jane telephoned the duty registrar to come and have a look at him.

As it turned out, David's condition that evening was largely due to his anxiety about the forthcoming tests and he had been in no immediate danger. Nevertheless, coronary heart disease was confirmed several days later and, after leaving the hospital, he was placed on a medication regime and given advice about diet and exercise. The psychologist attached to David's GP saw him a week later and reached the conclusion that he had been suffering from severe job-related stress. She also discovered that he had a tendency towards bouts of anxiety since childhood. Several months later, following deterioration in his condition, David was admitted for surgery. It was felt by the psychologist that his recovery from surgery might be inhibited to some extent by his generally high level of anxiety.

In contrast, Gary was diagnosed as suffering from a relatively minor occurrence of Da Costa's syndrome and was advised to stop smoking and limit his caffeine intake. It was not felt that any further treatment was necessary, but he was advised to return to his GP if the symptoms recurred.

The concept of personality

Why study personality?

Box 7.1 clearly demonstrates that the personal characteristics of the patient and of the nurse can have a significant role in the patient's illness as well as in his or her response to treatment. In Box 7.1, David and Gary are very different – David's history of anxiety and his inability to cope with stress have probably contributed significantly to the onset of his illness. What is more, these personality characteristics seriously affect his experience of hospitalization and may also influence the outcome of his planned surgery.

The personality of the nurse is also significant. Sue's sensitivity was especially important in helping her see that David needed special attention when he was admitted. However, she seems more vulnerable to the stress of the job than Jane. Jane's resilience seems to have given her extra resources and now she is coping far better with the pressures than Sue.

It is clear that a study of personality can help the nurse to increase her understanding both of the nature of illness and also of a patient's response to treatment. Furthermore, the study of personality can help her learn more about her natural approach to caring for her patients and make her more able to cope with a highly demanding professional job. This chapter will look at these issues in more depth, focusing in particular on:

- The evidence for the proposition that personality can significantly influence the course of illness.
- The ways in which the nurse's personality can influence her approach to patient care.
- The ways in which concepts drawn from personality can guide the nurse in her self-development.

First, though, we shall examine the concept of personality itself in more depth.

DISCUSSION POINT
Re-read Box 7.1. Which personality traits do you think are associated with being a good nurse? Do you think it is possible for health professionals to care for the emotional and physical needs of patients without being at risk of emotional exhaustion? If so, how can this be achieved?

What is personality?

The term personality refers to those patterns of behaviour, feelings and attitudes a person has that are relatively enduring and relatively predictable in a given situation. At its most general and most simple, the term refers to the ways in which individuals differ; indeed, the study of personality has been subsumed by psychologists under the more general field known as 'individual differences'.

Perhaps the most important word in the definition of personality is 'predictable'. It is assumed that some property of a person's internal state or internal functioning has an effect on how that person behaves such that the person will, to some degree, behave predictably when faced with a particular set of circumstances. The underlying assumption is that the person's present internal state is determined in one way or another by his or her past history, where the term 'history' may include that person's genetic history. This assumption allows that personality may either be genetically determined or may have arisen as a consequence of the person's interaction throughout life with his or her physical and social environment. Although the issue of which of these two influences is the stronger has exercised the minds of psychologists in the past, it is of rather less relevance for the purpose of applying knowledge about personality to practical human situations. In principle, if we know that an individual's behaviour is predictable, then we can put that predictability to good use.

It must be emphasized though that to say that a person's behaviour is predictable is not to say that any one person will behave consistently in every situation. A person who behaves spontaneously and uninhibitedly in one situation may well behave in just the opposite way in another. What may, however, be true is that the person's behaviour will show consistency across situations of any given type. This idea is referred to in terms of the *interaction between person and situation*. Thus, it has been argued that how a person behaves in a given situation will to some extent be determined both by enduring traits of personality which are influential across a wide range of situations and by specific features of each and every situation (Anastasi, 1988; Lanyon and Goodstein, 1982 (in Further Reading)). For example, if I am generally self-confident, then on balance I should be self-confident in the majority of situations. However, if I have had some unpleasant experiences in the past when talking about work with my boss, this might be one situation in which I would be less self-confident than most people would be in a similar situation.

To be able to make predictions about a person's behaviour, one needs to know about that person's general behavioural tendencies across all situations (traits) and then add to that specific knowledge about how he or she has previously behaved in the sorts of situation in which we are interested. Information within the former category is normally obtained by use of a personality questionnaire (see below). Information of the latter category is rather more difficult to obtain and would normally be gained only by direct observation of, or in interview with, the person.

Illustrative theoretical approaches to the description of personality

Since the beginning of the twentieth century, many different approaches to the theoretical description of personality have been proposed. In this section, we shall briefly summarize three of the better known.

The Behavioural Approach
The behavioural approach to personality is based on the pioneering work of the learning theorists of the early and middle part of the twentieth century (See Box

---

BOX 7.2 **THE BEHAVIOURAL APPROACH TO PERSONALITY**

Pavlov's work on classical conditioning (Pavlov, 1927) established that specific responses of the autonomic nervous system (largely involuntary) could become associated with specific, normally neutral, environmental stimuli. This occurs by a process of pairing of those stimuli with other stimuli which have either pleasurable or noxious properties. For instance, if on a number of occasions a bell was sounded immediately before food was presented to an animal (food being a stimulus which would normally produce the autonomic nervous system response of salivation), then eventually the sound of the bell alone would also come to produce salivation. This idea was then applied to the development of human behaviour by Watson and Raynor who demonstrated how a phobia of white, furry objects could be conditioned in a young child by the pairing of such objects with an aversive stimulus such as a loud noise (Watson and Raynor, 1920). Skinner's later work on instrumental conditioning (1938) demonstrated that the likelihood of occurence of specific *voluntary* behavioural responses could be increased by arranging for those responses to be followed either by pleasurable (reinforcing) or aversive (punishing) stimuli.

7.2). It was presumed that the occurrence of almost all human behaviours, with the exception of the most instinctive ones, could be explained by one or other conditioning process. Personality to the behaviourist, therefore, was interpreted as the consequence of the sum total of a person's conditioning experiences, and this point of view minimized the importance both of inherited personality traits and the notion that personality would show consistency across situations of different types. Among the most prominent writers in this tradition in more recent times are Dollard and Miller (1950), Skinner (1971), Bandura (1977) and Mischel (1973).

The Personal Construct Approach

George Kelly (1955) believed that differences between people could be explained largely in terms of differences in the way each individual perceives (or 'construes') his or her world. According to Kelly, we each make use of a set of personal dimensions or 'constructs' which we apply in our perception of the world and which serve as a basis for evaluating, categorizing and distinguishing between things we deal with in our world. Thus, for one individual, the construct *KIND–UNKIND* might be of primary importance in evaluating, categorizing and distinguishing between people. To another person, the construct *INFLUENTIAL–NOT INFLUEN-TIAL* may be of primary importance.

Kelly argued that each individual uses his or her construct system to anticipate and make predictions about events in the world. That this is possible is largely because of the complex network of interrelationships among an individual's personal set of constructs. Thus, for the first person, the construct *KIND–UNKIND* may be inversely related to the construct *STRONG–WEAK*: i.e. to be kind implies also to be weak. In the framework of Kelly's theory, such a person might therefore have difficulties in showing kindness to others since in doing so he must inevitably perceive himself also as being weak. Thus, 'personality' was understood by Kelly to refer ultimately to the differences between individuals' construct systems. To the extent that each individual construes the world differently and to the extent that there are differences between individuals in the relationships among their constructs, then there will be differences between people, both in how they experience the world and in how they behave.

The Factor Analytic Approach

The factor analytic approach to personality is typified by the work of Raymond Cattell (e.g. Cattell, 1965). Cattell's approach was essentially atheoretical. He did not wish to be guided by preconceptions about the structure of personality, nor by pre-existing ideas about what specific concepts or dimensions might be most useful in describing differences between people. Rather, his strategy was to investigate the natural structuring of human behaviours by applying a mathematical technique, factor analysis, to the study of the interrelationships between personality concepts as used by his research subjects.

Put simply, this technique involves collecting data from questionnaires and ratings scales and finding the correlations (see Box 7.3) between each individual item. Thus, it might be found, for instance, that a correlation exists between ratings on a questionnaire item about whether a person likes going to parties and a further item which asks about whether she has many friends. If a group of such items is discovered in which each item correlates with every other item in the set, then it may be inferred that there is likely to be some underlying reason for these correlations.

It might, for instance, be proposed that some underlying dimension of personality exists, let us call it property X, such that if a person has a lot of property X, then he

---

BOX 7.3 **CORRELATION**

To say that two things are correlated means that there is a relationship between them, such that a change in one is reliably associated with a change in the other. For example, we would normally expect the height and the weight of a sample of men to be correlated. To some extent, taller men will weigh more than shorter men. However, this is not a perfect relationship. Height and weight are not perfectly correlated. Short, heavy men and tall, light men, for instance, would be considered as exceptions to the general rule. A rather stronger correlation might be expected to hold between the speed at which a pump rotates and the amount of water delivered per second. If the speed of the pump is doubled, then we would expect the rate of water delivery to increase by a more or less proportionate amount. And if we found that there was a *perfect* relationship between these two variables, then we would say that there was a *perfect correlation* between them.

In just the same way, we might apply the concept of correlation to the relationships between people's responses to individual items from a questionnaire. If two items are correlated, we would expect that if a person gives a positive response to one of the items, then there will be an increased possibility of them giving a positive response to the second.

or she will tend to score high on each item in the set. If the person has relatively little of property X, then he or she will tend to score low on each item in the set. The mathematical technique of factor analysis essentially deals with only the first part of this process: namely, the identification of clusters of items which might reflect underlying dimensions. The subsequent process of identifying precisely what these underlying dimensions might be is a rather more subjective affair, which depends very much on the intuition and insight of the factor analyst. Over several decades of research, Cattell and his colleagues have identified what they believe are sixteen fundamental dimensions of personality (see p. 141) which they believe are sufficient to provide an efficient and effective general description of the range of human behaviour.

How is personality assessed?

In order to understand further how psychologists have theorized about personality, it helps to know a little about the ways in which personality is assessed. The most common means of assessing personality is by a written questionnaire. Typically, a personality questionnaire will contain between 50 and 200 questions (items) refer- ring to the test taker's interests, attitudes, preferences and behaviour in specific situations. Most commonly, the questionnaire items will be in multiple-choice for- mat, in which a choice must be made from several possible response options. The following examples illustrate two common formats:

1. On a Saturday evening, I would rather:
   (a) go out for a meal with some friends,
   (b) uncertain,
   (c) stay at home with a good book.
2. I am known as a person who is practically minded:
   (a) strongly disagree,
   (b) disagree,
   (c) neither agree nor disagree,
   (d) agree,
   (e) strongly agree.

The test taker indicates the appropriate responses on a standard answer sheet. Responses to individual items are usually summed to produce scores on several subscales representing different dimensions of personality. These 'raw scores' are then compared with scores obtained by representative groups from the population and are thus transformed into 'standardized scores' which indicate the extent to which the test taker falls above or below the mean (average) score for the com- parison group on each personality dimension assessed by the test.

Not all forms of personality assessment use standardized scoring systems as in the above example. So-called 'projective tests' require the test taker to give his or her interpretation of an ambiguous stimulus such as an inkblot, e.g. the Rorschach

BOX 7.4   **RELIABILITY AND VALIDITY**

The advantage of standardization in both questionnaire format and scoring procedure is that the reliability of the assessment is thereby increased. Reliability in this context essentially refers to the ability of a test to produce consistent results from one occasion to another. The advantage of standardization is that this will help to eliminate as far as possible errors due to variations in administration or interpretation of specific responses. Nevertheless, reliability of personality questionnaires will still often remain a long way short of perfect. This is largely due to the difficulty of finding unambiguous and simply interpretable items that uniformly measure the personality dimensions of interest.

Reliability of assessment, however, does not of itself guarantee that the test will measure what it is supposed to measure (i.e. that inferences drawn on the basis of the person's responses will be *valid*). Reasonably good levels of both reliability and validity *can* be achieved if sufficient care is devoted to the development of the questionnaire. However, the results of a personality assessment should still always be treated with caution and should be seen only as a general indication which must be confirmed by other means wherever possible.

(Aronow and Reznikoff, 1976), or a picture, e.g. the Thematic Apperception Test (Murray, 1938). The scoring of the person's responses is not a straightforward matter in these tests, relying as it does on the test administrator's subjective interpretations and also usually dependent on the assumptions of the underlying theoretical models of personality. The usefulness of such tests will therefore depend greatly upon the experience and skill of the test administrator and inevitably will be limited by the relatively low reliability (see Box 7.4) across different administrators.

Questionnaires and projective methods are not, however, the only means by which personality may be assessed. More or less any means by which information can be gained about a person's typical behaviour in specific situations could, in principle, serve as a measure of personality. To illustrate, a variety of assessment methods are currently used to assess personality-like dimensions in the context of personnel selection. These include role-play assessments, team-work exercises, problem-solving exercises and, of course, the interview. The usefulness of these methods will depend ultimately on the objectivity of the method (usually a matter of how standardized are the assessment procedure, the recording of observations and the means by which interpretations are made) and the validity of the inferences that are drawn (a question largely of the extent to which generalizations can be made from the behaviour recorded in the assessment situation to real-life situations).

Illustrative personality questionnaires

Two of the most widely used personality questionnaires in the United Kingdom are the Sixteen Personality Factor Questionnaire (16PF) (Cattell, Eber and Tatsuoka,

Table 7.1   *Dimensions of the Sixteen Personality Factor Questionnaire*

Thinking Style

I	TOUGH-MINDED	TENDER-MINDED
	Realistic, down-to-earth, takes a realistic approach, objective.	Intuitive, less realistic and objective, depends more on insight and feeling.
M	EXTERNALLY ORIENTED	INTERNALLY ORIENTED
	Oriented to external realities, prefers doing rather than thinking, focused on the here-and-now.	Focused on internal thoughts and feelings, less oriented to external realities, tends to be imaginative and creative.
N	NOT SOCIALLY ANALYTICAL	SOCIALLY ANALYTICAL (SHREWD)
	Straightforward in his/her approach, takes a 'natural' approach to people, not concerned to analyze what's going on in a situation.	Socially aware and astute, likes to understand what's going on in a situation, likes to 'handle' situations and people.
Q1	CONVENTIONAL	INNOVATIVE
	Prefers the tried-and-tested. Prefers not to experiment with new methods.	Likes to innovate. Enjoys solving problems. Easily bored by routine tasks.

Social Interaction

A	RESERVED	OUTGOING, SOCIABLE
	Reserved when with others. Tends to be more interested in facts than in relationships. Enjoys working alone.	Oriented towards people and relationships. Interested in people's feelings. Values relationships.
E	UNASSERTIVE	ASSERTIVE
	Does not find it easy to be assertive. Finds it difficult to stand up for his/her own point of view.	Assertive. Sticks up for his/her own point of view. Can be forceful and persuasive.
H	SHY	SOCIALLY CONFIDENT
	Is often anxious in the company of others. May find it difficult to mix. Does not enjoy being the centre of attention or having to perform in public.	Confident when with other people. Does not mind being the centre of attention. Is not worried about performing in public.
L	TRUSTING	CAUTIOUS OF OTHERS
	Trusts other people. Does not doubt their motives. Does not suspect others or their intentions.	Tends to be suspicious of other people's motives. Does not trust people easily.

Q2	DEPENDENT	SELF-SUFFICIENT
	Enjoys working with groups. Prefers group decisions to his/her own. Likes to know what others think before taking a decision.	Enjoys working alone. Prefers own decisions to those of the group. Enjoys taking responsibility.

Emotions

C	AFFECTED BY FEELINGS	NOT AFFECTED BY FEELINGS
	Can be affected by his/her feelings. Can feel upset when things aren't going well. Finds it hard to keep emotions under control.	Manages to suppress emotions where necessary. Tries to see that feelings don't interfere with his/her judgements or actions.

O	SELF-CONFIDENT	LACKING IN SELF-CONFIDENCE
	Has strong sense of belief in him/herself. Has high self-regard. Not worried by doubts about self or his/her worth in front of other people.	Lacks self-confidence. Does not have high self-regard. May doubt his/her worth and/or abilities.

Q4	CALM AND RELAXED	ENERGETIC, DRIVEN OR TENSE
	Takes life casually and easily. Tends to be 'laid back'. Approaches situations calmly. Does not expend energy unnecessarily.	Restless and tense in many situations. May have high activity level. Works best in high-activity environments.

Controls

F	CAUTIOUS IN ACTING AND THINKING	QUICK TO ACT AND THINK
	Tends to think before acting. Slow in reaching decisions. Prefers to be cautious and not take risks.	Makes decisions quickly. Thinks and acts with spontaneity. Responds to situations enthusiastically.

G	UNCONCERNED WITH DUTY AND OBLIGATION	CONCERNED WITH DUTY AND OBLIGATION
	Is not greatly concerned about rules and regulations. Does not feel particularly strong regard for or ties to the establishment. Does not have a strong sense of 'duty'.	Has a strong sense of duty. Has a regard for authority. Thinks it is important to do what is expected of him/her.

Q3	CASUAL	SELF-DISCIPLINED
	Does not find it easy to respond to demands imposed by self and others. Does not develop sense of self-discipline easily. May find it difficult to meet standards set by others.	Does what is required of him/her. Imposes sense of discipline on his/her life and actions. Careful about standards of behaviour and appearance. Tries to do things well.

1988) and the Myers–Briggs Type Indicator (MBTI) (Myers, 1987). The 16PF contains some 200 questions and produces scores on sixteen personality dimensions, including a rough-and-ready (and so not absolute) assessment of the person's intelligence level. The sixteen dimensions are given in Table 7.1.

The MBTI provides scores on only four dimensions (see Table 7.2). Note that the MBTI dimensions are rather different in nature from the 16PF dimensions. The philosophy underlying the MBTI is that each of the four dimensions represents a *preference* for one mode of functioning rather than another (Myers, 1987; Myers and Myers, 1980) . Thus to describe a person as a *sensing type* (i.e. one whose score lies to the left of the SENSING–INTUITION dimension) is to say that that person prefers operating in the sensing mode, even though at times and according to

Table 7.2 *Dimensions of the Myers–Briggs personality indicator*

E–I	EXTRAVERT	INTROVERT
	Externally oriented. Attention directed towards the outside world of people and things. Enjoys relating to people. Likes to keep active and enjoys doing rather than thinking.	Internally oriented. Interested in the inner world of thoughts and ideas. Happy with own company. Enjoys thinking about things more than doing them. Can get absorbed with ideas.
S–N	SENSING	INTUITION
	Depends on information that can be apprehended by the senses. Accurate with and has good memory for facts and figures. Likes the tried and tested. Prefers conventional ways of doing things. Looks for evidence to back up assertions. Tends not to be interested in creativity.	Likes to read between the lines. Does not depend only upon raw sensory information. Concerned with possibilities and with what could be rather than what is. Tends to be creative and possibly radical. Less good with facts and figures.
T–F	THINKING	FEELING
	Decisions are based on reason and logic. Tends to be analytical. Tries not to let subjective feelings get in the way of reasoned judgement. Tends not to act on gut reactions.	Decisions based on feeling and gut reaction. Tends to be less interested in the logical and analytical. Concerned about and sensitive to the feelings of other people.
H–P	JUDGING	PERCEPTION
	Prefers to plan and to be well organized. Monitors progress towards goals and aims for task completion. Likes to anticipate contingencies and plan for emergencies. Does not like to have to change plans.	Prefers not to organize and plan. Prefers to leave decisions until they are necessary. Likes to act spontaneously. Good at dealing with unplanned contingencies and emergency situations.

circumstance, he or she may feel it both appropriate and possible to adopt the alternative, *intuitive* mode of functioning.

It is also central to the philosophy of the MBTI that individuals' preferences are not static. Through a process of self-development, one may learn to develop the characteristics of one's non-preferred mode of functioning on each dimension and so expand the possibilities of one's personality (see Myers and McCauley, 1985). Also central to the philosophy underlying the MBTI is that in most work situations people from both sides of each dimension are needed. Thus, every team needs *judging* types to organize and plan and to see that tasks get completed, as well as *perceiving* types, who are able to adapt to changing circumstances and react to emergencies. Precisely the same principles will apply to each of the other three MBTI dimensions. The way in which these principles have been applied in self-development programmes and in team-building at work will be discussed at the end of this chapter.

DISCUSSION POINT

Taking the four dimensions of the Myers–Briggs Type Indicator, how might each side of the four dimensions be valuable to patient care?

Personality and the patient

Let us now turn to the question of how an understanding of personality can be applied to nursing practice. The first issue is how the personality of the patient can influence the development and course of his or her illness.

There is a growing body of evidence that the personality characteristics of the patient have at least a modifying, if not a causal, effect on illness. One difficulty in interpreting much of this work is that it is not always clear whether to interpret the current state of the person in terms of the individual's 'personality' or in terms of relatively transitory mental states resulting from emotional or psychiatric disorders. Nevertheless, it does seem to be clear that disturbed emotional functioning for whatever reason can influence the development of illness. Rutter *et al.* (1993), for instance, conclude that both depression and anxiety show significant general associations with both increased morbidity and increased mortality when all kinds of illness are taken into consideration.

One area in which this connection has been well researched is that of coronary heart disease (CHD). Booth-Kewley and Friedman (1987: 358) conclude in relation to CHD patients that 'the true picture seems to be one of a person with one or more negative emotions: perhaps someone who is depressed, aggressively competitive, easily frustrated, anxious, angry or some combination' (see also Friedman and Booth-Kewley, 1988; Mathews, 1988; Smith, Follick and Korr, 1984; Chapter 15, this volume). In the field of gastroenterology too, there is evidence of the involvement of personality factors. Bennett (1989) has reviewed evidence which indicates an association between irritable bowel syndrome and the personality traits of anxiety, depression and hypochondriasis, and between peptic ulcer disease and the traits of anxiety, emotional instability, hypochondriasis and low assertiveness.

Almost by definition, one would expect that psychosomatic disorders (i.e. physical disorders thought to be of psychogenic origin) would be associated with individual differences in psychological functioning. Indeed, there has long been a number of clinically-based accounts of the typical psychosomatic patient. Gildea (1949), for instance, describes psychosomatic patients as lacking in assertiveness, possessing obsessive compulsive traits, finding difficulty in becoming aware of bodily feelings and being less able to express emotion. These traits may not be restricted to patients suffering from psychosomatic disorders, however, since Smith (1983) found ·them equally typical of patients suffering from a variety of other conditions.

A fundamental question in all this work is whether the personality factors involved *cause* the illness or *are consequences of* the illness. Establishing the direction of the causality is not easy, although some authors have attempted to set out a chain of causal events. Rutter *et al.* (1993) have reviewed evidence of the effects of personality variables and emotional state on the outcome of pregnancy. They see these as interacting with life experiences to determine the woman's 'coping style' (see Chapter 15, this volume) in response to pregnancy. They conclude that:

> Life events and lack of support lead in turn to emotional problems, including lowered self-esteem, stress, anxiety and depression while poor education and lack of access to information produce a corresponding range of cognitive problems, including a lack of knowledge and a set of beliefs and attitudes that lead the woman to see herself as vulnerable to illness and complications but helpless to prevent them. . . . The emotional and cognitive effects combine, we argue, to produce a set of coping styles and strategies that are characterised by hopelessness and a willingness to take potentially serious risks. From there, it is a short step to inappropriate behaviours and thence to negative outcomes. (Rutter *et al.*, 1993: 101–2).

In their study, Rutter *et al.* showed that depression, low self-confidence, a sense of being unable to cope with life, feeling worried and being subject to variations of mood were all significantly related to 'satisfaction with the birth experience'.

Coping style also appears to be of relevance at a more fundamental physiological level. For instance, Greer, Morris and Peetingale (1979) found that recurrence-free survival after surgery for early breast cancer was more common in patients who had previously reacted with either 'denial' or 'fighting spirit' (75 per cent of subjects alive and well after five years) rather than with 'stoic acceptance' or 'helplessness' (35 per cent of subjects alive and well after five years). This suggests the possibility of a connection between coping style and the immune system; evidence for this possibility has been discussed by Marteau (1989) and Harvey (1989). Further connections between personality and immune system functioning have also been established by Kiecolt-Glaser *et al.* (1985), who demonstrated that high scores on the Depression scale of the Minnesota Multiphasic Personality Inventory were associated with worse DNA repair after X-ray irradiation.

DISCUSSION POINT

How might a nurse intervene to help a patient whose coping styles are maladaptive?

Related to coping is the concept of hope. Grimm (1991) considers hope as a personal attribute which has both 'state' properties (i.e. it can be a relatively transient phenomenon) and 'trait' properties (i.e. it can also be a relatively enduring phenomenon). This is how Grimm defines hope:

> Hope implies a future orientation. The difficult present is made tolerable through the anticipation of what is to come. To hope is to have expectations of the future, and the expectations have the possibility of being met. Hope implies the setting of future goals in order to enhance the meeting of one's expectations. To hope is to take action to achieve these goals. Hope is an interpersonal process. It is created through trust and is nurtured by trusting relationships with others, including God. (Grimm, 1991: 510)

Figure 7.1 illustrates Grimm's model of the relationship between hope as a trait and mechanisms of appraisal and coping. First, a person's appraisal of illness is influenced by the trait aspect of hoping. The appraisal itself then influences the current state of hope in relation to the current illness. This in turn influences the coping strategies employed to deal with the illness. In one of Grimm's studies investigating cancer patients, she found that the more hopeful the patients, the more positive their affect and the less psychological distress they experienced as a consequence of their illness (Grimm, 1991).

Not unrelated to hope is the concept of hardiness. Kobasa (1979) proposed that people who (1) view life as a challenge, (2) feel committed to and involved with their lives, their work, other people and themselves, and (3) feel a sense of personal control over their lives will remain healthier than people who lack these characteristics. The reasoning behind this proposition was that these characteristics lead to the use of more effective coping strategies when the individual is confronted by

Figure 7.1 *Grimm's model of the relationship between hope and appraisal (from Grimm, 1991)*

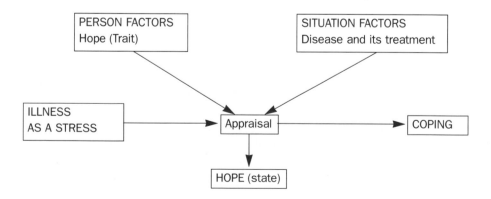

illness. The three characteristics were jointly conceived of under the label of 'hardiness'. Among other findings, Kobasa and her colleagues have shown that male executives who scored high on hardiness reported significantly fewer illnesses over the prior five years than those low on hardiness, thus demonstrating a further connection between personality and illness (Kobasa, Maddi and Courington, 1981).

It would seem, therefore, that the personality of the patient is clearly involved in the development and course of the patient's illness, although the causal relationship between symptomatology and psychological factors appears to be complex and may operate in both directions.

Personality and the nurse

Let us turn now to the nurse's personality. Lewis (1983) examined the personality of 964 British student nurses. The nurses differed from a comparison group of undergraduates in the following ways. First, female nurses showed higher scores on Factor F and lower scores on Factor Q1 of the 16PF. In other words, the female nurses appeared to be more spontaneous and quick to act, but less inventive and creative than the undergraduates. In contrast, the male nurses were more conscientious (Factor G) and less socially analytical and shrewd (Factor N) than the undergraduates.

DISCUSSION POINT
Why do you think that nurses differ from undergraduates? Can you think of explanations for the different findings for male and female nurses?

Other studies have investigated the relationship between 'burnout' in nurses and Kobasa's personality dimension of hardiness. The term 'burnout' refers to a severe stress reaction associated with work, evidenced by low morale, lack of energy and inability to respond to the demands of the job. Keane, Ducette and Adler (1985) found that hardiness in staff nurses in a large university hospital was significantly related to indices of burnout but, surprisingly, not to work location (i.e. intensive care versus general medical and social wards). Similarly, Topf (1989) found that high commitment – one of Kobasa's three dimensions of hardiness – was indicative of lower levels of burnout in a sample of intensive care nurses. These findings suggest that the personality of the nurse can be important in determining how well she or he will respond to the very demanding nature of the job (see also Chapters 1 and 16).

Lewis's study also looked at the personality differences between those nurses who completed their training and those who did not. The completers were found to be more socially confident, more self-confident and more group-oriented (Factors H, O and Q1) than the non-completers. This finding is useful in pointing to the dimensions which discriminate between good and poor performance at the job. The observed differences between completers and non-completers does not of itself tell us this, but it does suggest that the three characteristics of social confidence, self-confidence and group dependence may be necessary for a nurse to complete her initial years of training successfully. The relevance of these three characteristics should not be surprising. Nursing is not only about the application of procedures. It is also about caring for people. Furthermore, it is about being able to relate effectively as a professional to other professionals in a caring environment. Nurses must have the skills to relate to their patients with understanding and sensitivity. They must be perceptive to their patients' needs and must be able to express their understanding with warmth, compassion and human genuineness.

The importance of these three characteristics has long been recognized as central to all helping relationships (Rogers, 1961; Sundeen, 1991) and it seems that their importance is also recognized by those who train nurses. A study of UK nursing tutors' perceptions found that interpersonal qualities were rated as being more important that intellectual qualities when considering the suitability of applicants for both traditional and Project 2000 courses (Cater, 1993). For the traditional courses, tutors judged the most important characteristics required of the applicant to be (in order) 'good communication skills', 'being a good listener' and 'an ability to get on with people'. For the more academically-oriented Project 2000 courses, the three most important qualities (again in order) were 'good communication skills', 'an ability to get on with people' and 'an understanding of the [technical] rationale behind his/her work'.

Naturally, many nurses will enter the profession possessing these more social and human of skills in abundance. Indeed, it is probably because they do possess them that they are attracted to nursing in the first place. However, no matter how much social skill a nurse may possess on entry, there will always be room for improvement; indeed, it will be the nurse's responsibility as a professional to ensure that she does whatever is needed to maximize both the technical and human skills she applies in her work with her patients. For this reason, the concept of 'development' is central to the progression of nurses throughout their careers. Development means not only development of technical knowledge and skills but also development as a person; and it is here that the issue of personality is again of importance. Much attention has been given in recent times to the question of personal development (perhaps more so in commercial organizations than in the caring professions). And much of this effort has been guided by models of development informed by personality theory. The theory and philosophy underlying the MBTI referred to earlier has been a particular driving force. With its emphasis on the possibility of personal change and with its equal valuing of all personality types, it is especially relevant to the development of training programmes for both individuals and work teams in organisations (see Hirsh, 1987). So far, relatively little training of this sort has taken place in the nursing profession, but clearly this is an area ripe for expansion.

Personality and the nurse manager

Nurses are, of course, not only providers of care. Those who are successful in their profession soon take on additional responsibilities for the supervision and management of other staff. Especially relevant here is the concept of 'leadership' (see also Chapter 4).

Hersey and Duldt (1989) define leadership as a process of influencing the activities of an individual or a group in efforts toward goal achievement in a given situation. They argue that leadership is a style, where the term 'style' is defined as 'a pattern of behaviour that is consistent as perceived by others' (*ibid.*: 9) and is therefore equivalent in their view to the term personality. They refer to Hersey and Blanchard's definition of leadership style as 'the consistent behaviour patterns they [leaders] use when they are working with and through other people as perceived by those people' (Hersey and Blanchard, 1988: 146) and argue that leaders may differ in terms of their ability to employ four fundamental leadership styles ('telling', 'selling', 'participating' and 'delegating') and also in the degree to which leaders are able to change the style they use in accordance with the requirements of the situation. For instance, 'telling' (i.e. providing clear, specific directions) is appropriate only where the subordinate is both unable and unwilling to take personal responsibility for a task. In contrast, 'delegating' is for people who have greater ability and willingness in relation to the task in question. In relation to nursing:

> To become a leader in nursing requires a change of perspective: one must change from being responsible for clients having health problems and needing help to being responsible for people who are capable of caring for themselves and others as well . . . they are commissioned not only to continue indirectly taking care of an even larger number of clients than before, but also to oversee and manage the nursing staff who provide the nursing care. . . . Former ways of being successful now need to be replaced with new perspectives and behaviours. (Hersey and Duldt, 1989: 49)

Hersey and Duldt define the nurse leader in terms of several distinct roles:

- As a person with autonomy, in the sense of having higher levels of self-discipline, freedom and accountability in nursing practice.
- As a provider of expert nursing care.
- As a colleague, in relation with peers, both within nursing and from other health care professions.
- As a consultant who is able to provide specialist advice to other nurses and to professionals from other disciplines.
- As a scholar possessing specialist academic knowledge.
- As a person who is able to influence the quality of nursing care and its knowledge base through theory or research-based practice, teaching and administration.

In terms of tasks rather than roles, they propose that the nurse leader contributes at the technical level (clinical assessment, planning, implementation and evaluation of treatment), at the organizational level (e.g. in relation to nursing care, equipment usage and supplies, infection control, staff scheduling, etc.), at the educational level (orientation, education and development of nursing staff) and at the administrative level (recording of health care, committee membership, dealing with staff problems, and so on).

The implication of Hersey and Duldt's suggestions is that the personality of the nurse-manager will be critical to her/his success as a leader within the profession. Self-development and training will be obvious pathways the nurse may follow in order to develop the qualities necessary for a leadership role. However, the possibility of identifying those nurses who already possess these qualities at a high level should lead to an enhancement of the quality of nursing management and, as a consequence, to an enhancement of the quality of service provided by the profession as a whole. This brings us to the final consideration in this chapter: staff selection.

In recent years, considerable efforts have been placed on improving the quality of staff selection in the commercial and industrial sectors and also in some parts of the public sector. The rationale underlying this movement, expressed at its most simple, is that 'people are an organization's most valuable resource' (see also Chapter 1). Thus, if an organization invests only in its buildings, its equipment and its techniques and not in its people, then it is failing to maximise the value and usefulness of this most precious resource. The move has been to improve methods of selection in order to get the best people for the job, to develop methods of appraisal in order to identify the strengths and weakness of individual employees and to develop training systems to ensure that each individual is able to offer his or her very best to the organization within the limits of his or her potential.

Personality assessment has been of growing importance in the first of these stages. Instruments such as the 16PF and MBTI, along with more recent instruments such as the Occupational Personality Questionnaire, and the Rapid Personality Questionnaire have been used extensively both in the United Kingdom and the United States to attempt to improve the fit between person and job. The use of these instruments is normally preceded by a *job analysis*, which involves an analysis of the tasks involved in a given job and then the specification of the Knowledge, Skills, Abilities and Traits (KSATs) which are thought to be essential for good performance in the job. Along with other methods of assessment, such as structured interviews, exercises, role-play and group discussions, psychological tests of both ability and personality have been used to ensure as far as possible that the person selected is psychologically fitted to the job in question. In relation to personality tests alone, the validity of these instruments has now been clearly established in terms of their ability to predict future on-the-job performance.

So far, relatively little of this new approach to selection and assessment appears to have been taken up in the health professions and especially not in nursing (Cater, 1993, personal communication). However, it is clear that there is considerable potential for the use of such methods in both initial selection for nurse training and also for selection to higher positions within the profession. Clearly, the task of selection is one of the major responsibilities of senior nurse managers and it is to be hoped that they will soon see the value of an initiative in this field.

Summary

It should be apparent that the study of personality is of particular importance for nurses. Personality seems to be clearly implicated in a number of illnesses and an awareness of this can help nurses to adapt their own caring styles to the particular needs of each patient. Furthermore, the personality of nurses is relevant to how they as individuals approach the care of patients and how well they will respond to and cope with the demands of their work.

Seminar questions

1. Discuss from a practical point of view, the ways in which an understanding of personality can guide the nurse's approach to patient care.
2. Can an understanding of yourself and your own personality provide you with an insight into how you approach your work as a nurse?

Further reading

Ewen, R.B. (ed.) (1993) *An Introduction to Theories of Personality*, 4th edition. Hillsdale, NJ: Lawrence Erlbaum. An easy introduction to the topic which covers a wide range of theories of personality.

Lanyon, R.I. and Goodstein, L.D. (1982) *Personality Assessment*, 2nd edition. New York: John Wiley. A more thought-provoking discussion of 'personality' as a concept.

Nunnaly, J.C. (1978) *Psychometric Theory*, 2nd edition. New York: McGraw-Hill. For the technically-minded only.

Smith, M. and Robinson, I.T. (1993) *The Theory and Practice of Systematic Personnel Selection*, 2nd edition. Houndmills: Macmillan. A good general introduction to a variety of approaches used in modern-day personnel selection.

Schuler, H., Farr, J.L. and Smith, M. (1993) *Personnel Selection and Assessment: Individual and organizational perspectives*. Hillsdale, NJ.: Lawrence Erlbaum. Deals with some of the broader issues which arise in personnel selection.

References

Anastasi, A. (1988) *Psychological Testing*, 6th edition. New York: Macmillan.

Aronow, E. and Reznikoff, M. (1976) *Rorschach Content Interpretation*. Orlando, Fla.: Grune & Stratton.

Bandura, A. (1977) *A Social Learning Theory*. Englewood Cliffs, NJ: Prentice Hall.

Bennett, G. (1989) 'Gastroentecology', in A.K. Broon (ed.) *Health Psychology: Processes and Applications*. London: Chapman & Hall.

Booth-Kewley, S. and Friedman, H.S. (1987) 'Psychological predictors of heart disease: A quantitative review', *Psychological Bulletin* **101**, 343–62.

Cater, C. (1993) *An Exploratory Study of Student Nurse Selection.* Unpublished master's dissertation, University of Hertfordshire.

Cattell, R.B (1965) *The Scientific Analysis of Personality*. London: Penguin Books.

Cattell, R., Eber, H. and Tatsuoka, M. (1988) *Handbook for the 16PF*. Champaign, Ill.: Institute for Personality and Ability Testing.

Dollard, J. and Miller, N.E. (1950) *Personality and Psychotherapy: An analysis in terms of learning, thinking and culture*. New York: McGraw-Hill.

Friedman, H.S. and Booth-Kewley, S. (1988) 'Validity of the type A construct: A reprise', *Psychological Bulletin* **104**, 381–4.

Gildea, E.F. (1949) 'Special features of personality which are common to certain psychosomatic disorders', *Psychosomatic Medicine* **11**, 273–81.

Greer, S., Morris, T. and Peetingale, K.W. (1979) 'Psychological response to breast cancer: 'effect on outcome', *Lancet* **ii**, 785–7.

Grimm, P.M. (1991) 'Hope', in J.L. Creasia and B. Parker (eds.) *Conceptual Foundations of Professional Nursing Practice*. St Louis: Mosby Year Book.

Harvey, P. (1989) 'Stress and health', in A.K. Broom (ed.) *Health Psychology: Processes and applications*. London: Chapman & Hall.

Hersey, P. and Blanchard, K. (1988) *Management of Organizational Behavior: Utilizing human resources,* 5th edition. Englewood Cliffs, NJ: Prentice Hall.

Hersey, P. and Duldt, B.W. (1989) *Situational Leadership in Nursing*. Norwalk, Conn.: Appleton & Lange.

Hirsh, S.K. (1987) *Using the Myers-Briggs Type Indicator in Organizations: A resource book*. Palo Alto, Calif.: Consulting Psychologists Press.

Keane, A., Ducette, J. and Adler, D. (1985) 'Stress in ICU and non-ICU nurses', *Nursing Research* **34**, 231–6.

Kelly, G. (1955) *The Psychology of Personal Constructs*, Vols I and II. New York: W.W. Norton.

Kiecolt-Glaser, J.K., Stephens, R.E. Lipetz, P.D. *et al.* (1985) 'Distress and DNA repair in human lymphocytes', *Journal of Behavioural Medicine* **8**, 311–20.

Kobasa, S. (1979) 'Stressful life events, personality and health: An enquiry into hardiness', *Journal of Personality and Social Psychology* **37**, 1–11.

Kobasa, S., Maddi, S. and Courington, S. (1981) 'Personality and constitution as mediators in the stress–illness relationship', *Journal of Health and Social Behaviour* **22**, 368–78.

Lewis, B.R. (1983) 'Personality and intellectual characteristics of trainee nurses', in B.D. Davis (ed.) *Research into nurse education*. London: Croom Helm.

Marteau, T.M. (1989) 'Health beliefs and attributions', in A.K. Broom (ed.) *Health Psychology: Processes and applications*. London: Chapman & Hall.

Mathews, K.A. (1988) 'Coronary heart disease and type A behaviors; Update on and alternative to the Booth-Kewley and Friedman (1987) quantitative view', *Psychological Bulletin* **104**, 373–80.

Mischel, W. (1973) 'Toward a cognitive social-learning reconceptualization of personality', *Psychological Review* **80**, 252–83.

Murray, H.A (1938) *Explorations in Personality*. New York: Oxford University Press.

Myers, I.B. (1987) *Introduction to Type*, 4th edition. Palo Alto, Calif.: Consulting Psychologists Press.

Myers, I.B. and McCauley, M.H. (1985) *A Guide to the Development and use of the Myers-Briggs Type Indicator.* Palo Alto, Calif.: Consulting Psychologists Press.

Myers, I.B. with Myers, P.B. (1980) *Gifts Differing.* Palo Alto, Calif.: Consulting Psychologists Press.

Nunnaly, J.C. (1978) *Psychometric Theory*, 2nd edition. New York: McGraw-Hill.

Pavlov, I.P. (1927) *Conditioned Reflexes: An investigation of the physiological activity of the cerebral cortex.* New York: Oxford University Press.

Rogers, C.R. (1961) *On Becoming a Person.* Boston: Houghton Mifflin.

Rutter, D.R., Quine, L. and Chesham, D.J. (1993) *Social Psychological Approaches to Health.* Hemel Hempstead: Harvester Wheatsheaf.

Schuler, H., Farr, J.L. and Smith, M. (1993) *Personnel Selection and Assessment: Individual and organizational perspectives.* Hillsdale, NJ: Lawrence Erlbaum.

Skinner, B.F. (1938) *The Behavior of Organisms: An experimental analysis.* New York: Appleton-Century-Croft.

Skinner, B.F. (1971) *Beyond Freedom and Dignity.* New York: Knopf.

Smith, G.R. (1983) 'Alexithymia in medical patients referred to a consultation liaison service', *American Journal of Psychiatry* **140**, 99–101.

Smith, T.W., Follick, M.J. and Korr, K.S. (1984) 'Anger, neuroticism, type A behaviour and the experience of angina. *British Journal of Medical Psychology* **57**, 249–52.

Sundeen, S.J. (1991) Interpersonal communication, in J.L. Creasia and B. Parker (eds.) *Conceptual Foundations of Professional Nursing Practice.* St Louis: Mosby Year Book.

Tett, R.P. Jackson, D.N. and Rothstein, M. (1991) 'Personality measures as predictors of job performance: A meta-analytic review', *Personnel Psychology* **44**, 703–36.

Topf, M. (1989) 'Personality hardiness, occupational stress and burnout in critical care nurses', *Research in Nursing and Health* **12**, 179–86.

Watson, J.B. and Raynor, R. (1920) 'Conditioned emotional reactions', *Journal of Experimental Psychology* **3**, 1–14.

CHAPTER 8

Memory, information and meaning

NEVILLE AUSTIN

Chapter outline

Introduction

This chapter has two aims. The first is to explain a number of the distinctions about the contents of memory and the processes that give access to them which are key to understanding modern interpretations of its operations. The second is to illustrate these points with examples of research on phenomena which may be of particular interest to the reader and which display some of the methods for investigating memory. Readers who wish to pursue these and related matters in greater depth should consult the sources listed in the Further Reading at the end of the chapter.

Moment by moment, the senses are continually bombarded with stimulation. Certain of the sound waves reaching the ears become converted in the nervous system to experiences of words and meanings, light reaching the eye generates experiences of an external world of objects in space. Of all the input to our senses, and of all the internally generated activity of thought, very little appears to leave a permanent effect. Very little is remembered, at least in the sense that it can be recalled or can be shown to influence thought or action. It would be convenient if it could be concluded that the significance or personal importance of an experience was the crucial factor in whether it left a permanent record of its occurrence.

Clearly, however, even casual observation shows that it would be stretching credibility to argue that all significant experiences are remembered or that all the trivia that can be brought to mind have personal significance. Memory is a complex issue and no simple intuition gives a key to understanding how it operates.

Memory is a store of many different sorts of information. The mechanism by which information is processed to enter memory is called encoding. Information which has been *encoded* and *stored* may be *retrieved* in a variety of ways. *Forgetting* is a failure to recover information when wanted. It may be that the information is no longer in store, although it is hard to be certain that once stored information has been wiped clean. It may be that once stored information has been modified by subsequently encoded information and so is no longer present in its original form. It may be, and perhaps most commonly is, the result of a more or less temporary failure to retrieve stored information which may be recoverable at other times or in other circumstances.

After gaining a picture of some of the different types of information that are stored in memory we shall go on to consider the problem of remembering, of how and when stored information can be recovered for use. In the course of these discussions I shall address questions of the reliability and accuracy of memory, and I shall pay particular attention to how a person's pre-existing store of memories and understanding of the world affects what aspects of experience become embodied in memory.

The contents of long-term memory

The store of a person's experience is his or her long-term memory. Its contents are very varied. They include records of particular happenings in a person's life; knowledge and beliefs about the general characteristics of people, objects and situations that she or he has either heard about or come across; knowledge of facts and ideas and the meanings associated with words and non-linguistic signs; the knowledge about how to do things which underlies the ability to perform skilled actions as varied as riding a bicycle or adding up a shopping list. The research literature on memory distinguishes between the different types of content of which memory appears to be composed.

1. *Episodic* memories are a type of memory that people often think of when the topic of memory arises – that is, memory for particular episodes or events in a person's life. They are memories of what occurred at a particular time and place given in response to questions such as 'What did she say yesterday?' or 'What happened after your operation?'
2. *Generic* memories are general knowledge about types of experience. These are memories for the common characteristics of objects and situations. Examples might include knowledge of how to act in restaurants or of what you expect to get when you order a hamburger. An experience of a particular restaurant or hamburger will have its own episodic characteristics, but it is easy to imagine

your surprise if these characteristics deviated a lot from your general ideas about such matters.

3. *Semantic* memories encompass a great variety of content and are the foundation for our understanding of the world in which we live. They range from knowledge of individual facts ('Harvey discovered the circulation of the blood'), to systematically organized concepts (the word penicillin refers to the antibiotic 'penicillin'; antibiotics are a type of drug and drugs achieve their effects by . . . etc.). Some theorists include generic memories as a variety of semantic memory.

4. *Procedural* memories are memories of how to achieve particular goals. Some, such as your knowledge of how to ride a bicycle, cannot effectively be put into words, while others, such as the skills of mental arithmetic, can.

DISCUSSION POINT

Think of some of the procedural knowledge (knowledge of how to perform skilled actions to achieve a goal) that you have acquired in your training. Try to put some of it/them into words. What difficulties do you experience in trying to do so? What implications do these difficulties have for devising effective training procedures for these skills?

Access to memory

Intention and the retrieval of memories

In addition to distinguishing between types of memory content it is important to distinguish between modes of access to memory. This section draws attention to the role of intention in memory retrieval.

Explicit and implicit retrieval

Explicit retrieval refers to a focused and conscious attempt to bring something specific to mind. Success or failure of explicit retrieval is usually taken as the hallmark of so-called good or bad memory. Until quite recently, nearly all the research into the operation of memory was research on explicit retrieval.

Implicit retrieval is a more elusive idea, but may well be a more significant aspect of the workings of memory than explicit retrieval. It signifies a demonstrable influence of past experience on some current activity without there being any deliberate effort to relate that experience to the activity or any conscious realization that it is doing so.

Every interaction that a person has with the world is influenced by the content of his or her memory. It may seem odd to say that when drivers stop at a red light they are drawing on their memory of the meaning of red lights to know that they should stop, or that their memory of how to behave in a restaurant guides their actions when they go out to dinner, but in both cases it surely does. In neither case is it likely that much if any attempt at deliberate or conscious recollection takes place, but then memory exerts its influence as much when someone is aware that it is happening as when they are not. One of the most active areas of current memory research is aimed at achieving a deeper understanding of implicit retrieval and of its dependence on properties of the physical brain (Roediger, 1990).

Amnesia and the explicit/implicit distinction

The complexity of human memory and the subtlety of the investigative procedures that are needed to investigate it are well illustrated by studies of the memory deficits of individuals who are amnesic. Amnesia may arise from a variety of causes. Korsakoff's syndrome results from brain damage due to prolonged heavy drinking coupled with reduced eating and a consequent deficiency of thiamine. Viral encephalitis and some surgically produced brain lesions are other causes. One of the most striking features of these amnesics is that they may be unable to recall anything about recent events despite the fact that in other respects their behaviour and conversation may seem unaffected. They may, for example, be unable to recognize someone they have met only moments before. They are, however, quite capable of learning difficult procedural skills, such as learning over a series of practice sessions to trace round a pattern on paper when they can view only the pattern and their hand reflected in a mirror, or becoming increasingly fluent at solving a jigsaw puzzle with repeated practice. Each practice attempt must have contributed to the growth of a procedural memory. Yet, consistent with their general symptoms, in each practice session they say that they cannot remember having come across the task before. They learn the skill but cannot recall ever having practised it (Baddeley, 1990; Parkin, 1993). But the situation is more complicated still.

If amnesiacs are asked to recall a list of familiar words that they were shown only moments before, as one would expect, they are unable to do so. Normal adults can recollect it quite well. But, is the amnesiacs' problem one of storage or one of retrieval? Is it a problem of learning or recollection?

In a further test both normal and amnesic individuals were shown a list of word stems corresponding to the words from a list that they had recently studied, e.g. if 'computer' had been part of the list, then 'comp----' would be its word stem. It should be noted that 'Company' and 'composer' also have this same stem. They were all then asked to do one of two things: either attempt to recall the original words explicitly using the stems as hints; or, crucially, say the first words that came into their minds that had the stems as their first letters – an implicit memory task. When asked to use the stems as explicit recall cues the amnesiacs remembered much less well than the normals, so as usual they could not recollect recent events. But the results of the implicit word completion test were dramatically different. There are legitimate answers to that test, but otherwise no answer is 'right' or 'wrong'. However, the answers that are given may or may not be words from the studied list. The word completions that were given by both the normals and amnesiacs were very similar and in both cases they were generally words from the studied list. It is clear that the amnesiacs must have stored the studied list as an episodic memory and that it was this memory that was responsible for the fact that they completed the word stems with the just seen list words rather than with alternative, legitimate completions.

One can conclude that the amnesiacs suffer a retrieval deficit but one which is limited to explicit recall. Neither motor skill practice nor spontaneous word completion involves a focused attempt to bring a specific past episode to mind. So implicit retrieval appears to be unaffected. This is an important conclusion as it suggests that the reason that these amnesiacs cannot remember their past life may be that they have somehow lost the ability to recover memories to order, but they may not have lost the memories themselves. Forgetting must be due to retrieval failure rather than the erasure of old memories (or a general failure to record new experiences in memory). This conclusion cannot, however, be the whole story. It cannot, for example, explain why amnesiacs may still be able spontaneously to recall very old memories reasonably well (Parkin, 1993). A comprehensive theory linking all the characteristics of amnesia is still in the future.

Context interpretation and retrieval

It is easy to suppose that episodic memories are literal records of experience, as if they were videos or a series of snapshots. This is a mistaken view. To understand remembering one must consider the way that an experience was understood, which aspects of it were attended to and what interpretation was made of them. Success in recovering or retrieving a memory will then depend on whether the circumstances under which retrieval is attempted are sufficiently similar in crucial respects to the content of the original mental record to enable it to be located and distinguished from similar memories. A memory may be 'available', in the sense that a record may be present in the mind (or, if you like, in the brain), but remembering depends on creating circumstances under which that memory is 'accessible'. The significance of these points will become clearer with examples.

State-dependent retrieval

Godden and Baddeley (1975) conducted a very simple experiment in which they asked people to learn a list of unrelated familiar words and to recall them without any hints a little later. The special feature of the study was that some people undertook the original learning on land while others did so underwater (Baddeley is interested in diving). Then half of each of these original groups attempted recall in the same place in which they had earlier learned the list while the other half made their attempt in the other environment. When people switched locations between learning and recall they were able to bring fewer of the words to mind than if both took place in the same location. Whether people were able to remember the content of a learning experience depended on whether the environment at recall was the same or different from that in which the original experience took place, despite the fact that neither location had any bearing on the meaning or significance of the focal content of that experience, the list of words. State-dependent effects have also been found when the change in location is less dramatic than the one above (Bjork and Richardson-Klavehn, 1989). There is some evidence to suggest that imagining the circumstances in which information was learned may sometimes increase the likelihood that the information can be recalled. However, it is important to recognize that this is not the same as the experience of memories coming flooding back on revisiting a place one had lived in years ago. In that case, features of the place are intimately associated with the meaning of the events that took place there.

State-dependent memory effects have also been found when the state change is one induced by alcohol or other psychoactive drugs rather than one reflecting a change in the outside world (see also Chapter 10). Individuals in drugged states are generally believed to have less reliable memories when drugged than when not, but this is not always so. Events that occurred during a mild drugged state are generally better recalled when in a similar state than in a sober or undrugged state (Eich, 1980). A common interpretation of all these findings is that successful recall depends on accessing a stored memory of the specific episode in which the target content of interest took place, a finding that emphasizes the complexities of the remembering process.

Interpreting an experience: meaning in context

The target content for which memory was tested in most of the studies discussed so far has consisted of lists of words (almost invariably concrete nouns) which, though familiar in themselves, have no meaningful connection with each other (Baddeley, 1976: ch.1, gives some of the historical context for this research practice). More complex features of memory emerge with a shift of focus to content with more interconnected meaning, where the meaning attached to one element is influenced by that associated with others in the same context. As an example, consider the phrase 'the heart woman', which by itself could mean many things, but which in context might mean 'the surgeon', 'the patient', 'the lover', 'the researcher', etc. Although people can sometimes remember the exact words that they have heard, more often they remember just the meaning that they attached to them.

Consider a neat study by Anderson *et al.* (1976). People were asked to remember a long list of sentences which they were shown one by one. Each of the sentences had a matched alternative and any one person saw just one of the alternatives. An example is:

> The woman worked near the theatre.
> The woman worked in the theatre.

When it came to the memory test the participants were given hints (technically they are called *cues*). Each cue also had a matched alternative and any one person was given just one of them. For the example sentences the cues were 'woman' and 'actress'. The cue 'woman' was equally effective in reminding people of either sentence; however, the cue 'actress' reminded people much more of the 'in' sentence than it did of the 'near' sentence, and in fact for the 'in' sentence people found that 'actress' was a more effective cue than 'woman', the subject noun that they had in fact seen. What people had remembered was not so much the 'in' sentence that they had seen but the interpretation that they had unconsciously made of it. They had understood what the sentence meant by thinking of a highly likely sort of woman that it might be who would work 'in' the theatre.

It is interesting to speculate whether, if the people who had participated in the Anderson *et al.* study had all been nursing students, the cue 'nurse' would have had the same effect as 'actress' had for the original non-medical participants. If this turned out to be so, then it would be reasonable to suppose that the nurse students had understood 'theatre' to refer to an operating theatre rather than the playhouse which was what the original non-medical participants presumably understood it to mean.

What all this implies is not only that people tend to remember meanings rather than literal events, but also that the meanings that they remember depend on a complex interaction of two influences. The first is the context in which events take place, the second is the particular knowledge of the world that each person brings to their experience and which is responsible for the specific way in which they attach meaning to the experiences that they have. Episodic meaning is constructed by an interaction between input from the world and the contents of semantic memory. A further implication is that a cue or hint is effective only if it matches the way that someone has encoded an experience (Bransford, 1979; Parkin, 1993).

Interpreting an experience: comprehending related ideas

Experiences that are poorly understood are rarely easily remembered (Bransford, 1979). It might seem that people would know whether or not they understood something (and hence whether they think they are likely to be able to remember it). To some extent this may be true, but people often discover whether or not something has been understood only when they are asked questions about it. Medical students are taught both the causes and symptoms of an enormous range of pathological conditions, but it is very easy to become confused about which symptoms diagnose which condition. In those cases in which the causes of a condition are known in sufficient detail that they explain why particular symptoms are found, there is a reasoned basis for remembering the link between the two. When a student has failed to grasp such relations fully her/his ability to remember the connection is seriously impaired with possibly unfortunate consequences when it comes to making diagnoses (Feltovich *et al.*, 1984). At a more superficial level, it has been shown that people may read a passage which contains contradictory information and not even notice the contradiction (Glenberg, Wilkinson and Epstein, 1982).

What does it mean to say that some experience has been 'understood' or 'comprehended'? An apparently simple question, which is remarkably hard to answer.

To understand something is certainly to read into it more than is apparent on the surface. If someone at dinner asks you 'Do you have the salt?' they don't expect a 'yes' (or 'no') answer, yet you will grasp what they mean without thinking. Achieving understanding can often, however, require some effort. A thought-provoking study of this point has been reported by Franks *et al.* (1982), who were puzzled as to why some late primary age children are poorer readers than others. The less able readers were not illiterate as they could translate the squiggles on a page into spoken words. But equally they were not fully literate, as they were not very good at explaining what they had read. The investigators wondered whether the children's comprehension problem might lie as much in the characteristics of the text that they were asked to read as in their reading abilities.

Most text (and speech as well if one thinks about it) communicates only part of the message which a reader, or listener, is intended to get from it. The receiver is assumed to fill out the intended meaning by reference to their background knowledge of the topic of the communication (Sanford, 1987; Stevenson, 1993).

Each pupil was asked to read one of two versions of a text (see Box 8.1) which described two imaginary robots until they felt sure that they understood it well enough to answer some questions about it. One robot was designed to paint the outside of houses, the other to paint office buildings. An 'implicit' text listed only the parts of which the robots were built. A fully 'explicit' version included further information about each part to give a clearer idea of the way that they contributed to fulfilling the purpose for which its robot was designed. Memory for text content was tested by asking to which of the robots each of the properties belonged. Given the number of parts (18) that were described, it was thought unlikely that they could be learned by rote and that a pupil would be able to remember accurately only if they had understood the structure–function relations linking properties to robot design purposes. These links provide a reasoned basis for deciding to which robot a property belongs. The 'explicit' version provided this information; the 'implicit' version required the reader to work this out by drawing on their general knowledge.

Both skilled and less skilled readers who had read the 'explicit' version remembered it very well. Skilled readers also remembered the 'implicit' version well, but the less skilled readers did not. The skilled readers were individuals who realized that reading for understanding is a sort of problem-solving which requires them to work out how the different ideas that are mentioned are sensibly related to and connect with each other. The less skilled readers had problems when it came to understanding the significance of information when they had to work out the significance by themselves without any guidance in the text itself. Seeing how a set of ideas connect with each other is a large part of what it means to say that something has been understood.

The lesson from this and many other studies is that the initiator of a communication must take account of the knowledge and cognitive skills of the recipient if the intended meaning of the message is to get across. If the meaning is not communicated, it is hardly surprising that a recipient will not 'remember what they were

---

BOX 8.1   A WELL-WRITTEN TEXT IS MORE READILY REMEMBERED

Implicit 'Robots' Text (extract)

Billy went to visit his father at work. He saw the new robots that his father had made. Billy first looked at the robot that paints houses. It had a bucket on top of its head. This robot was carrying a roll of tape. It also had a sign with some words on it.

Fully Explicit 'Robots' Text (extract)

Billy went to visit his father at work. He saw the new robots that his father had made. Billy first looked at the robot that paints houses. It had a bucket on top of its head in order to carry paint. This robot was carrying a roll of tape to put on the windows to protect them from the paint. It also had a sign with the words 'Wet Paint' written on it.

Two versions of the beginning of an expository text cast in the form of a story acceptable to children. The fully explicit version describes how each of the robot's parts contributes to the function for which the robot was designed. The implicit version lists the parts without explaining them.

Source: adapted from Franks *et al.* (1982).

---

told'. The importance of this observation for effective health education is self-evident.

DISCUSSION POINT

Imagine that you are giving three different patients/clients the same piece of advice/instructions about their illness. One of the patients is a fully qualified nurse or doctor, another is an average intelligent adult, the last is a young adolescent.

Plan how you would communicate what you want to get across to each of these three individuals. How would you make sure that you had been understood? How would you help them to remember what they had been told?

Interpreting an experience: constructing false memories

Memory failures can be of two sorts. Forgetting, in everyday terms, is an omission, but recollections can be mistaken as well as incomplete. False memories, given in good faith, may arise for many reasons. One obvious reason is simple confusion; mixing up left and right is quite common and it is only too easy to get a PIN number wrong given the large number of otherwise meaningless number codes that one carries in one's head. But to a large extent they are the flip side of normal comprehension processes. Unless one is very observant, it is only too easy to suppose that things are as one might have expected them to be. Brewer and Treyens (1981), for example, asked students to wait in a research worker's office for a moment and then a little later asked them to describe it. Many of them claimed, quite reasonably, that they remembered seeing books although there were no books in the room; and a few said that they had seen a notepad on the desk, where one might have expected it to be, although in fact it had been left on a chair. Sometimes a false memory may be encoded into memory, as when one incorrectly interprets a person's action because of some prior knowledge or belief one had about that person, which leads one to see them in a particular light; at other times it may arise when trying to construct a sensible account of an experience from some rather fragmentary memories of it. Such processes are, of course, relevant to the observations that health professionals make of their clients/patients and highlight the need to make and to consult systematic records.

A further source of false memories comes from post-event information; that is, information that one learns about an event some time after it has taken place and that leads one to revise one's memory of it. This can take some quite subtle forms, as when one is asked what are called 'leading questions' about the past (a leading question is one that suggests a particular answer). Contrast the two requests: 'Tell me what sort of pain it was' and 'Tell me how awful the pain was'. The latter is a leading question; it suggests that the pain was undoubtedly awful and the only matter at issue is just how awful it was. Once asked, a leading question can leave a permanent impression on how one recollects an experience. Loftus and Palmer (1974) showed people a film of a car accident and then asked them a set of questions about it. One of the questions was phrased in one of two ways for different groups of observers. This was: 'How fast were the cars going when they collided/smashed into each other?' Unsurprisingly, the latter, leading question induced people to name a higher speed than the more neutral question. A week later the observers were asked further questions about the incident, and particularly: 'Do you remember seeing broken glass on the road afterwards?'. In fact, there hadn't been any, but many of the people to whom it had been suggested that the cars had 'smashed' thought there was – as did some of the 'collided' observers, but many fewer of them.

Memory early and late in the lifespan

It is beyond the scope of this chapter to attempt a full consideration of the characteristics of the memory of children and old people. The current state of our understanding of children's memory is reviewed by Kail (1990). One aspect of this research which is of particular concern at the moment is discussed below. The demographic change to an older population has given a strong impetus to research on ageing. Parkin (1993) discusses the current state of understanding of memory in old age. A brief account of some of the complexities in understanding the relation of memory to ageing is given below.

Accuracy and completeness of children's memory

There is considerable medico-legal concern about the extent of the reliability of children's memory. Reliability will, of course, depend on the age of the child, but there is a strong folk belief that children are both highly suggestible and unable to distinguish fantasy from reality. If this were true, then no weight could be attached to what children claim had happened to them in the past. It is by no means easy, however, to decide whether this is true or not, especially when the memory of concern is that of highly emotional episodes of stress or abuse in which they may have been involved and which may have occurred some time ago. In passing, one might wonder about the origins of this common belief. One can only speculate, but two possible bases come to mind. It is certainly true that children can typically recall experiences in much less detail than most adults can (Kail, 1990), and this may be one reason why adults have less overall confidence in children's memory. Another is that children are simply less experienced than adults in the ways of the world and so face more situations in which they are unsure about exactly what is going on. The problem in this case will arise when an adult's interrogation presses them to tell more than they have grasped. In such circumstances even adults can be provoked into imagining that they actually remember more than they first thought, especially in response to leading questions.

Standard studies which test children's memories for everyday events and of which they may have been only observers fail to address the issues of concern. Even when children falsely remember apparently routine everyday experiences the cause is just as likely to be an unsophisticated misunderstanding of what had happened as some sort of fantasizing. Not that they do recall such situations falsely to any great extent. What is needed is tests of memory for emotionally significant events in a child's life and for which there is independent evidence of exactly what went on to check against. One series of studies (Goodman, Aman and Hirschman, 1987) compared children's and adults' memory for relatively brief, carefully monitored, naturally occurring experiences in which they had been active participants. The experiences ranged from a stressful medical intervention (immunization or having a blood sample taken), to a non-stressful medical visit, to a play session. The youngest children, who were around 3 years old, recalled with fair accuracy in response to direct questions; recalled very little when they were asked to say what had happened without any prompting; and were quite inaccurate when they were pressed with leading questions. Older (6–7-year-old) children presented a much more promising picture on all three counts, being about as accurate as adults in response to direct questions, although still inferior in unprompted recall. They were much superior to the 3-year-olds in resisting the misleading implications of leading questions, although still a little short of adults. It is fair to conclude that children can remember what has happened to them with a dependable level of accuracy, but that as their spontaneous recall is quite limited, great care must be taken when posing direct questions to them so as not to suggest ideas to them in the way that questions are put (see also Chapter 19). A further result, and one of some considerable importance, is that there was no noticeable loss of accuracy in children's recall for stressful experiences as compared to their recall for those that were more benign. Although these are encouraging findings, they must nevertheless be treated with care until a wider range of studies has been reported (see Steward, 1993). There are

significant practical problems in assessing memory for realistically stressful experiences and ethical as well as humane considerations impose strict limits on research.
It should not be forgotten that adult memory is not always reliable and that in the
real world it is never easy to distinguish false memories reported in good faith from
deliberate dissembling.

Some problems in understanding memory in old age

The main problem of understanding memory in old age is that of understanding
ageing in general. The likelihood of degenerative decline increases with age and so,
for example, dementia (see Chapter 24) is becoming increasingly common as more
individuals survive to advanced years. Older people are typically retired people with
a less active engagement with the stimulus of the social, intellectual and practical
concerns of everyday life. In a rapidly changing world older people can find themselves at a considerable disadvantage in understanding events and ideas which are
radically different from those to which they were accustomed in the past. (This last
problem is not restricted to people of advanced years; analyses of the biographies of
famous scientists have shown that their best discoveries tend to be made quite early
in their careers, and everyone is familiar with relatively young stick-in-the-muds.) But
none of these is the inevitable consequence of ageing in and of itself. Hence it is
extremely difficult to make generalizations about the effect of ageing *per se* on a
mental function like memory (see Parkin, 1993, for current views).

It is worth adding that objective understanding of changes in mental performance
with age is only half the story. In a similar fashion to what was noted above in the
discussion of children's memory, we must also recognize that instances of slips or a
lack of mental sharpness by old people are generally interpreted more harshly (in a
more patronizing fashion?) than they would be if they were made by a younger
adult (see also Chapter 23). The mental status of an individual cannot usually be
estimated from a brief and restricted acquaintance (see Chapter 7).

Memory in the head and in the world

Anyone who has ever returned to a place where they spent time many years before
will have experienced a flood of returning memories of people and happenings and
emotions of that time. Although it is impossible to be sure that these memories are
accurate in every respect, it is certainly the case that the memories that come back
are more detailed and extensive than those that are recoverable by reflection in an
armchair back home. Exotic experiences like this remind us of the fragility of
remembering. In fact, we are all aware of the unreliability of memory in general and
to some extent of the circumstances in which this is most likely. We write out
shopping lists, keep clinical history records, take notes when studying, leave ourselves reminder notes on kitchen pin-boards, keep reference books to hand, and all

because we know that we need 'in the world' support to help us remember when necessary. There has been very little research on the effectiveness of different types of aid in different types of circumstance, and what there has been has not been very illuminating. But we may be sure that in the everyday world such aids are of great practical importance when accuracy is all-important.

Summary

Memory is at the centre of people's sense of who they are and of their relations with the world at large. This chapter has concentrated on some of the central ideas about how memory operates, focusing on the nature of what is stored and the circumstances under which stored information is retrieved. We now see that memory cannot be considered as a separate mental function but that it is intimately related to more general processes concerned with meaning and understanding. The fallibility of memory was emphasized and thus led to an account of the idea of memories 'residing outside the mind'. Particular attention was given to methods for investigating memory and the difficulties of doing so.

Seminar questions

1. In the specific case of the female contraceptive pill, would you merely advise a patient of the importance of remembering to take one pill each day, or do you think that there would be any merit in helping them not to forget by suggesting a particular time of day to take it? If the latter, then when? After brushing their teeth? With morning coffee? Before going to bed? Or when? Justify your opinion. What assumptions about an individual's lifestyle might you be making in formulating your recommendation?
2. Select a medical condition of which you have experience or knowledge. Consider the problems that might arise in providing good nursing care for a person with amnesia who requires treatment for this condition (see also Chapter 24).

Further reading

Baddeley, A.D. (1994) *Your Memory: A user's guide.* Harmondsworth: Penguin Books. Written for the general reader, but a serious work and lavishly and informatively illustrated.

Bransford, J.D. (1979) *Human Cognition: Learning understanding and remembering.* London: Wadsworth. One of the most intelligent and clearly written accounts of memory and related topics ever written. The ideas are still up-to-date despite its age.

Cohen, G., Kiss, G. and LeVoi, M. (1993) *Memory: Current issues*, 2nd edition. Milton Keynes: Open University Press. An impressive attempt to make major technical and theoretical issues comprehensible to students.

Parkin, A.J. (1993) *Memory: Phenomena, experiment and theory.* Oxford: Basil Blackwell. The clearest (and most elegant) analysis of current research into normal and pathological memory.

Rose, S.P.R. (1992) *The Making of Memory.* New York: Bantam. A Rhone-Poulenc prize-winning discussion of memory and the brain written by an active researcher in the field. 'Popular' science writing at its best.

Stevenson, R.J. (1993) *Language, Thought and Representation.* Chichester: John Wiley. Essential for anyone interested in the role of memory in human thought.

References

Anderson, R.C., Pichert, J.W., Goetz, E.T., Schallert, D.L., Stevens, K.V. and Trollip, S.R. (1976) 'Instantiation of general terms', *Journal of Verbal Learning and Verbal Behavior* **15**, 667–79.

Baddeley, A.D. (1976) *The Psychology of Memory.* New York: Harper & Row.

Baddeley, A.D. (1990) *Human Memory: Theory and practice.* Hove: Lawrence Erlbaum.

Bjork, R.A. and Richardson-Klavehn, A. (1989) 'On the puzzling relationship between environmental context and human memory', in C. Izawa (ed.) *Current Issues in Cognitive Processes: The Tulane Flowerree Symposium on Cognition.* Hove: Lawrence Erlbaum.

Bransford, J.D. (1979) *Human Cognition: Learning understanding and remembering.* London: Wadsworth.

Brewer, W.F. and Treyens, J.C. (1981) 'Role of schemata in memory for places', *Cognitive Psychology* **13**, 207–30.

Eich, J.E. (1980) 'The cue-dependent nature of state-dependent retrieval', *Memory and Cognition* **8**, 157–73.

Feltovich, P.J., Johnson, P.E., Moller, J.H. and Swanson, D.B. (1984) 'The role and development of medical knowledge in diagnostic expertise', in W. Clancey and E.H. Shortliffe (eds.) *Readings in Medical Artificial Intelligence: The first decade.* Reading, Mass.: Addison-Wesley.

Franks, J.R., Vye, N.J., Auble, P.A., Mezynski, K.J., Perfetto, G.A., Bransford, J.D., Stein, B.S. and Littelefield, J. (1982) 'Learning from explicit versus implicit texts', *Journal of Experimental Psychology: General* **111**, 414–22.

Glenberg, A.M., Wilkinson, A.C. and Epstein, W. (1982) 'The illusion of knowing: Failure in the self-assessment of comprehension', *Memory and Cognition* **10**, 597–602.

Godden, D. and Baddeley, A.D. (1975) 'Context-dependent memory in two natural environments: On land and under water', *British Journal of Psychology* **66**, 325–31.

Goodman, G.S., Aman, C. and Hirschman, J. (1987) 'Child sexual and physical abuse: Children's testimony', in S.J. Ceci, M.P. Toglia and D.F. Ross (eds.) *Children's Eyewitness Memory.* New York: Springer-Verlag.

Kail, R. (1990) *The Development of Memory in Children*, 3rd edition. New York: W.H. Freeman.

Loftus, E.F. and Palmer, J.C. (1974) 'Reconstruction of automobile destruction: An example of the interaction between language and memory', *Journal of Verbal Learning and Verbal Behavior* **13**, 585–9.

Parkin, A.J. (1993) *Memory: Phenomena, experiment and theory*. Oxford: Basil Blackwell.
Roediger, H.L. III (1990) 'Implicit memory: Retention without remembering', *American Psychologist* **45**, 1043–56.
Sanford, A. J. (1987) *The Mind of Man*. Hemel Hempstead: Harvester Wheatsheaf.
Stevenson, R.J. (1993) *Language, Thought and Representation*. Chichester: John Wiley.
Steward, M.S. (1993) 'Understanding children's memories of medical procedures: "He didn't touch me and it didn't hurt!" ' in C.A. Nelson (ed.) *Memory and Affect in Development: Minnesota Symposia in Child Psychology*, No. 26. Hove: Lawrence Erlbaum.

CHAPTER 9

Nursing and error

DONALD RIDLEY

Chapter outline

Introduction
Error classification
Individual causes of error
    Lack of knowledge
    Lack of training and skills
    Forgetting
    Paying insufficient attention to routine tasks
    Misdiagnosis or misunderstanding
Organizational causes of error
    Poor communication
    Role conflict
    Organizational resistance to change
Error minimization using the systems approach
Summary

Introduction

This chapter is directed at all health care professionals. The general aims of the chapter are to provide basic knowledge of the nature of error from both conceptual and practical points of view and to assist the review and planning of day-to-day activity at individual, group and organizational levels. Specifically, this includes an understanding of the complex nature of error, some ways in which error may be classified and an outline knowledge of the principles involved in systems analysis, together with general guidelines for the recognition and prevention of error.

Why should nurses and health care professionals be interested in error? There are two answers to this question, the first obvious, the second a little less so. First, they should be interested in error as an awareness of the nature and causes of error may help them reduce the likelihood of error in their professional activity. Second, and perhaps more importantly, the role of the health care professional is changing. They increasingly have managerial as well as patient care functions and the range of their duties is being extended into areas that were previously the domain of other professional groups. These changes bring increased responsibilities and managing the quality of the delivery of care is an important one, involving setting up effective systems that maximize performance and value for money.

No one is perfect, everyone makes mistakes, and to fail to acknowledge this fact in oneself, in one's organization or in a team of people for whom one is responsible is the first stage in a chain of events that can lead to poor performance at best and disaster at worst. It is very difficult, if not impossible, to eradicate error in any field of endeavour, but there is a great deal that can be done to reduce both the likelihood and consequences of error and much of it is quite simple. Errors offer an opportunity to learn about ourselves and the organizations in which they occur.

When errors occur, what should be done? The cheap option is often to blame the person at the front end of the system; thus the captain of the Boeing 737–400 that crashed on the M1 motorway in 1989 taking many lives was compulsorily retired and his first officer sacked. They had mistakenly turned off a healthy engine and flown a damaged one to the point of destruction. Certainly they did not perform ideally, but disposing of their services did not answer the question: 'Why and how did this happen?'. In fact, there were a number of contributory problems: for example, the engine that had failed was a new type that had not been tested properly. Such deficiencies were not the responsibility of the pilots but the responsibility of the organizational managements who designed and operated the aircraft. Dismissing the pilots addressed none of these issues, although it is quite likely that pilots are sensitive to this particular possibility, making repetition unlikely; the training and design deficiencies may still reside in the organizations concerned. Sacking the last people to touch a system, be they a pilot, train driver or nurse, will probably not solve the problem. The use of the term error precipitates a mantle of causality around those close to an untoward event and distracts attention from other antecedents which are often rather more important but harder to define. The message is this: organizational factors may have a big impact on the likelihood and consequences of error. Box 9.1 below asks the question 'What is error?'.

There have been extensive studies of error. Some rely on well-documented diary studies which examine day-to-day tasks such as tea- and coffee-making. These studies provide a great deal of information but tend to focus on simple errors which are not part of complex systems. Other methods are more pragmatic and analyze past events where errors are known to have occurred. These tend to deal with more complex events and provide some degree of insight, but suffer from the particular wisdom that is imbued by 20/20 hindsight. Reason (1990) provides more detail.

Errors have been analyzed for many occupations. These include pilots, nuclear power station operators, train drivers, shipmasters and radiographers. Examples may be found in Reason (1990). Work on error has been undertaken in the nursing field, but this has been somewhat limited and tends to be anecdotal, confined to general articles in the nursing press (e.g. Cobb, 1990) and concentrates on simple and highly tangible errors such as errors of medication (Forster, 1992). One of the difficulties in studying error in the health context stems from the fact that error contains a pejorative connotation. Imagine that you are a nursing manager or a

---

BOX 9.1 **WHAT IS ERROR? A DISCUSSION TASK**

What is error?

This is not as simple a question as might initially appear to be the case. The simple answer might be: doing something that is 'wrong'. But ask yourself the following questions in discussion groups:

1. Can you make an error while you are asleep?
2. Is intention a necessary prerequisite for error?
3. Do errors have to have negative outcomes? If there is no negative outcome, has an error been made?
4. The same piece of behaviour, or its absence, may be an error under one set of circumstances but not under others. How would you distinguish between the two?
5. Do errors always involve physical action or can errors occur without physical action?

Answers to some of the questions should indicate that 'error' is not a simple issue. The term error is actually a construct, a fusion of different ideas, which is often mistaken for actual behaviour (or its absence). Put another way, an error is a violation of an expectation, desire or intention, and one person's error might be another's desired outcome. Error is a very difficult term to define yet is much used. It has pejorative associations; when you say someone has made an error you are not just saying that they have done something that prevented a particular outcome being achieved, you are implying that they are to blame. To blame any individual or group for them without considering the 'system' in which they are operating leads to a neglect of the real causes of 'error'.

---

hospital administrator being approached by a keen researcher with the request to study error in your workforce. The temptation is to be cautious and respond that your organization is not in the business of making errors. This is understandable, as the final consumer of your service, the patients, will not wish to know that errors might occur. The faintest hint that 'error' might occur in your institution may damage its standing in the eyes of professional colleagues, of central funding agencies and also of the general public, often by way of press reports. In the case of nursing, this resistance is quite strong. There are occasional publications of error reports in the nursing press, but in general terms the possibility of error is not openly considered, although individual nurses indicate in conversation that errors are neither more nor less common than in any other field of endeavour.

Error classification

DISCUSSION POINT
List a minimum of ten errors that might occur in nursing and related health care functions and try to classify them before reading this section.

BOX 9.2   **TYPES OF ERROR CLASSIFICATION**

Type of Error	Comments
Slips and Mistakes	At the beginning of the 1980s Donald Norman and James Reason both developed a way of looking at error based on a distinction between *slips* and *mistakes*.
	Slips are errors of execution; thus, if you have the correct intention but fail to carry out an act correctly you have made a 'slip'. A simple example might be an attempt to give an intradermal injection and inadvertently 'overshooting' and giving a subcutaneous injection.
	Mistakes are errors of planning. They are more common than slips in virtually all domains and arise from such factors as misperceptions, misinterpretation or misdiagnosis, and lead to poor or inadequate planning. They are much harder to prevent than slips, as one of their characteristics is a misunderstanding of the situation. That is seductive in the sense that the perpetrator of a mistake will believe that what they are doing is correct and may have no reason to question their behaviour.
Errors of omission vs errors of commission	This is a simple distinction but an important one.
	Errors of commission are those errors that result from action; for example, administration of a particular medication to a patient who does not require any medication or who requires a different medication.
	Errors of omission are those errors that involve lack of activity. Failing to administer medication to a patient when it is required would be an error of omission.
Skill, Rule and Knowledge based Errors	The distinctions between slips and mistakes and errors of commission and omission are quite simple. Over the past ten years or so, it has been argued that a more sophisticated approach is needed. With this in mind the behaviour of people who interact with systems has been classified into three different types: *skill*, *rule* and *knowledge-based behaviour*. Put simply, skill-based errors are those that occur as a result of inappropriate application skills or where skills are not fully developed. An example might be failing to find a vein while drawing a blood sample. Rule-based errors are those that occur as a result of incorrectly or inappropriately supplied procedures; for example, failing to check a patient's recent oral intake prior to anaesthetic. Knowledge-based errors are errors that might arise through poor planning or misdiagnosis.
Latent errors	Latent errors are actions, omissions, plans and other activities that occur at one point in time and that may reside passively in a system until they

interact with a particular series of events or other contextual phenomena and cause an untoward occurrence. An example might be a fault in a GP's software package, so that it fails to indicate that a blood test should be taken in the morning after fasting and where an evening reading might give a spurious and misleading value. Latent errors are very difficult to prevent. They have been described as being like viruses waiting to become active at a later stage. The more complex a system is, and the more people who have responsibility for designing and operating a system, the more likely it is that latent errors will be present. As it is not possible to foresee every eventuality, it is not possible to eradicate latent errors. The favoured way of dealing with it is to ensure that a system is resistant to errors and allows recovery from those errors.

There are many different ways of viewing error; most of them have some merit. Before reading about some of them remember that they should be thought of as ways of thinking about error, helping you to develop a sophisticated appreciation of the nature of error. Box 9.2 summarizes some ways of classifying error.

While these approaches provide ways of understanding what has happened in the lead-up to error, it is important to ask what they tell us about preventing errors in the future. While it is true that they might provide some general exhortation such as 'don't forget to do this', or 'do A not B', it is fair to say that their utility is biased towards explanation rather than prediction. Unfortunately, the latter is necessary for error prevention. If this sounds negative then it need not be so, for underlying the use of these distinctions is a powerful notion; that errors are simply parts of planned actions that go wrong, or put another way, they are system failures that may result from a wide range of causes. The person who is 'closest' to an error might be the person who commits the error, but in reality the management who create the system in which the so-called perpetrator works and colleagues who have influenced the current scenario are all involved in the system, as indeed are the designers of any equipment that might be used (see Chapters 1 and 25 for further discussion of systems). Thus we move towards the idea of error as a distributed system failure. The idea of a distributed system failure provides us with a mechanism for looking at errors that have already happened which is both simple and effective. It also allows us to make credible attempts at preventing future errors, as we shall see later in the chapter. It helps us move away from a notion of error that precipitates a mantle of causality around those close to an event, allowing those at a distance to be removed from a causal chain. This approaches militates against the use of generic classification systems because a systems approach begs integration of context. As noted earlier, error is not a behaviour but a combination of context with a violation of that expectation, desire or intention. Errors cannot be separated from the contexts in which they occur. Error is normally a result of complex interactions between a range of causal factors.

Individual causes of error

Lack of knowledge

If someone does not know what they are supposed to do or lacks contextual knowledge that allows them to evaluate the likely outcomes of their actions, then they may make an error. Thus someone operating a new piece of equipment with which they are unfamiliar might not, initially, use it properly. Someone new to a ward, institution or, indeed, working for an agency may not realise that there are differences in, say, who is responsible for reviewing levels of medication between one institution and another.

Lack of training and skills

It is of course one thing to be able to recite or know the series of steps that make up a complicated series of events, but another to be able to undertake them successfully and efficiently, providing maximum effect with minimum inconvenience to the patient or other recipient. The difference between the two relates to the acquisition of skill (or in jargon, the development of appropriate competencies). This transition should occur as a result of training which will set up a basis of skill that will be developed under supervision in applied settings.

Forgetting

Forgetting to do things is a common error. People are prone to forget in all aspects of their lives and under normal circumstances the outcomes of forgetfulness are trivial or inconvenient. But occasionally they can be fatal. Some people have a predisposition to be more forgetful than others and it is possible to counter this tendency by the use of checklists and the design of tasks and jobs that provide automatic points where the person concerned is forced to make some form of positive acknowledgement before proceeding further. Inaccurate recall is a type of forgetting, as is mistaking the intention to do something for actually doing it, i.e. mistaking a prior intention for prior action (see Chapter 8). This type of forgetting is dangerous as it automatically renders ineffective any error protection that may have been set in place.

Paying insufficient attention to routine tasks

No doubt at some stage in your life you will have started doing something, daydreamed a little and then found yourself doing something else. A common example is driving down the route that you normally take to work when you are actually going somewhere else. You are paying insufficient attention to what is going on and routine, automatic behaviour takes over. This type of error is common when undertaking routine tasks.

Misdiagnosis or misunderstanding

Where someone incorrectly assesses or misperceives a situation and then bases their subsequent actions on this information, their plan of action may be inappropriate, leading to errors.

Organizational causes of error

Poor communication

Organizations are groups of individuals working together for ostensibly common goals (see Chapter 1). To share goals and work together on tasks, they must communicate effectively. Failure to do so will lead to suboptimal organizational performance, and one of the ways in which this might be manifested will be in so-called errors. If the communication structure is deficient, this may contribute towards the subsequent error.

Information flow, and hence communication, in organizations may be classified into two types: vertical information flow and horizontal information flow. Vertical information flow refers to the flow of information up and down an organizational hierarchy; thus a manager may give instructions to a supervisor who will instruct team members to undertake particular tasks. In a similar manner, team members might pass information back up the hierarchy. Note that there are two aspects to this, one which is functional and relates to the nature of the job, the other which is managerial and relates to the management of staff. This dual function for the vertical communications systems can help cause errors and make error prevention more difficult. The managerial aspect of the vertical reporting chain makes vertical information flow more salient and this means that the importance of horizontal information flow is often neglected. Horizontal information flow is the transfer of functional information between team members which allows them to do their jobs effectively as a group. If we were to measure the amount of information moving around organizations, the vast bulk would probably turn out to be functional information, transmitted horizontally.

Given the foregoing it is not difficult to identify errors that might relate to a breakdown in horizontal communication. These might result from:

- A colleague not telling you something.
- A colleague not telling you that they expect you to do something.
- A colleague assuming, without checking, you will do something.

■ Personal feelings about colleagues causing either positive or negative perceptions. For example, you might discount the technical importance of the information some people might give you because you do not value their opinions, ideas or views.

Breakdown of functional communication can occur within a group (e.g. a ward team) or between groups – for example, with nursing staff from other wards or other nursing activities, with other paramedical professionals such as radiotherapists or with doctors. This is an interesting source of error as each of the different specialities has its own vertical reporting structure which tends to be unique to that part of the health care profession and may make functional information more difficult to 'transmit'. Consequently, it is particularly important to check that it has arrived.

Changes in patient care mean that particular attention needs to be paid to functional communication, e.g. where patients are returned home more quickly after operations and where people with certain types of condition that might have previously been institutionalized are now cared for in residential centres.

Role conflict

In all organizations there comes a point where the technical specialist of one kind or another becomes more of a manager and less of a technical specialist. It is quite often the case that those rising through the ranks to managerial position are in fact by dint of training and experience poorly prepared for undertaking their new tasks. The relevance to error is a subtle one and is brought about by role conflict. Managers will have responsibility for making sure that the part of the organization that they are responsible for (or indeed the whole organization, if appropriate) functions effectively. Put simply, a manager will often have to wear two hats, that of a specialist and that of the manager, and the outcomes of decisions made may vary depending on which hat is being worn at the time. This conflict is a subtle but pervasive factor, which will affect the decision-making and planning behaviour of the manager concerned. It may lead to condoning shortcuts on the unstated basis that it has always been all right before. It may lead to conflicting messages to staff, insisting, for example, that patient care is always the highest priority but offering some form of informal disapproval for following procedures correctly, where this may delay achievement of routine objectives. Conflicting goals also affect staff at an operational level, e.g. which patient to see first. Conflicting goals produce errors because they increase uncertainty and uncertainty leads to the formulation of poor plans.

Organizational resistance to change

An important issue is organizational resistance to change. As noted earlier, no manager wishes the organization to be held up as an example of an organization that makes errors, and it is fair to say that people would like those who are responsible for treating their maladies to be infallible. This, combined with professional ethos manifested by the different professional bodies associated with medical professions, leads to overt denials that error goes on in health care settings, and that even if it does, it can be sorted out internally. This only adds to the usual resistance of management to change and makes the discussion of error and its prevention in medical settings a no-go area. In other words, there tends to be a lack of positive critique and an overemphasis on personal responsibility, a tendency to see clinicians (including nurses) as the sole agent rather than just the visible part of a much larger system.

DISCUSSION POINT
To what extent does your experience agree with this analysis of what causes error?

Error minimization using the systems approach

Preventing error has exercised the minds of many groups of people including professionals of many different types (e.g. engineers, pilots, doctors, psychologists), regulatory bodies and professional associations. The most important part of error prevention is the realization that errors are unavoidable and provide an important source of feedback on system performance and are rarely issues of personal culpability. This viewpoint fosters a culture where people are more likely to talk about the difficulties they experience, sharing this with others, identifying possible improvements in procedures and identifying training and other personal development needs. Organizational systems should be error-tolerant and allow recovery from errors, allowing 'graceful degradation' of system performance without catastrophic failure.

The first task when attempting to prevent error is to conduct a 'systems' analysis. This grandiose term in reality is simply a detailed analysis of the particular activities of an individual or group of people. A detailed account of task and systems analysis can be found in found in Kirwan and Ainsworth (1992). There are a number of key phases in a systems analysis. The first is to describe the system, and it is important to undertake a thorough data-gathering exercise from a representative sample of people who operate a system and others who might have relevant experiences or views, such as the recipients of a service or those responsible for managing the system. Data-gathering can be by interview, questionnaire or systematic observation. Once gathered, your data need to be presented in a manner that helps you meet the goals of your analysis. The most common way of doing this is by flowcharting or hierarchical subdivision of the overall activity into its component tasks. Such a process might subdivide a task, e.g. taking blood pressure or administering medication, into a number of levels of depth of analysis. This is the basis of what is termed hierarchical task analysis (HTA). Another way of representing data is to use a tabular format with task elements at the left-hand side of the table, which

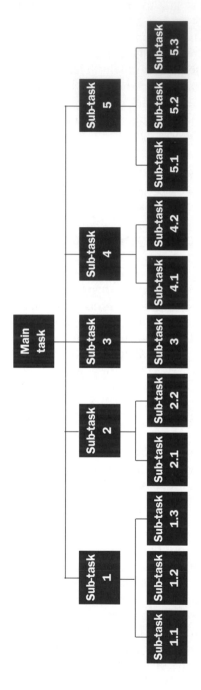

Figure 9.1 *Possible format for hierarchical task analysis*

Figure 9.2 *Possible format for failure mode effects analysis*

Task element	Type of error	Probability	Consequences	Recovery
Sub-task 1				
Sub-task 1.1				
Sub-task 1.2				
Sub-task 1.3				
Sub-task 2				
Sub-task 2.1				
Sub-task 2.2				
Sub-task 3				
Sub-task 3.1				
Sub-task 4				
Sub-task 4.1				
Sub-task 4.2				
Sub-task 5				
Sub-task 5.1				
Sub-task 5.2				
Sub-task 5.3				

extends across beneath a range of possible headings, which might include error type, probability of error, consequences of error and ways of recovering from that error. This is known as a failure mode effects analysis (FMEA). Detailed accounts of both HTA and FMEA are given in Kirwan and Ainsworth (1992) and are illustrated in Figures 9.1 and 9.2, which use the same logical task structure.

It is important to check or validate your findings by obtaining feedback from other people who are involved in the system you are analyzing. Organizational factors are more difficult to incorporate into such an analysis, but this should not deter you from attempting to include them as they are often very important. It is probably best to practise a systems analysis on a simple non-crucial task to develop your skills

---

BOX 9.3 STAGES IN CONDUCTING A SYSTEMS ANALYSIS

1. Characterize organization, system or subsystem of interest

1.1 Knowledge elicitation/data-gathering
From self and other experts using techniques such as interviews, questionnaires, documentation analysis.

1.2 System representation/description
Using HTA, FMEA and other techniques such as flowcharting, identification of decision points, identification of functional information requirements for task completion, identification of points of high workload, identification of high-risk events, identification of high hazard events, identification of other pertinent issues as appropriate. Use techniques such as prepared, goal-directed structured interview, questionnaires.

2. Identify likely errors from 1.2
Classify errors according to slips/mistakes, omissions, unwanted actions, skill/rule/knowledge-based errors, latent errors. Remember that these classes of error are not mutually exclusive and you should expect to have a degree of redundancy in your analysis.

3. Identify probability of errors in 2 and potential consequences
Some formal methods for identifying probabilities do exist but are complex and of dubious reliability. The best way of dealing with estimating probabilities of various types of error is by estimation in, say, four qualitative categories: e.g. hardly ever, unlikely, likely, near certain. Use of event records may be very useful in dealing with probabilistic estimations of error occurrence. Care should be taken to ensure that estimates are gleaned from a range of experienced practitioners and not just one individual. Error probabilities are normally estimates and this should be borne in mind when making planning decisions based on this information.

4. Identify possible interventions
These might include job redesign, training, changes to procedures, reallocation of responsibility for various tasks. Interventions may be resource-intensive and sometimes take time to have any effect. Resistance to change may be met from a variety of quarters. It is not uncommon for a series of interventions to be employed. Changes should only be for well-defined reasons, with clearly defined goals.

5. Assure quality of analysis
This is essential. In its simplest form, it should be done by taking the view of all interested parties, who should be required to make positive critiques of the analyses and planned intervention. This should include operational staff (e.g. ward nurses) as well as those with managerial responsibilities.

in gathering data and representing them in a useful manner. Finally, remember that systems analysis is an iterative process and you will be unlikely to achieve perfection at the first attempt. Note that it is rare for any two systems analyses of the same task to contain identical elements as tasks of any complexity can normally be described in a number of different ways. Systems analyses tend to converge not in the analysis phase but when the results of the analysis are used as a basis for implementing improvements.

If you are trying to prevent error, you might be in a position to undertake a complete systems analysis by yourself. However, it is more likely that you will have detailed knowledge of only part of the system but not the whole, and so will have to gather data from other people as well. This allows personal viewpoints to be checked against the views of others avoiding subjective biases and invites a range of different perspectives. Once an analysis has been completed it can then be reviewed, step by step, looking for potential failures of the system under study. Some failures will be obvious, others less so. Some failures will be highly unlikely, others potentially quite common. To identify the weak links in a system you must pay attention to the likelihood of a particular part of the system failing and the consequences of that failure.

There is a range of possible outcomes from a systems analysis. It may be that your analysis of a task illustrates fundamental flaws in the design of the system with which you are involved, necessitating a fundamental redesign of the system or the activities within it (jobs or particular tasks). Deficiencies in training may be identified. Effective training requires an accurate specification of training needs, directive inculcation of *skills* and follow-up to ensure that the training has been effective. Training for error reduction depends on a clear specification of situations and scenarios where error might occur (the systems analysis) and identification of parts of the job that might be responsive to training. These need not involve a course or other exotic intervention but might well be something that can be undertaken in a work setting on an intermittent basis. Checklist, guidelines and procedures may also

---

| BOX 9.4 **QUALITY** |

Quality

One of the best ways of reducing errors in any setting is to ensure that the quality of the final product – be it patient/client care, administrative effectiveness or staff training – is of the best possible quality. This, by implication, means that there will be fewer errors as the interventions that will improve quality will reduce errors (among other benefits). It is helpful to provide a brief introduction to 'quality'.

The notion of quality arises from two sources. The first is the idea of quality control, i.e. measuring organizational output of goods and/or services against some defined standard. Waiting list length is the type of measure that might be used in the case of hospital performance, although there are many others, which may give conflicting indications. Quality measurement has led to extensive schemes for quality control. If quality measurement indicates that a system is not performing well, this raises the question what to do about it. From this the notion of Quality Assurance (QA) developed; that is, all the parts of a system that contribute towards the final product or service must perform as well as possible. Thus in order to assure quality, it is important to ensure that such activities in all parts of a system meet certain standards. If this is achieved, then the need for quality measurement inspection, which is often very expensive, will be reduced and overall quality will improve. This change in emphasis leads to the idea of QA. One of the ways in which quality may be assured is by reference to fixed standards, and the modern world is well served with both national and international standards that organizations attempt to comply with. For example, BS5750 and ISO9000 address administrative quality procedures in organizations.

The second approach to quality comes from a different direction, and is termed Total Quality Management (TQM). TQM originated with American ideas implemented in Japan after the Second World War (and not in the US incidentally). Put simply, the key insight was that people do not operate systems, they are part of them and they bring human qualities to the system. These may be beneficial (e.g. flexibility and innovation) as well as detrimental (e.g. not bothering to do things as well as they could and being capable of being demotivated). This view led to the inclusion of the people involved in an organization in the running of that organization. This participation was not an exercise in industrial democracy, but in functional optimization. It involves asking people who run a system what they think about the development of the bits that they are familiar with, and using this information in a productive way. So from one view point, managers manage, design teams design, production teams produce, and rather than each having a set of individual goals or targets, they are consulted, by mechanisms such as quality circles, on their goals, the organization's overall goals and the best ways of integrating these goals and achieving them. The idea is to create a 'brave new world' where the entire organization shares commitment, where discretion and responsibility are distributed appropriately throughout an organization, and where customer needs are seen as one of the prime driving forces for the organization. This leads to so-called Total Quality Management, and is often manifested visibly by the public display of missions statements and commitments to quality.

It is important to note that both QA and TQM can be very useful, but it can also be abused. If you adhere to a set of poorly specified or inappropriate quality standards, then this may impair your function rather than facilitate it. TQM is concerned with flexibility and openness and needs to be adopted by management as well as the workforce and not used simply as a public relations tool. This does not always happen, yet without management commitment TQM will fail. As far as error prevention is concerned, the use of standards should help to assure the quality of individual systems components and the integration of different parts of the system, thereby reducing the likelihood of error. The difficulties arise when there is no suitable standard published for a particular activity. If this is the case, it is possible to prepare operational standards that relate to such an activity. Procedures exist for undertaking this type of analysis and in general they should be based on a detailed task analysis, should be achievable rather than excessively optimistic and should be simple and easy to understand.

be derived from the systems analysis. They normally address complex series of actions and planning where the detail of the activity concerned is such that it renders errors likely. This might apply to a procedure that is carried out very infrequently or one that is complex and has a number of different potential outcomes. A good checklist will be easy to use, will describe operations clearly and visibly and will indicate key decision points.

This overview of systems analysis is only a starting point in error minimization and can be extended into more sophisticated interventions. Two common types of intervention are the implementation of quality systems (see Box 9.4) and of operational feedback systems (see Box 9.5). Quality systems aim to optimize the function of both part of an organization and of the organization as a whole. Operational feedback systems glean information about errors and 'near misses' and feed them back into the organizational management process without attributing blame to the individuals concerned. Although these approaches are not mutually exclusive, they are detailed in separate boxes.

BOX 9.5   OPERATIONAL FEEDBACK SYSTEMS

Learning from errors in the workplace is termed event reporting.

Much can be learned from the mistakes that we all make, but it is not unusual for this valuable source of information to be neglected. Quite often we make errors from which we recover and the insight gained from such errors can be very useful for preventing future errors. There is, of course, a natural reluctance to tell your line manager about the errors you have made as this is likely to colour your line manager's perception of your performance. Many organizations profess to have open error reporting systems, and require staff to report errors through their line management. Quite often if such reports filter through to middle and senior management, the open-minded encouragement to report such errors can be lost in a flurry of anger, culminating in informal or formal disciplinary action.

There are two ways in which this type of problem might be addressed, both of which are known as procedures for 'near miss reporting'. The first and the most obvious is an anonymous reporting system where staff are provided with a form designed in a way that allows them to give details of their own near miss in a way that highlights the details and how the near miss came about. Feedback is anonymous and is collated centrally and disseminated to all interested parties. One of the problems with this type of system is that in small organizations the details of an incident can identify the perpetrator. An alternative is the appointment of an 'operational feedback officer' who sits outside the management structure, who debriefs people who wish to share their near misses and passes on the accumulated wisdom in a general manner to those who need to know. For such a post to be successful two clear criteria must be met. First the operational feedback officer must win the trust of the staff, and second management must accept that confidentiality has to be respected. Such schemes work successfully in a range of different types of activity.

Summary

This chapter has illustrated the complex nature of error, showing how what might be considered an error is completely dependent on the context in which the so-called error occurs. Errors are a useful source of feedback for the success of a range of different interventions, including training, job design, operational procedures and indeed of management strategy. Errors are unavoidable and within certain limits the issue of personal culpability is not one that is useful, although there are circumstances where this might not apply; for example, coming to work under the influence of alcohol. The first step in error minimization is to conduct a thorough-going analysis of all the factors that impinge on the required behaviour. This may be simple when considering, say, taking blood pressure using a sphingomanometer or more complex when considering the safe running of a psychogeriatric ward. No systems analysis is ever complete, as there will always be factors that impinge on performance which are difficult to characterize in a systematic way. One of the signs of a good cogent analysis is if it renders a complex series of tasks into what can be described as 'common sense'. Once potential errors and their probabilities have been identified, steps can be taken to reduce the likelihood of their occurrence. One of the byproducts of a systems analysis is the way in which it induces the analyst to consider all parts of a system in an iterative and eclectic manner. This normally leads to a broader perspective on the system in question, leading to a range of potential improvements, not all of which might be directly related to error.

If a systems analysis helps identify potential errors, it is important to work out how to proceed further by way of organizational interventions. These may take many forms. The use of operational feedback systems coupled with a 'no blame culture' and the implementation of quality systems have been outlined above. Other interventions include providing procedures for activities where errors are likely, identifying and training key skills and job redesign. Further reading on these topics is recommended at the end of this chapter. Bear in mind the fact that error is difficult to consider in the abstract, as this chapter attempts to do. You should gain insight from considering errors that might be made in day-to-day activities such as cooking a meal, programming a video cassette recorder or driving a car. More specific insight might be gained from the Seminar Questions below. Finally, you might usefully consider your own work-based activity. Properly conducted error analyses can form part of risk assessments relating to both patient/client care and health and safety at work and provide useful insights into ways of increasing work efficiency as well as reducing error.

Seminar questions

1. Using a friend or colleague, elicit the stages of the process involved in taking blood pressure using a sphingomanometer and produce an error analysis detailing possible errors, the approximate probabilities of such errors and

possible ways of reducing such errors. Compare your results with your colleagues'. You should use the templates for HTA and FMEA illustrated in Figures 9.1 and 9.2.

2. Using friends or colleagues, elicit the stages of the process involved in managing a general medical ward and produce an error analysis detailing possible errors, the approximate probabilities of such errors and possible ways of reducing such errors. Compare your results with those of colleagues.

3. Compare the types of error found in 1 above with the types of error found in 2 above. State, giving reasons, which types of error are easier to mitigate.

Further reading

Reason, J. (1990) *Human Error.* Cambridge: Cambridge University Press. A thorough grounding in error. The book's strong point is its wide range of practical examples. Do not be deterred by the theoretical treatment of error, which has a tendency to over-complicate issues.

Patrick, J. (1992) *Training Research and Practice.* London: Academic Press. This is a comprehensive consideration of training and addresses both theoretical and applied issues. It is of interest as training is probably the most effective way of preventing error in reasonably designed systems, and training is not easy to do effectively. The book details training needs specification, delivery and training evaluation. It contains a useful introduction to systems and task analysis.

Kirwan, B. and Ainsworth, L. (eds.) (1992) *A Guide to Task Analysis.* London: Taylor & Francis. An extensive practical guide to task and systems analysis, detailing many techniques for collecting and using data, with extensive case studies.

Singleton, W.T. (1989) *The Mind at Work.* Cambridge: Cambridge University Press, especially Chapters 1, 2 and 6. An easy to read book, which provides a good introduction to error and human reliability issues.

Berry, L.M. and Houston, J.P. (1993) *Psychology at Work.* Oxford: Brown & Benchmark, especially Chapters 9 and 13. A good general introduction to psychology in the workplace with useful chapters on organizational issues.

References

Cobb, M. (1990) 'Dealing fairly with medication errors', *Nursing* **20**(3), 42–3.
Forster, C. (1992) *Medication Administration Error.* MSc thesis, University of Hertfordshire.
Kirwan, B. and Ainsworth, L. (1992) *A Guide to Task Analysis.* London: Taylor & Francis.
Reason, J. (1990) *Human Error.* Cambridge: Cambridge University Press.

CHAPTER 10

Psychopharmacology

ELIZABETH A. SYKES

Chapter outline

Introduction: the domain of psychopharmacology

Psychopharmacology deals with a particularly interesting group of drugs, those that primarily affect the central nervous system, and especially the brain, and hence how people think, feel and behave. The term psychopharmacology is a combination of 'psychology' and 'pharmacology'.

'Psychoactive' or 'psychotropic' drugs have various chemical structures, actions and uses, both clinical and social. They include some that are very ancient, such as opiates and alcohol, as well as, at the other extreme, a profusion of recently discovered drugs, including neuroleptics, antidepressants and 'cognitive enhancers' for possible use in dementia. Then there are drugs which are not normally used medically, but have become fashionable partly because of the social myths that have grown up around some of the more spectacular (and illegal) ones – LSD and cocaine, for example. Nurses and others working in the health field are liable to come across most kinds of psychoactive drugs in the course of their day-to-day activities.

This chapter is intended to provide a framework for understanding psychopharmacology, including basic principles of drug action. More details can be found in pharmacology texts, such as Katzung (1992), Laurence and Bennett (1992), Rang and Dale (1991), Snyder (1986) and, to a lesser extent, Hopkins (1992).

Background

Unfortunately there is little space for going into the fascinating history of psychopharmacology (but see Ayd and Blackwell, 1970; Jarvik, 1977). The first modern drug for treating schizophrenic patients, chlorpromazine, was introduced into psychiatric hospitals in the early 1950s, with spectacular consequences (Swazey, 1974). In Europe, its proprietary name was Largactil, allegedly because of its *large* number of *actions*, including antihistaminic, antiemetic and the lowering of blood pressure and body temperature. Although the mechanism was not understood, it reduced the symptoms of mania and schizophrenia most efficiently.

The enthusiasm generated sparked off a pharmacological revolution in psychiatry. The large group of benzodiazepines, which includes diazepam (Valium) and chlordiazepoxide (Librium), for example, was developed and came to replace most of the more toxic and more addictive barbiturates. Other drugs which had appeared unpromising were re-examined, and as a result imipramine (Tofranil), the first tricyclic antidepressant, was discovered. The mood-enhancing effects of iproniazid, given to tuberculous patients to combat their disease, were noticed, and this led to the development of the large group of monoamine oxidase inhibitor antidepressants (McKim, 1991).

The enormous expansion in the development of psychoactive drugs in the 1950s and 1960s transformed the treatment of the mentally ill. Many patients who had failed to respond to other therapies responded well to pharmacological treatment, and this helped to generate the immense and continuing interest in the relationship between brain biochemistry and behaviour. Today, the paramount value of psychoactive drugs for treating mental disorders is generally accepted and drugs are sometimes used in combination with psychotherapy.

Basic psychopharmacology

Definition of 'drug'

In the context of hospitals or a doctor's surgery, a drug is normally understood to mean a medicine and is assumed to be beneficial. The World Health Organization (WHO) defines a drug as 'any substance or product that is used or intended to be used to modify or explore physiological systems or pathological states for the benefit of the recipient'. However, in popular use, the term is often applied only to drugs of addiction or abuse, such as heroin, LSD, cocaine, cannabis and so on, while alcohol may not be regarded as a drug at all (see also Chapter 12). The lack of precise definition can result in misleading interpretations.

Clearly, therefore, care must be taken when trying to define the term. If, for example, a drug is defined as a substance which, by interaction with a biological system, changes it, then it is necessary to exclude such naturally occurring chemicals in the body as hormones and the endorphins, as well as food.

Thus, *a drug may be defined as a non-food substance, which modifies one or more biological systems when it is administered in small amounts and when it is manufactured outside the body.* This definition, although clumsy and by no means watertight (there are still a number of grey areas; for example, trace elements, vitamins), draws out the common factors in all drugs, whether of recognized medicinal value, of homeopathy, of abuse or of all three.

It is important that nurses in particular are aware of the different possible interpretations of 'drug', so that patients and clients are not unnecessarily alarmed by their own, possibly negative, understanding of the word. Therefore 'medicine' and 'tablets' are normally preferred as substitute terms.

Determinants of drug effects

Generally, the effect of a drug is related to its concentration in the body rather than the absolute amount of drug administered. The effect of a drug is primarily determined by:

1. the concentration of the drug at its site of action.
2. the rate of accumulation of the drug at that site of action.

These two factors are affected in turn by:

3. dose, which is the quantity of drug administered at any one time, normally expressed as unit of drug per unit of body weight, e.g. milligrams per kilogram (mg/kg). Most human doses are based on the 'typical' 70 kg man.
4. the route of administration. Injected drugs usually reach their site of action more quickly than drugs taken orally, because of rapid transport via, for example, the bloodstream. They are also likely to have a greater site concentration, since drugs taken by mouth are often partly broken down by the digestive processes; it is estimated that about 90 per cent of an oral dose of mescaline is removed by the liver before it reaches the central nervous system (CNS). Other routes, such as the inhalational, intramuscular, rectal and sublingual, similarly affect a drug's speed of action and site concentration.
5. individual differences. The same doses do not necessarily have the same effects, even within the human species, let alone between species; for example, the same dose of alcohol may make one person feel pleasantly disinhibited

whereas it makes another depressed or aggressive. There can be large differences in the rate and degree of a drug's absorption, distribution, metabolism and excretion, not only between individuals but within the same individual at different times and ages. Older patients are often prescribed lower doses; as metabolism slows with increasing age, so the plasma half-life of the drug may be extended. Diazepam is a particularly good example of this, with a roughly four-fold change between the ages of 20 and 70, requiring a considerable adjustment of dose to compensate. An instance of a drug reversing its effects depending on age is seen with amphetamine, which is a powerful stimulant for adults but is used to 'calm' hyperactive children suffering from attention deficits.

The effects of psychoactive drugs are particularly influenced by expectation, mood, personality and the environment; for instance, a person's response to an illegal dose of morphine may be very different from the same dose of morphine given post-operatively. Where blood concentrations of psychoactive drugs have been correlated with intensity of psychological effects, agreement, except at the extremes (either very low or very high), tends to be poor. For some useful, commonly used terms, see Box 10.1.

BOX 10.1 **PSYCHOPHARMACOLOGY: SOME USEFUL TERMS**

The following terms may be useful in discussing psychopharmacology. They are not definitions, merely indications of the way these terms are used.

Extrapolation (from animals to humans). The process of deriving conclusions from animal behaviour which predict effects in humans even though the two kinds of behaviour may qualitatively have little in common. The only requirement in extrapolating is that the changes in animal behaviour predict changes in humans empirically and reliably.

Dose response curve. A graph showing the relationship between the dose of a drug and the response produced in living tissue. The responses may be behavioural and shown by whole animals, or physiological and shown by isolated living tissue (e.g. gut). The relationship can sometimes be complex.

Tolerance to a drug is said to develop when the dose required to produce a given effect needs to be increased on successive administrations (tolerance is frequently observed with administration of the opiate analgesics and of barbiturates). Another indication is that the duration of the effect of the same dose becomes progressively shorter.

Cross-tolerance. Tolerance (see above) to one drug that extends to drugs of a similar chemical group or pharmacological action (e.g. opiate analgesics).

Tachyphylaxis. The progressive *rapid* diminution of response to frequently repeated doses. It often occurs with drugs acting on the central nervous system (e.g. doses of nicotine repeated at short intervals have less effect than the first dose). Difference between tachyphylaxis and tolerance (see above): in tachyphylaxis, sensitivity to the drug is reduced very quickly, often in a matter of minutes, while tolerance usually describes a more gradual decrease in sensitivity to the drug, taking days or weeks to develop. The distinction between the two terms is not a sharp one.

Withdrawal/abstinence syndrome. A set of distinct signs and symptoms which appear when repeated (self or prescribed) administration of certain drugs is discontinued; the symptoms can be reversed by resuming the addictive drug. 'Precipitated withdrawal' occurs when an antagonist (see below) is given (e.g. the opiate antagonist naloxone given to animals or patients dependent on opiates).

Agonist. A biologically active substance (e.g. neurotransmitter, hormone, drug) which, on combining with a receptor (see below), induces a change in the receptor which initiates a biological process.

Antagonist. A biologically active substance which reduces or neutralizes the effect of an agonist (see above), by chemical, functional or pharmacological means.

Receptor. A specific molecular 'recognition site' for a specific agonist (see above) or series of agonists. When the appropriate agonist binds to the receptor, a biological process is initiated. Receptors in the central nervous system are often found on or in the post-synaptic membrane.

Neurotransmitter. A biologically active substance released from the end of a neuronal axon (see Synapse), which causes an electrical change in the post-synaptic cell via a receptor.

Synapse. A junction between the end ('terminal button') of an axon of a neuron (nerve cell) and the membrane of another neuron.

Potentiation means 'endowing with power', i.e. *any* increase in the effect of one drug which is due to administration of another, e.g. alcohol taken with barbiturates or benzodiazepines can increase the depressant effects of those drugs and so potentiate them; benzodiazepines given simultaneously with barbiturates increase barbiturate sleeping time by potentiation.

Drugs and receptors

Biologically active chemicals of the body which are capable of binding to receptors are often known as ligands, and comprise hormones, neurotransmitters, neurohormones and neuromodulators. Receptors are large molecules, usually composed of protein. When a ligand occupies a receptor, it is said to be 'bound' to it; if this 'binding' triggers activity, the receptor is 'activated'. When the ligand leaves the receptor, it 'dissociates' from it. Some ligands have the ability to remain bound to a receptor for a considerable time; they are then said to have an 'affinity' for it. The capacity of a ligand to activate a receptor is known as 'intrinsic activity'. A ligand which has both an affinity for and an ability to activate a receptor is known as an 'agonist'.

The difference between a ligand and a drug may be summarized as follows: whereas both compounds are capable of activating a receptor, a ligand is endogenous (synthesized within the body) and a drug is exogenous (produced outside the body). Both ligands and drugs usually act at specific sites. Since many drugs act in a similar manner to ligands, they may also be called agonists. In some cases, the drug does not combine directly with the receptor but increases the amount of endogenous ligand available for the receptor. In this case it is known as an 'indirect agonist' (see Box 10.2). Other drugs exert their effects by blocking the action of agonists and are therefore known as 'antagonists'. (For further discussion of types of agonist, see Laurence and Bennett, 1992.)

A common analogy for the interaction of ligands and drugs with receptors is that of key and lock. A drug (the key) fits a matching receptor (the lock) and starts the required biological response. Several slightly different drugs (keys) may fit the same receptor (lock) and each is capable of causing a response, the strength of which depends on the affinity of the drug for the receptor (for example, in the opiate group of drugs, different members of the group have varying degrees of affinity for opiate receptors).

The terminology may seem confusing at first, but it helps us to understand the action of a drug. For example, the drug naloxone is a relatively specific opiate antagonist and can block the effects of opiates; it is therefore used in treating cases of opiate overdose, when it will, among other things, rapidly reverse respiratory depression. It will also cause withdrawal symptoms in opiate-dependent patients. In both cases, naloxone has blocked those receptors which an opiate would normally activate (see Box 10.2).

The impression so far is that receptors are stable entities. This unfortunately is not the case. The number of receptors on the cell surface can change, as can their availability and sensitivity to a ligand or drug. These changes depend on circumstances (for example, the long-term administration of a drug) and can be complex and profound. They are probably linked to homeostasis; that is, the body's need to achieve a stable internal equilibrium.

Dose–response relationships

A drug's actions depend on the amount of drug available which, in turn, depends upon its dose. The relationship between the dose and the response observed is expressed as a dose–response function. In order to get a true picture of the effect of a drug, it is necessary to study a range of doses. This range should cover a dose so low that there is no detectable effect and a dose so high that further increases in dose will have no further effect. This sort of information is obtained by working with groups of subjects, in the initial stages usually laboratory animals, e.g. frogs or mice. Each group is given a different dose of the drug and the percentage of

---

BOX 10.2 **NEUROTRANSMITTERS AND THE SYNAPSE**

Synapse The nerve impulse travels down the neuron, triggering the release of the neurotransmitter into the synapse. Some molecules lock onto receptors, others are taken back into the original neuron by a reuptake mechanism to be 'recycled'.

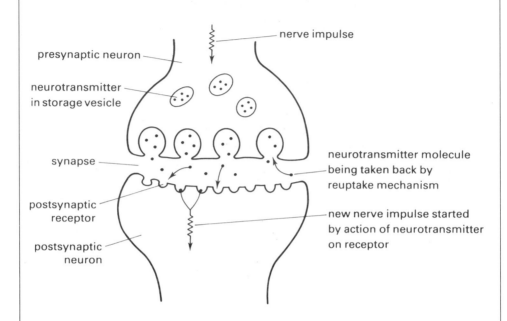

Drugs can affect neurotransmission in a number of ways, of which the following are examples particularly relevant to this chapter:

1. crowding neurotransmitters out of storage vesicles, e.g. amphetamines (indirect agonists) and noradrenaline.
2. blocking neurotransmitter re-uptake, e.g. tricyclic antidepressants and serotonin re-uptake inhibitors.
3. blocking enzymes that degrade neurotransmitters, e.g. MAOIs and noradrenaline/ serotonin.
4. binding to the postsynaptic receptors and blocking neurotransmitters, e.g. neuroleptics and dopamine; naloxone and endorphins/opioids; chlorpromazine and dopamine.

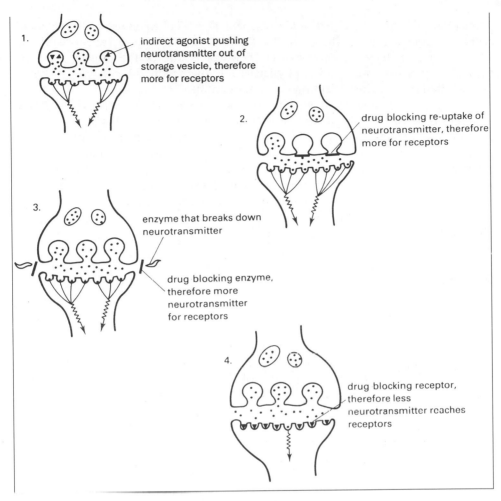

1. indirect agonist pushing neurotransmitter out of storage vesicle, therefore more for receptors

2. drug blocking re-uptake of neurotransmitter, therefore more for receptors

3. enzyme that breaks down neurotransmitter

drug blocking enzyme, therefore more neurotransmitter for receptors

4. drug blocking receptor, therefore less neurotransmitter reaches receptors

subjects in each group that shows a predetermined effect is then plotted. The resulting graph shows the ED_{50} or median effective dose; that is, the dose that is effective in 50 per cent of the individuals tested.

When new drugs are being developed it is common to establish the LD_{50}; that is, the dose that is lethal for 50 per cent of the test animals. (Recently, the use of LD_{50} has become controversial on ethical grounds, and substitute methods are being developed.) Other effective and lethal doses may also be calculated: ED_{99} is a dose that is effective in 99 per cent of cases, whereas LD_1 is the dose that kills 1 per cent of the test animals. Obviously, the further the lethal dose is from the effective dose, the safer the drug. The safety of a drug is often described by the 'therapeutic index' (TI), which is the ratio of the LD_{50} to the ED_{50}; thus $TI = LD_{50}/ED_{50}$. The higher the index, the safer the drug. For example, the TIs for the benzodiazepine group of drugs (chlordiazepoxide TI = 93 and oxazepam TI = 5,714 when used as anticonvulsants) are considerably higher than the TIs for the barbiturates (phenobarbitone TI = 9 when used as an anticonvulsant), which is one of the reasons why the benzodiazepines are preferred by physicians; it is much more difficult for patients to take a lethal dose, either intentionally or accidentally.

It must be remembered, however, that the therapeutic index provides only a crude measure of the safety of any drug used in clinical practice: first, it is based on data obtained from animals, and second, it fails to take account of idiosyncratic toxic reactions in humans. Nevertheless, the TI remains a useful, if general, pointer. Similarly, a dose–response curve is not a perfect predictor of an individual's response, since it does not take individual variations into account. Nevertheless, it provides valuable information as to *probable* response, and the bigger the groups used to provide the data for that curve, the more reliable it is likely to be; a range of 20–50 per group is considered acceptable.

Placebos

What is a placebo?

A placebo (Latin *placebo*: I shall please) is normally defined as a pharmacologically inert substance which is given to benefit or please a patient. In a wider context, a placebo is also seen as any component of therapy that is without specific (biological) activity for the condition being treated or evaluated (Laurence and Shaw, 1984).

There is a strong element of suggestion in any form of treatment (see also Chapter 15), especially in treatment with psychoactive drugs. The efficacy of a placebo is likely to be enhanced by its colour (preferably red, yellow or brown), its size (either very large and thus effective, or very small and therefore potent), its taste (bitter or highly flavoured) and its route of administration (injection rather than oral). The effectiveness of placebo injections may in part be due to the presence of a nurse or physician, because of the respect felt by most people for health professionals (Laurence and Bennett, 1992).

Placebos have many of the characteristics of an active drug. A placebo may show a time–effect curve, although its onset may be later, its effect smaller and its duration shorter than its active counterpart (see Figure 10.1). It may also mimic the cumulative effects shown by repeated doses of an active drug, as well as tolerance. It may even produce unwanted side-effects, for example, urticaria, nausea, and so on (Kornetsky, 1976).

It is possible to increase placebo effects further, by using an 'active' placebo. The active placebo will mimic some of the side-effects of a known drug (e.g. drowsiness), without possessing any of the therapeutic effects. One of the newest non-benzodiazepine anxiolytics, buspirone, seems to have lost some credibility with patients because it does not make them drowsy, unlike benzodiazepines.

Figure 10.1 *Per cent of patients reporting complete relief of postpartum pain at various intervals after administration of either aspirin or placebo (adapted from Lasagna, 1959)*

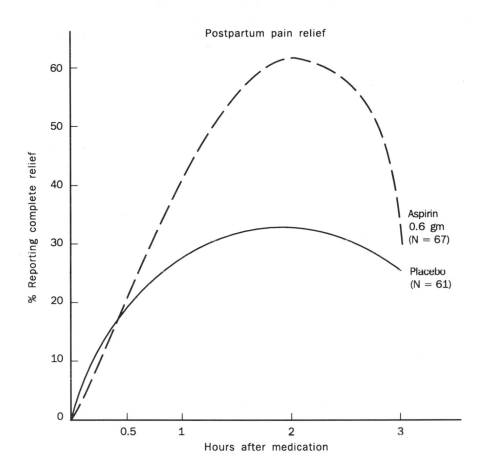

Uses of placebos

Why should one want to use placebos? Placebos are usually given to patients with mild psychological disorders who prefer to attribute their symptoms to physical disease. On other occasions, a placebo can act as a temporary substitute when further doses of an active drug may be harmful, thus retaining the patient's confidence until the active drug can again be given or the condition subsides. Placebos may also be used to reduce addiction to a medicine; in the 1960s, people who became addicted to Drinamyl (amphetamine + barbiturate, also known as 'purple hearts') could be given Drinamyl-X, identical in appearance but pharmacologically inert.

So far placebos have been considered only as inert pharmacological substances. It &has been argued, however, that placebo effects are more wide-ranging and apply to *any* interaction between physician or nurse and patient. The personal attention and the expectations of the professional may play a large role in the positive response of a patient to treatment. It has therefore been suggested that *all* forms of medicine rely, in part, on the patient's expectation of being made better.

In a different role, placebos (better called dummies in this context) are frequently used as controls in the scientific evaluation of drugs ('clinical trials'). A double- or triple-blind procedure can be used to remove any unconscious doctor or patient bias (the patient, the doctor and those involved in evaluating the patient's response are kept ignorant of who receives a drug or a dummy; this is revealed only when the results have been analyzed).

The phenomenon of placebo reaction is well known, though its underlying mechanisms are as yet little understood. Despite recent research reports, modern texts on psychopharmacology usually mention placebos only briefly. See Kornetsky (1976), Jarvik (1977) and Shapiro (1978) for interesting chapters on placebos.

DISCUSSION POINT
How far do you think that your own expectations might affect patients'/clients' responses when you give them prescribed drugs?

Psychoactive drugs

Psychoactive drugs can be roughly divided into those that are predominantly stimulant and those that are predominantly depressant, a classification which is primarily functional and therapeutic rather than chemical or pharmacological, although chemistry can often parallel psychological effects. The result, while convenient, is oversimplified: the classification does not take into account the complexity of the effects of drugs, nor the wide individual variations in responses. Antidepressants, for example, do not normally elevate the mood of those who are just sad; they do, however, elevate the mood of those who are clinically depressed. Small doses of barbiturates may make elderly patients confused but will usually sedate others.

Another problem is that a drug's effects may change from depressant to stimulant, depending on the dose or, perhaps, on the target behaviour. A drug may decrease the frequency of one behaviour and increase the frequency of another at the same time; for example, some tricyclic antidepressants elevate mood while depressing activity by promoting sleep. Similarly, a drug may raise mood at one dose and depress it at another. At low doses, the barbiturates and alcohol can increase activity and raise mood – hence their reputation as stimulants; at higher

Table 10.1 *Examples of psychoactive drugs and their predominant modes of action*

Depressant	*Stimulant*
Anticonvulsants	*Cerebral Stimulants*
Anaesthetics	Caffeine
	Amphetamine
Anxiolytics	Nicotine
[Barbiturates in small doses, e.g. amylobarbitone]	*Hallucinogens*
Benzodiazepines:	Mescaline
Chlordiazepoxide (Librium)	Lysergic acid diethylamide (LSD-25)
Diazepam (Valium)	(Lysergide)
Non-barbiturates:	Cannabis
Meprobamate	*Antidepressants*
Hypnotics	MAO inhibitors (MAOIs):
Barbiturates	Phenelzine (Nardil)
Benzodiazepines:	Isocarboxazid (Marplan)
Nitrazepam (Mogadon)	Tricyclics (TCAs):
Neuroleptics	Imipramine (Tofranil)
Phenothiazines:	Amitriptyline (Tryptizol)
Chlorpromazine (Largactil)	Tetracyclics:
Butyrophenones:	Mianserin (Norval)
Haloperidol (Haldol)	Serotonin re-uptake inhibitors (SSRIs):
[Reserpine]	Fluoxetine (Prozac)
Analgesics	Reversible inhibitors of MAO (RIMAs):
Opioid analgesics:	Moclobemide (Manerix)
Morphine] antagonized	(Lithium)
Codeine by	
Pethidine naloxone	
Methadone]	
Alcohol	

doses, both groups of drugs do the opposite. Nevertheless, and bearing these caveats in mind, the depressant/stimulant dichotomy is a useful, if coarse, method of classification, and it is the one that will be used here (see Table 10.1).

Depressants

The largest and most important group of psychoactive drugs is made up of those that depress some part of the central nervous system. Although all drugs that act on the central nervous system (e.g. anaesthetics and anticonvulsants) belong to the realm of psychopharmacology, in practice there is most concern with those drugs that have subtler psychological effects. Consequently, anticonvulsants and ana-esthetics will not be discussed.

It is likely, although not certain, that depressants act mainly upon the cerebral cortex, the limbic system and the reticular formation. They probably lower the overall level of arousal of the brain, especially by damping down the reticular formation which is primarily responsible for the sleep–wake cycle and for cortical arousal. They may also interfere directly with particular cortical neurotransmitter pathways.

Anxiolytics and hypnotics

The terms anxiolytics, sedatives and minor tranquillizers are often used inter-changeably for drugs which soothe or calm without inducing sleep or impairing consciousness. 'Anxiolytic' is nowadays preferred for all three. *Anxiolytics* are used to treat disorders where the main symptom is anxiety, for instance, in neuroses, and they also help the person to sleep because of the reduction in anxiety. *Hypnotics*, on the other hand, are primarily sleep-inducing rather than anxiety-reducing. Some drugs perform both functions: they are anxiolytic in smaller and hypnotic in larger doses; for example, certain members of the benzodiazepine group.

Anxiolytics and hypnotics are frequently used to treat insomnia caused by stress and anxiety, and it is now known that long-term use of these drugs may lead to tolerance and dependence. Insomnia should be considered as a symptom, not a disease; it is often indicative of anxiety or depression, or may be caused by pain. In either case, treatment of the underlying cause should relieve the insomnia in the long term, although the anxiolytic–hypnotic action of drugs may tide the patient over. Furthermore, it should be remembered that the sleep induced by hypnotics does not mimic natural sleep in all respects; the amount of dream sleep is reduced, for example. Consequently, patients may not be as rested or relaxed by an un-broken night's sleep as they should be.

The older drugs of the nineteenth century which were used to treat anxiety and insomnia (bromide, paraldehyde, sulfonal, chloral hydrate), although still occasion-ally used, were largely replaced by the barbiturates in the early 1900s, by meproba-mate (1955) and by a few other non-barbiturate sedatives. Since the 1960s and 1970s, the barbiturates have been displaced by the benzodiazepines, although some are still used as preanaesthetics and short-acting anaesthetics and in the treatment of severe insomnia. Tolerance can develop within 14 days, as can dependence. They also interact with many other drugs, including alcohol, and can form a lethal cock-tail. The TIs (see above) for the barbiturates are low, so that it is relatively easy for a confused patient to take a lethal overdose.

The large chemical group of drugs known as benzodiazepines contains both hypnotics and anxiolytics; they also have muscle relaxant actions (Garattini, Mus-sini and Randall, 1973). They are thought to act by reducing the excitability of the cerebral cortex: they increase the amount of the inhibitory neurotransmitter gamma-aminobutyric acid (GABA), which in turn binds to GABA receptors and thus prevents those particular neurons from responding to stimulation. Specific benzodiazepine receptors have been found in the brain, which interact with the GABA receptors and this interaction seems to be responsible for the decrease in cortical arousal. Unlike barbiturates, benzodiazepines interact much less with other drugs and have high TIs, and so are considerably safer. In addition, they are said to bestow 'alert tranquillity' on the patient, in contrast to the barbiturates which, in anxiolytic doses, are apt to induce drowsiness. Although on the whole benzodiazepines have few side-effects, dependence is possible and it is usually recommended that no benzodiazepine should be used continuously for more than four weeks. Withdrawal symptoms following dependence can be troublesome and prolonged.

Although the majority of the benzodiazepines fall into the hypnotic/anxiolytic category, this chemical group has a wide range of actions and includes, for example, an antipsychotic (clozapine) and an antidepressant (alprazolam).

DISCUSSION POINT
How would you explain to a client the difference between an anxiolytic and an hypnotic?

Neuroleptics/antipsychotics

The neuroleptics are used primarily to treat schizophrenia and, occasionally, other agitated states; probably the first and best known is chlorpromazine (Largactil). These drugs come from six main chemical groups and are bound together by function rather than by chemical similarity; virtually all are antagonists of the neurotransmitter dopamine in the central nervous system.

According to available evidence, schizophrenia affects about 1 per cent of the UK population; it is a serious illness, with a strong genetic component (see review by Crow, 1982a). The symptoms are usually of two kinds: the 'positive', which include hallucinations (frequently auditory), delusions and thought disorders, and the 'negative', which include flattened affect, refusal to speak, catatonia and loss of motivation. Crow (1982b) has suggested that there are two categories: Type I and Type II. Type I, sometimes referred to as acute, has a rapid onset and a good prognosis, and appears to be caused by a biochemical malfunctioning; the main symptoms are 'positive'. Type II, by contrast, is chronic, has a slow onset and a poor prognosis, and is accompanied by loss of brain tissue; here the symptoms are often 'negative'. It is the chronic schizophrenic patients who constitute a large proportion of long-term patients in psychiatric hospitals.

Type I schizophrenic patients on the whole respond well to neuroleptics, which are thought to restore the dopamine balance by blocking dopamine receptors and so reducing the amount of dopamine reaching the post-synaptic neurons (see Box 10.2). The neuroleptic drugs are particularly effective in reducing 'positive' symptoms, but 'negative' symptoms respond less well. It is interesting that acute attacks may respond almost immediately to medication, whereas chronic states may take three or more weeks to respond.

The side-effects of the older drugs (for example, chlorpromazine (Largactil) and haloperidol (Haldol)) include Parkinson-like movement disorders; one form, tardive dyskinesia, can be irreversible. Newer drugs, such as sulpiride (Dolmatil or Sulpitil) and clozapine (Clozaril), seem to be less hazardous as regards dyskinesia, but not necessarily so on other counts; clozapine, for example, causes agranulocytosis in 1–2 per cent of patients, making regular blood-count monitoring essential (Laurence and Bennett, 1992; Meltzer, 1992).

A convenient form of treatment for long-term maintenance in schizophrenia is by monthly intramuscular depot injections of, for example, fluphenazine decanoate (Modecate). This method also ensures compliance in outpatients.

Stimulants

Stimulants, as their name suggests, stimulate the central nervous system. By far the most important group, medically speaking, are the antidepressants, although it is questionable whether they should be classified as stimulants, since their actions are considerably more complex than the implied 'arousal of the central nervous system'. Caffeine and nicotine are perhaps the most widely used legal social stimulants, while the hallucinogens are an interesting group in their own right.

Xanthines
Three xanthines – caffeine, theophylline and theobromine – occur in plants and are similar, except in potency. Coffee and cola drinks contain caffeine, tea contains caffeine and theophylline, and chocolate has caffeine and theobromine. Theophylline is a more potent CNS stimulant than caffeine and is primarily used as a bronchodilator in severe asthmatic attacks. Theobromine is weak and unimportant clinically (Gilman *et al.*, 1991).

Caffeine is probably the most widely used social drug in the world, although most people would not consider it to be a drug at all. The average daily consumption in tea and coffee drinking countries is about 200 mg. It has a marked stimulant effect, reducing fatigue and, in moderate amounts (200 mg), improving both mental and physical performance (Rang and Dale, 1991). It can disturb sleep and heart rhythm in older people, if taken in large quantities. Withdrawal symptoms of lethargy, irritability and headache may be seen in heavy coffee drinkers if they reduce their daily intake drastically.

Nicotine
Nicotine, which occurs only in tobacco, can act either as a stimulant of the central nervous system or as a relaxant, depending on the dose, the interval between doses and the psychological state of the person. Thus it may relieve boredom (stimulant) or anxiety (depressant). The pharmacological actions of nicotine are complex, but it apparently doubles the metabolic rate during light exercise, which partly accounts for the weight gain experienced by some people on giving up smoking. Nicotine is

the only pharmacologically active ingredient in tobacco smoke, although, in heavy smokers, carbon monoxide may also be involved since it causes a lack of oxygen. In doses used in smoking, nicotine causes the release of monoamine neurotransmitters (for example, serotonin, noradrenaline, dopamine) in the central nervous system; in higher doses, it also affects the peripheral nervous system, including the neuromuscular junctions, and at very high doses it can cause paralysis. It is not clear how nicotine gives pleasure to smokers; it is addictive (although nicotine given i.v. does not entirely replicate the effects of smoking) and tolerance to some of the more unpleasant effects, such as nausea, quickly develops. Some tolerance to nicotine is also as quickly lost, which is why the first cigarette of the day has a more pronounced effect than do successive ones (see 'tachyphylaxis', Box 10.1). Heavy smokers may suffer from withdrawal symptoms such as depression and tremors if they try to stop smoking too abruptly (see, e.g., McKim, 1991).

Amphetamines

Amphetamine and dexamphetamine are the principal cerebral stimulants. In normal volunteers (usually medical students) they have been shown capable of improving skilled performances, inducing an euphoric mood and prolonging wakefulness. During World War II they were used by soldiers to stay awake (Canadian Government Commission of Enquiry, 1971). When this was rashly tried by students working for examinations, results were sometimes disastrous: long periods without sleep made examinees confused and unable to perform (Rang and Dale, 1991).

Amphetamines act by releasing the neurotransmitter noradrenaline stored in nerve endings in both the central nervous system and the periphery (see Box 10.2). They were probably the first drugs to be seriously used clinically as antidepressants, but their effects were more energizing than antidepressant, and there were also cases of dependence and acute overdose with toxic excitement and confusion, not unlike acute schizophrenia. As a result, and because of the arrival of potent antidepressant drugs, the use of amphetamines has become obsolete except in special cases; for example, for narcolepsy and in some hyperactive children with attention difficulties (Canadian Government Commission of Enquiry, 1971; Rang and Dale, 1991).

Hallucinogens

Substances which induce hallucinations and other bizarre mental phenomena have been found in morning glory seeds, cactus buttons (mescaline), magic mushrooms (psilocybin) and the ergot fungus (ergot is chemically related to LSD-25) which grows on rye. LSD-25 (lysergide) itself was discovered fortuitously in the course of Swiss laboratory work about forty years ago; it is not known to occur in nature. All these drugs also have chemical structures which resemble those of three major neurotransmitters: noradrenaline, serotonin and dopamine. The mechanisms by which hallucinogens act differ from one another, although all result in disordered perception and hallucinations, not unlike a schizophrenic state.

A second group of hallucinogens, although structurally unrelated to the monoamine neurotransmitters, has similar effects; the best-known example is probably cannabis. This in its dried form (marijuana) is normally smoked and the effects resemble those of the other hallucinogens, although they are possibly milder. Medicinal uses include alleviating pain and glaucoma.

Despite their name, hallucinations are probably not the major effects of hallucinogens. Behaviour seems to be profoundly affected and it has been known for underlying psychoses to become full-blown as a result. Terms such as 'psychotomimetic' (mimicking psychotic behaviour) and 'psychedelic' (revealing the psyche) have been used to describe these drugs.

The clinical uses of hallucinogens are limited. Psychiatrists have taken LSD-25 in order to try to understand their schizophrenic patients' experiences (Hoffer and Osmond, 1967). Psychiatric patients have also been given small doses of the drug to help them gain insight if other treatments, such as psychotherapy, are 'stuck'. There are great individual differences in reaction, depending on the individual's history, personality and current circumstances. LSD is effective in oral doses of 30 micrograms which makes it a highly potent and hence scientifically interesting substance; it seems to work through reducing the activity of serotonin, though its precise mode of action is not clear. Tolerance to LSD develops quickly, with cross-tolerance between it and many other hallucinogens. However, following dangerous abuse, manufacture of and research on LSD was stopped by the makers in the 1960s.

Antidepressants

Forms of depression are among the commonest mental disorders and, although their classification is still debated, it is usual to distinguish the following:

1. endogenous (occurring without apparent cause) vs reactive (triggered by an upsetting event) although some people have a mixture of the two; and
2. unipolar (depression) vs bipolar (depression alternating with elation and mania).

Endogenous depression affects about 1 per cent of the population, distributed equally between the sexes; reactive depression is found in 3–10 per cent of the population, affecting women more than men and increasing with age (Rang and Dale, 1991). Both endogenous and bipolar depression are thought to be the result of biochemical abnormalities in the brain, which are probably inherited. The symptoms of major depression, which embraces all categories, may be found in the *Diagnostic and Statistical Manual of Mental Disorders (DSM-IV)*.

Monoamine oxidase inhibitors (MAOIs) are a class of antidepressants which increases the level of monoamine neurotransmitters (particularly serotonin and to a lesser extent noradrenaline and dopamine), by blocking the action of monoamine oxidase, the enzyme responsible for breaking them down (see Box 10.2). Consequently, all successful antidepressants are thought to remedy a deficiency in monoamine neurotransmission, although by somewhat different mechanisms. This is known as the 'monoamine hypothesis', which states that, in depression, the levels of monoamine neurotransmitters, particularly noradrenaline and serotonin, are too low because their release from their parent neurons is inhibited; in mania, the release is excessive (Schildkraut, 1965). This hypothesis was supported by the finding in the 1950s that reserpine (which *lowers* noradrenaline levels and was used as a hypotensive drug), also induced depression, not only in patients but in normal people and in animals (Squires, 1978). However, the original hypothesis is now regarded as an oversimplification; if it were correct, antidepressants should work within 30 minutes of administration. In fact, they take days or weeks to have an effect, suggesting that a complex readjustment of the receptor mechanisms is taking place (Bradley, 1989). Among the side-effects of this group of drugs is the 'cheese reaction' between MAOIs and foods containing tyramine, which can lead to severe hypertension.

Tricyclic antidepressants (TCAs) are structurally related to the phenothiazines and are so-called because they have three benzene rings or 'cycles'. They prevent the re-uptake into neuronal stores of released monoamines, primarily noradrenaline and serotonin (5-HT) and so increase their availability (see Box 10.2). Although the TCAs are effective clinically and appear to be faster-acting and safer than the MAOIs, there are side-effects (dry mouth, constipation, occasional blurred vision, possible cardiac risk); these side-effects are probably due to the anticholinergic action of the TCAs, where acetylcholine receptors are blocked at cholinergic synapses in the parasympathetic nervous system (McKim, 1991).

The search for more effective antidepressants with fewer side-effects, lower acute toxicity in overdose, faster action and greater efficacy has resulted in an 'atypical' heterogeneous group of drugs which bear little chemical relationship to the more traditional tricyclic antidepressants. Mianserin (a tetracyclic), for example, has less cardiac risk and hence may be more suitable for people who are elderly; however, drowsiness and weight gain are common. The mechanism by which this group of drugs acts is not yet fully understood, although they appear to block the re-uptake of noradrenaline.

Since the late 1980s, specific serotonin re-uptake inhibitors (SSRIs) have attracted much attention, especially as a result of the success of newer antidepressants such as fluoxetine (Prozac). In this case, the drug prevents the free serotonin from being reabsorbed (and thence recycled) by the presynaptic neuron and consequently raises the amount of serotonin available (see Box 10.2). Although the mechanism is different from that of the MAOIs and the TCAs, this group contains some very effective antidepressants. In addition, the side-effects are less, with little anticholinergic activity, cardiotoxicity, sedative effects or weight gain.

Reversible inhibitors of monoamine oxidase A (RIMAs) are a new class of antidepressants, of which the best known is moclobemide (Manerix). Available in the United Kingdom since March 1993, moclobemide is similar to the classic MAOIs in that it blocks the action of the enzyme monoamine oxidase. However, the MAOIs inhibit the enzyme irreversibly and their potentially hazardous interactions with tyramine and the TCAs are a drawback; they also have a long duration of action. By contrast, moclobemide's binding to the enzyme is reversible, its duration of action is shorter, it has virtually no tyramine interaction and it has a much lower overdose risk. This reversibility also means that a long, drug-free interval is not needed if other antidepressants are to be used subsequently. So far, moclobemide has a very good profile as regards side-effects and safety, but its long-term efficacy has yet to be demonstrated.

Lithium is unlike any other antidepressant (indeed, some refer to it as a 'mood stabilizer' rather than an antidepressant, e.g. Julien, 1992). It is an alkali metal, whose therapeutic value for the affective disorders was discovered, more or less by accident, in 1949 (Cade, 1970). Its mode of action is not clear, but it seems to modify receptor responses to the monoamine neurotransmitters by a complex mechanism. Clinically, lithium is probably the most effective drug for the treatment of manic-depressive (bipolar) disorder, in particular alleviating the manic episodes. It may also be used in combination with other antidepressants for treating or preventing depression (e.g. Dinan, 1993). Its main drawback is that it has a low therapeutic index, so that the therapeutic and toxic doses are close; hence patients on lithium should have their blood plasma concentrations regularly monitored.

All antidepressants have a delay of about two or more weeks before they are fully effective, and it seems that about 70 per cent of patients can be expected to respond (Buckett, 1992). Success rates do not differ between the different groups of drugs; the main advantage of the later generation antidepressants (e.g. SSRIs, RIMAs) is that they have fewer side-effects. On the other hand, there can be great individual differences in the responsiveness of different patients; it is therefore valuable to have a selection of drugs to choose from. Antidepressants have greatly improved the prognosis for depressed patients, although in suitable cases, ECT (which acts quickly), amphetamine and cognitive psychotherapy should not be discounted. One group of antidepressants (SSRIs) has also been found to be useful in panic attacks (Sheehan *et al.*, 1988).

DISCUSSION POINT
A patient is starting antidepressant drug therapy. What would you tell him/her to expect?

Drug interactions

These are becoming increasingly widespread as so many powerful new psychoactive drugs are being introduced. Many drug interactions appear almost entirely undesirable and potentially harmful, and it is perhaps surprising that they were not properly recognized long ago. Alcohol, for example, interacts with most psychoactive drugs and especially with those that have depressant actions; it is only fairly recently that general warnings about interactions between it and other drugs have become prominent.

Particularly interesting, however, is the finding that multiple therapy can be highly beneficial and bestow effects and benefits which cannot be attained by any dose of the separate constituent drugs alone. Examples include Parkinson's disease where a combination of levodopa and selegiline, which prevents the enzymatic breakdown of dopamine and so extends the action of levodopa, is being found more therapeutic than levodopa alone; similarly, the metabolism of levodopa outside the central nervous system is slowed if it is given with carbidopa, which means that smaller amounts of levodopa can be used and so side-effects reduced (Rang and Dale, 1991). Combinations of some antidepressants with lithium seem to be better at preventing and counteracting bipolar depressions than either drug alone for reasons that are not entirely clear (Dinan, 1993).

Doses in combinations need to be worked out particularly carefully and unexpected and sometimes paradoxical effects allowed for. More laboratory work needs to be done if their special benefits and dangers are to be fully mapped (see, for example, Steinberg, 1990). Clinical trials with combinations pose special problems of dose regimes and control groups. Nevertheless, the convenience of one tablet instead of two, with its improved patient compliance especially in elderly people, is another reason why such trials are worthwhile.

Various fixed-ratio psychoactive drug combinations are marketed, e.g. Limbitrol (Roche), which is a combination of the anxiolytic chlordiazepoxide (Librium) and the tricyclic antidepressant amitriptyline (Tryptizol), for people with mixed anxiety–depressive states. Some physicians, however, prefer administering the two kinds of drug separately, since this allows greater control over doses. Certain fixed-dose combinations are inappropriate (and even dangerous), e.g. if the time courses of the two drugs are very different. However, particular patient needs can be effectively met with sensible and wise combinations.

The development of new drugs

A recent estimate put the cost of developing a new drug from the chemist's bench to use in patients at £100,000,000 over ten years (Buckett, 1992). A potential new drug undergoes varied and intense testing. The evidence from these tests is scrutinized by official bodies. In the United Kingdom this is carried out mainly by the Committee for the Safety of Medicines, before the drug can be used therapeutically in patients.

Testing begins in the laboratory. Initially, potential psychoactive drugs are usually tested on animals, mostly rats and mice. Apart from undergoing standard laboratory tests such as ED_{50} and LD_{50}, and acute and chronic toxicity, tests are also conducted for relatively simple behaviour such as sleep and wakefulness, and increased, reduced or disorganized locomotor activity (see Figure 10.2); later, more complex behaviour – for instance, learning various tasks in order to obtain food – is studied.

The standard procedure for a drug that survives these early investigations may be divided into four stages:

1. *Clinical pharmacology*: using between 20 and 50 healthy volunteers, the pharmacokinetics (absorption, distribution, metabolism and excretion) and pharmacodynamics (biological effects, including tolerance, efficacy, safety) are established as far as possible.
2. *Clinical investigation*: pharmacokinetics and pharmacodynamics are further investigated in patients (usually between 50 and 300); dose ranges are also explored.

Figure 10.2 *A simple method for determining ataxia in rats and humans. (1) Prints of the hind feet of a rat walking following an injection of saline [left] and an amphetamine-barbiturate mixture [right] (Rushton, Steinberg and Tinson, 1963); (2) Prints of a human subject walking under control conditions [left] and after a dose of cyclobarbitone [right] (Besser and Steinberg, 1967). Labels A and B (fig. 1) and C and D (fig. 2) indicate the points from which measurements were taken, in mms and cms respectively. The irregularity of the prints has been found to give a good quantitative measure of drug-induced ataxia in both species.*

fig. 1   fig. 2

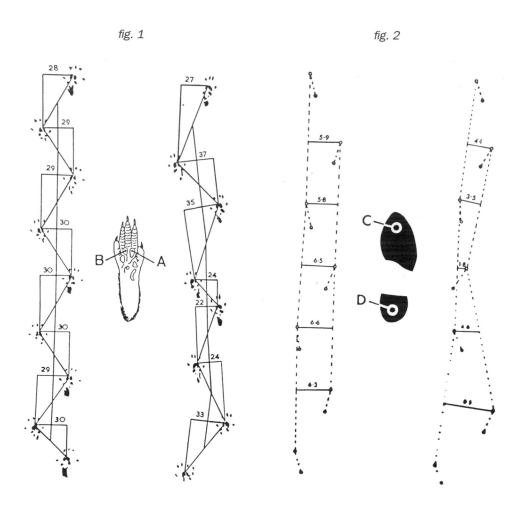

3. *Formal therapeutic trials*: randomized controlled trials, on 250–1,000+ patients, are conducted; the new drug is compared with established drugs and undergoes additional efficacy and safety tests.
4. *Marketing/post-licensing studies*: formal therapeutic trials are continued, with samples of 2,000–10,000+ patients.

Thus a new drug may be tested on thousands of patients before it is agreed to be a medicine by a regulatory authority and is licensed for general prescribing. Equally, the testing may be abandoned at any stage if negative effects are found. Tests of this kind have been developed by pharmacologists, experimental psychologists and clinicians and follow strict rules of reliability and validity. Drugs that may enhance learning and so improve cognitive function in elderly people, are being especially targeted by the pharmaceutical industry.

Drug dependence

Addictive behaviours are discussed in Chapter 12 and opiate drugs in Chapter 13 in relation to the relief of physical pain. Here it should be added only that, from the psychopharmacological point of view, a minimal set of criteria for a drug to be regarded as dependence-inducing should include the following:

1. The effect should be pleasurable and therefore lead to repetition.
2. If the drug becomes unavailable, there should be disagreeable withdrawal symptoms, which can be relieved by reinstating the drug.
3. 'Tolerance' should develop with repetition; thus the pleasurable effects of the same dose become progressively smaller and shorter-lasting.

Additional characteristics for opiates are that the drug should raise pain thresholds and that its effects should be counteracted by opiate antagonists, for example, naloxone.

The search for analgesics that do not have addiction potential continues, but it is possible that the effectiveness of opiates and similar drugs in reducing severe pain is partly due to the pleasurable mood they induce, and therefore this search may fail. Much recent interest has been aroused by the discovery of endorphins, the body's own opiates, which are mobilized in times of pain and stress (Steinberg and Sykes, 1985). This has led to the expectation that other drugs acting on the central nervous system may turn out to owe their actions to mimicry of endogenous substances; such drugs could be used to restore a natural equilibrium which, for whatever reason, has become unbalanced.

Summary

Psychopharmacology is concerned with drugs which selectively affect the central nervous system and therefore emotion, thoughts and behaviour. Some of these drugs are very ancient. Modern psychopharmacology began after World War II with the discovery of the neuroleptic chlorpromazine. The modes of action of drugs are usually complex and partly depend on their absorption and distribution, the underlying drug–neurotransmitter–receptor relationships, and on expectation and suggestion. The main groups of psychiatric drugs in current use are anxiolytics, hypnotics, neuroleptics and antidepressants. Each group contains a number of drugs, some of which may be linked by similar chemistry. Combinations of psychoactive drugs may have beneficial effects and are gaining credence, but caution is needed. Some widely used drugs, such as benzodiazepines, can lead to dependence, as can opiates, alcohol and nicotine (see also Chapter 12).

Psychopharmacology is one of the most rapidly growing and successful subjects which bridges psychology, pharmacology and psychiatry and it has transformed the outlook for innumerable patients.

Seminar questions

1. By what criteria would you judge a new drug to be psychoactive?
2. How would you explain to a new student the relationship between psychoactive drugs and neurotransmitters?
3. How far can psychoactive drugs be said to alleviate symptoms rather than cure them?
4. List the characteristics that an ideal antidepressant would have to have.

Further reading

Barondes, S.H. (1993) *Molecules and Mental Illness.* New York: Scientific American Books. Written by a leading biologist and psychiatrist, this is an excellent book which links the principles of neuroscience and psychopharmacology to recent research into psychoactive drugs and treatment for mental illness. Plenty of clear, helpful illustrations.

Healy, D. (1993) *Psychiatric Drugs Explained.* London: Mosby Year Book. A useful and highly readable book by a practising psychiatrist, which considers the effects and side-effects of psychotropic drugs and highlights the diversity of responses to medication.

Hopkins, S.J. (1992) *Drugs and Pharmacology for Nurses*, 11th edition. Edinburgh: Churchill Livingstone. A useful, well-written and up-to-date guide to the actions and clinical applications of a wide range of drugs in daily use.

Jarvik, M.E. (ed.) (1977) *Psychopharmacology in the Practice of Medicine.* New York: Appleton-Century-Crofts. A useful book, with a particularly interesting (though short) chapter on the placebo phenomenon.

Julien, R.M. (1992) *A Primer of Drug Action*, 6th edition. New York: W.H. Freeman. A non-technical, concise and readable guide to the psychoactive drugs, with plenty of references and a useful glossary.

References

Ayd, F.J. and Blackwell, B. (eds.) (1970) *Discoveries in Biological Psychiatry*. Philadelphia: J.B. Lippincott.

Barondes, S.H. (1993) *Molecules and Mental Illness*. New York: Scientific American Books.

Besser, G.M. and Steinberg, H. (1967) 'On psychopharmacology', *Potential*, UCL Physiological Society **11**, 3–8.

Bradley, P.B. (1989) *Introduction to Neuropharmacology*. London: Wright.

Buckett, W.R. (1992) 'New directions in the development of anxiolytic and antidepressant drugs', in J.M. Elliott, D.J. Heal and C.A. Marsden (eds.) *Experimental Approaches to Anxiety and Depression*. Chichester: John Wiley.

Cade, J.F.J. (1970) 'The story of lithium', in F.J. Ayd and B. Blackwell (eds.) *Discoveries in Biological Psychiatry*. Philadelphia: J.B. Lippincott.

Canadian Government Commission of Enquiry (1971) *The Non-medical Use of Drugs (Interim Report)*. London: Penguin Books.

Crow, T.J. (1982a) 'Schizophrenia', in T.J. Crow (ed.) *Disorders of Neurohumoral Transmission*. London: Academic Press.

Crow, T.J. (1982b) 'Two syndromes in schizophrenia?' *Trends in Neurosciences* **5**, 351–4.

Diagnostic and Statistical Manual of Mental Disorders (DSM-IV) (1994, 4th edition). Washington: American Psychiatric Association.

Dinan, T.G. (1993) 'Lithium augmentation in sertraline-resistant patients: A preliminary dose-response study', *Acta Psychiatrica Scandinavica* **88**, 300–1.

Garattini, S., Mussini, E. and Randall, L.O. (eds.) (1973) *The Benzodiazepines*. New York: Raven Press.

Gilman, A.G., Rall, T.W., Nies, A.S. and Taylor, P. (1991) (eds.) *Goodman & Gilman's The Pharmacological Basis of Therapeutics*, 8th edition. New York: McGraw-Hill.

Healy, D. (1993) *Psychiatric Drugs Explained*. London: Mosby Year Book.

Hoffer, A. and Osmond, H. (1967) *The Hallucinogens*. New York: Academic Press.

Hopkins, S.J. (1992) *Drugs and Pharmacology for Nurses*, 11th edition. Edinburgh: Churchill Livingstone.

Jarvik, M.E. (ed.) (1977) *Psychopharmacology in the Practice of Medicine*. New York: Appleton-Century-Crofts.

Julien, R.M. (1992) *A Primer of Drug Action*, 6th edition. New York: W.H. Freeman.

Katzung, B.G. (1992) *Basic and Clinical Pharmacology*, 5th edition. Connecticut: Appleton & Lange.

Kornetsky, C. (1976) *Pharmacology: Drugs affecting behavior*. New York: John Wiley.

Lasagna, L. (1959) Discussion, in H.K. Beecher, *Measurement of Subjective States*, in D.R. Laurence (ed.) *Quantitative Methods in Human Pharmacology and Therapeutics*. London: Pergamon Press.

Laurence, D.R. and Bennett P.N. (1992) *Clinical Pharmacology*, 7th edition. London: Churchill Livingstone.

Laurence, D.R. and Shaw, I.C. (1984) *A Pharmacologist's Glossary* (printed at University College London).

McKim, W.A. (1991) *Drugs and Behavior: An introduction to behavioral pharmacology*, 2nd edition. Hillsdale, NJ: Prentice Hall.

Meltzer, H.Y. (1992) 'Dimensions of outcome with clozapine', *British Journal of Psychiatry* **160** (Suppl. 17), 46–53.

Rang, H.P. and Dale, M.M. (1991) *Pharmacology*, 2nd edition. Edinburgh: Churchill Livingstone.

Rushton, R., Steinberg, H. and Tinson, C. (1963) 'Effects of a single experience on subsequent reactions to drugs', *British Journal of Pharmacology and Chemotherapy* **20**, 99–105.

Schildkraut, J.J. (1965) 'The catecholamine hypothesis – a review of the supporting evidence', *American Journal of Psychiatry* **122**, 509–22.

Shapiro, A.K. (1978) 'The placebo effect', in W.G. Clark and J. del Giudice (eds.) *Principles of Psychopharmacology.* New York: Academic Press.

Sheehan, D.V., Zak, J.P., Miller, J.A. and Fanous, B.S.L. (1988) 'Panic disorder: The potential role of serotonin reuptake inhibitors', *Journal of Clinical Psychiatry* **49** (suppl.), 30–6.

Snyder, S.H. (1986) *Drugs and the Brain.* New York: Scientific American Books.

Squires, R.F. (1978) 'Monoamine oxidase inhibitors: Animal pharmacology', in L.L. Iversen, S.D. Iversen and S.H. Snyder (eds.) *Handbook of Psychopharmacology*, Vol. 14. New York: Plenum Press.

Steinberg, H. (1990) 'Rodent behaviour tests and antidepressant activity', in B.E. Leonard and P.S.J. Spencer (eds.) *Antidepressants: Thirty years on.* London: Clinical Neuroscience Publishers.

Steinberg, H. and Sykes, E.A. (1985) 'Introduction to symposium on endorphins and behavioural processes: Review of literature on endorphins and exercise', *Pharmacology and Biochemistry of Behavior* **23**, 857–62.

Swazey, J. (1974) *Chlorpromazine: The history of a psychiatric discovery.* Cambridge, Mass.: MIT Press.

CHAPTER 11

Brain damage

JANE M. PIERSON

Chapter outline

Introduction
Functional neuroanatomy of the brain
Causes of brain damage
   Stroke
   Head trauma
   Other causes of brain damage
Psychological effects of stroke and head trauma
Changes in personality and emotionality
   Disturbances of attention
   Language problems
   Memory deficits
Recovery and rehabilitation
Summary

Introduction

Damage to the brain, most commonly as a result of a stroke or a traumatic head injury, may have profound physical and psychological effects. After such damage, the patient's physical deficits, such as partial paralysis or loss of vision, are often the immediate focus of concern. However, it is the psychological problems which, in the longer term, are often the most distressing and problematic for patients, their relatives and the nurses and other health professionals involved in their care. This chapter begins with an outline of the structures and functions of the brain that are relevant for an understanding of the psychological consequences of brain damage. The sections that follow discuss the major causes of brain damage, some of the psychological effects of brain damage and recovery of function in brain-damaged people. The section dealing with the effects of brain damage focuses on stroke and head trauma and is necessarily selective and clinically oriented. Each subsection emphasizes the abnormalities of behaviour which are most likely to complicate acute and long-term care and management and are thus most relevant to students of nursing and other health professions. Details from the case history of a head-

---

BOX 11.1   **HEAD INJURY – A PERSONAL TRAGEDY**

In *The Man with a Shattered World* (1972) the eminent Russian neuropsychologist A.R. Luria gives a moving account of one head-injured person's struggle to surmount his difficulties over 25 years. L. Zasetsky, was a college student who was called to serve in the army during World War II and sustained a bullet wound to the brain. What follows are excerpts from Luria's description of his first meeting with Zasetsky, in a rehabilitation hospital, three months after he was wounded.

> I asked how he was getting on, and after some hesitation he replied shyly 'Okay.' What town was he from? 'At home . . . there's . . . I want to write but I just can't.' Did he have any relatives? 'There's . . . my mother . . . and also – what do you call them?' I then asked him to raise his right hand. 'Right? Right? . . . Left? . . . Where's my left hand?' He made a desperate effort to answer my questions and acutely sensed each failure. I [then] suggested 'Tell me what you remember about the front.' '. . . the attack. I clearly remember it . . . for then, then . . . then I wounded.' It was painful for him to describe what was still fresh in his memory; he simply could not find the words with which to begin. I asked him if he knew what month it was. 'Now? What's the word? . . . It's, it's . . . May!' And he smiled. Finally, he had come up with the right word. When I asked him to list the months of the year, he managed to do this with relative ease and again felt reassured. But when I asked him to list them in reverse order, he had endless difficulties. What did these desperate, futile attempts to remember mean? His response to nature was as keen as ever. He enjoyed the quiet and calm of his surroundings, listened intently to the sounds of birds, and noted how smooth the lake's surface became on a still day. He wanted very much to respond, to accomplish whatever was asked of him. Each failure only renewed his sense of loss. He had no trouble listing the months of the year. Why, then, couldn't he tell me what month precedes September, or indicate his left and right hands? Why was he unable to add two simple numbers, recognize letters, write, remember common words or describe a picture? In short, what type of brain injury had damaged these faculties, yet spared not only his immediate grasp of the world but his will, desire, and sensitivity to experience, allowing him to evaluate each and every failure? (pp. 17–20)

injured patient are given in Box 11.1 to illustrate later discussion and also to provide a preliminary reminder of the profound personal tragedy which lies behind the material in this chapter.

Functional neuroanatomy of the brain

Figure 11.1 shows the central nervous system (the brain and spinal cord) and some of the major divisions of the brain including the *cerebellum*, the *brain stem*, the *thalamus* and the *cerebral hemispheres*. While damage to any part of the central nervous system can result in disturbances of function, it is damage to the cerebral

Figure 11.1 *The central nervous system, with some of the major divisions of the brain indicated. Note that the thalamus, most of the brain stem and other brain structures not indicated here are hidden from view in the intact brain by the massive cerebral hemispheres*

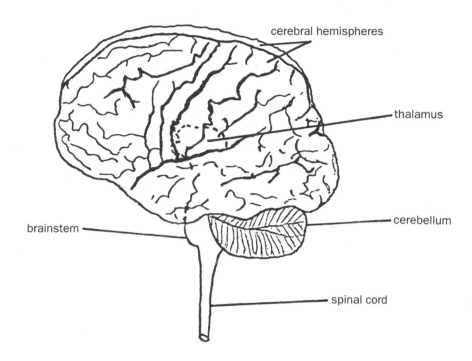

hemispheres and closely associated structures which is most often involved in the psychological deficits discussed later in this chapter. The left and right cerebral hemispheres are virtually identical in structure, although, as explained below, they differ somewhat in function. As can be seen in Figure 11.2, each has an outer layer of *cortex* (part of the grey matter of the brain) and a number of subcortical structures including the *fiber tracts* (white matter). The fiber tracts can be divided into intrahemispheric fibers, which interconnect areas of cortex within each hemisphere, and interhemispheric fibers, which run between the hemispheres. The major band of interhemispheric fibers is the *corpus callosum*. The cortex, fiber tracts and other underlying structures of each cerebral hemisphere are conventionally divided into four *lobes*: the *occipital*, *temporal*, *parietal* and *frontal*. Within each of these lobes are areas of *primary cortex*. Figure 11.3 shows the boundaries of each lobe and the primary cortical areas.

Knowledge about the different functions of each lobe has been derived from a number of sources including the study of brain-damaged patients and the correlation

Figure 11.2 A vertical section cut through the middle of the brain showing the cortex and underlying fiber tracts of the cerebral hemispheres. Note that the corpus callosum, the large tract connecting the two hemispheres, is also indicated. The plane of section is shown by the dashed line in the inset on the lower right (adapted from Dowling, 1992)

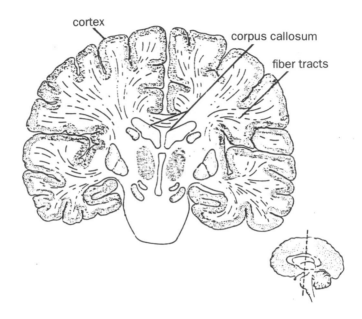

of their behavioural deficits with areas of damage seen post-mortem or in a *computerized axial tomography* (CAT) scan of the living brain (e.g. Andreasen, 1988). Other important sources of evidence include studies using cortical electrostimulation (Penfield and Jasper, 1954), the *electroencephalograph* (EEG), which records the brain's electrical activity, and experimental studies using *positron-emission tomography* (PET) (e.g. Petersen *et al.*, 1988).

The occipital lobes at the back of the brain are principally involved in vision. The *primary visual cortex* within each lobe receives information from the eyes via subcortical regions, including the thalamus. The rest of the occipital lobes are largely responsible for elaboration of visual information.

The lateral surface of each temporal lobe has a *primary auditory cortex*, which is the main target for information coming from the ears via areas within the brain stem. Areas on the medial surface of the temporal cortex and a closely associated region, the *hippocampus*, have been linked to some aspects of memory function. However, localization of memory function within the brain is controversial (Squire and Zola-Morgan, 1991).

Figure 11.3 *A lateral view of the left hemisphere indicating the boundaries of each lobe and the primary areas within each lobe*

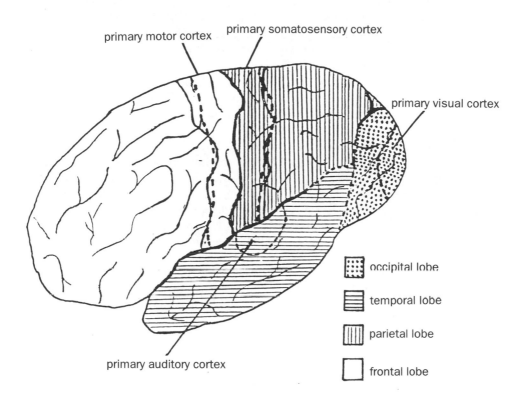

The *primary somatosensory cortex* of the parietal lobes is involved in the sense of touch and receives information (via the thalamus) from sensory receptors close to the surface of the skin and within body tissues. The functions of other areas of the parietal lobes are not well established. They may, however, be involved in processing spatial information such as that conveyed by a map (De Renzi, 1982). Recent research has also suggested that parietal areas may integrate spatial information from the visual, auditory and tactile (touch) modalities (Farah *et al.*, 1989; Pierson-Savage *et al.*, 1988). Areas of the parietal cortex may also be involved in the orienting of attention (Posner, 1990).

The *primary motor cortex* of the frontal lobes initiates movements of all parts of the body and functions in conjunction with other brain areas involved in movement control (see Schmidt, 1988). The rest of the frontal lobes, including the *pre-frontal cortex*, seem to be involved in some of the most sophisticated human behaviours, including the planning of complex sequences of actions, abstract thinking, problem-solving and inhibition of behaviour which does not conform to social rules (Eisenberg and Benton, 1991; Pribram and Luria, 1973).

While the functions discussed above are largely common to both cerebral hemispheres, there are a number of differences between them. Each hemisphere receives input only from the opposite half of the visual field. Thus both visual fields are seen by both eyes but the right visual field is represented in the visual cortex of the left hemisphere and the left visual field in the right visual cortex. The somatosensory cortex in each parietal lobe receives sensations only from the opposite side of the body and the motor movements of each side are largely initiated by the motor cortex in the opposite cerebral hemisphere. This crossed arrangement of projections explains why people with damage confined to one hemisphere often have paralysis and loss of sensation in the limbs on the side of the body opposite to the side of hemispheric damage. They may also have loss of vision, which is confined to areas within the opposite visual field. Note that, in contrast to the visual and sensorimotor projections, the neural pathways between the ears and the auditory cortex are predominantly bilateral and too complex for discussion here. A clear discussion of the auditory system is provided by Moore (1989).

In addition to the differences just discussed, there are also asymmetries in the higher, cognitive functions for which each hemisphere is specialized. In most right-handed people, speech production is controlled by an area in the frontal lobe of the left hemisphere adjacent to the primary motor cortex; the corresponding area in the right hemisphere has no apparent role in speech. Other areas of the left hemisphere have been linked to speech comprehension, reading and writing. However, the extent to which the right hemisphere may also contribute to these language processes is controversial (Baynes, Tramo and Gazzaniga, 1992; Bishop, 1988). In contrast to the verbal specialization of the left hemisphere, the right hemisphere is regarded as being relatively specialized for visuospatial tasks such as judging the orientation of lines or appreciating implied three dimensionality in a two-dimensional drawing. The pattern of hemispheric specialization outlined here appears to be characteristic of almost all right-handers and also of the majority of left-handers, although functional asymmetries may generally be weaker in members of the latter group and in a small minority the pattern may be reversed (Bradshaw, 1989). A further account of many aspects of functional hemispheric asymmetry is provided by Springer and Deutsch (1989).

Causes of brain damage

Stroke

A stroke or *cerebrovascular accident* (CVA) occurs when there is a sudden disruption of the brain's blood supply. Strokes are often a complication of atherosclerosis and hypertension and thus their frequency of occurrence increases with age. In cases of *cerebral ischaemia* blood flow is interrupted because a vessel becomes narrowed or blocked, usually by atherosclerotic deposits or a blood clot. In other cases a vessel may rupture resulting in an *intracerebral haemorrhage*. While the rupture may be a direct consequence of atherosclerosis and hypertension, in other (often younger) people it may be due to a congenital aneurysm which weakens part of the vessel wall. Ischaemia and haemorrhage deprive the neurons in the affected area of oxygen and glucose, and the cells die within a few minutes. In cases of haemorrhage there may be additional disruption of function because the accumulation of blood or *haematoma* exerts pressure on adjacent neural tissue. The ruptured vessel also floods nearby neurons with excessive calcium causing overstimulation.

Head trauma

Traumatic head injury does not have to involve penetration or even fracture of the skull to result in severe brain damage. A *closed head injury* (where there is no skull penetration) may occur when the brain is subjected to strong kinetic forces, either by a direct blow to the head or because of rapid deceleration of a vehicle during a traffic accident. These forces may rotate the brain and tear the protective structures which normally tether it in place, driving the brain against the inside of the skull. The rotation and impact with the skull may damage neural tissue directly and also rupture blood vessels. Blood from such injuries often accumulates in the *subdural space* between the *dura mater* and the *arachnoid mater*, two of the *meninges* or membranes which cover the brain. The pressure produced by the accumulated blood damages and disrupts the function of the underlying neural tissue. Frequently, the force of a blow to one side of the head causes the brain to strike the inside of the skull on the opposite side resulting in a *contrecoup injury*. The forces produced by rapid deceleration of a motor vehicle (and the blow to the head which often follows) may result in multiple areas of damage. However, the frontal lobes seem particularly vulnerable to damage in these circumstances (Walsh, 1987).

Other causes of brain damage

Tumours may form on the meninges or within the brain itself. *Meningiomas* are almost always benign and encapsulated; they damage the brain through the pressure they exert on underlying neural tissue. Other causes of brain damage include degenerative diseases such as Alzheimer's dementia, infections such as meningitis, anoxia (often as a result of a heart attack), exposure to neurotoxic drugs and over-consumption of alcohol. Some of the psychological consequences of these forms of brain damage and those of strokes and traumatic head injury can be similar. However, the remainder of this chapter will focus on the effects of stroke and head trauma. Dementia is discussed in Chapter 24.

Psychological effects of stroke and head trauma

Accounts of the psychological effects of brain damage usually discuss each of the common syndromes independently of each other. These accounts are based largely on people who have very limited areas of brain damage as a result of surgical removal of neural tissue, a localized tumour or an ischaemic stroke which affects only a small, circumscribed area of the brain. Such people may, for example, exhibit an isolated problem with one aspect of language or memory function but have no other impairments. However, cases of this kind are relatively rare. As noted above, those with head injuries often sustain damage to several areas of the hemispheres and as a consequence they may have multiple problems with language, memory, attention and social behaviour. A similar clinical picture is also seen quite often in cases of stroke, particularly where there has been a cerebral haemorrhage.

An appreciation of the multiplicity of interrelated psychological problems which may beset an individual brain-damaged person is vital for the development and implementation of effective care and rehabilitation programmes. Nevertheless, understanding the nature of the deficits themselves is aided greatly by examining them separately. This approach is facilitated by classification of syndromes and in this section some of the common consequences of stroke and head trauma are grouped broadly into changes in personality and emotionality, disturbances of attention, language problems and memory deficits. These groupings are somewhat arbitrary and the distinctions between deficits in each of these categories are not clear cut. It is worth noting in this context that the criteria for classification of neuropsychological syndromes are a matter of debate and the theoretical and clinical utility of extensive neuropsychological taxonomies is questionable (Caramazza, 1984).

Changes in personality and emotionality

Damage to the pre-frontal cortex may be associated with marked changes in personality (see Chapter 7). So called 'frontal patients', who are often young victims of traffic accidents, may become highly irritable and abusive and may be unable to cope with the routines and rules of a medical or rehabilitation ward. They may also experience disinhibition of impulses which profoundly affects their social behaviour. For example, such patients often swear continually and may make unwanted sexual advances toward other patients and staff or urinate in the middle of a crowded corridor. As well as being problematic in themselves, such severe behavioural disturbances also complicate attempts to remediate the patient's other deficits such as language or memory problems, even when these impairments are relatively mild. The interview extract in Box 11.2 provides examples of some of the typical symptoms of frontal damage, as well as the grief and suffering which such symptoms cause for those who are close to the patient.

Management of a behaviourally disturbed, brain-damaged patient is extremely difficult and patients with severe problems often have to be placed in psychiatric

---

BOX 11.2 **THE AFTERMATH OF FRONTAL LOBE DAMAGE**

'I just don't know what to do', sobbed Mrs W. 'He's my husband and I love him but I don't reckon I can stand it any longer. It's like he's a . . . stranger. Before it [the accident] happened he was always pretty easy going but he always had everything organized. Now he gets angry at the slightest thing and he swears all the . . . time – even in front of the kids and he would never have done that before. He's always making these big plans – we'll move to a new house . . . we'll go on a holiday and then five minutes later he's changed his mind before he's even thought about the . . . details, you know. He's still determined to ride his [motor] bike even though he knows he won't be allowed to and I'm dead scared he'll have another accident. He'd never even been booked for speeding or anything before, but now he just doesn't seem to care about the laws and that. . . . Most of our friends have stopped visiting him and I'm not surprised. Last time C came he tried to undo her shirt! I was so embarrassed. . . . I just keep waiting for the old J to come back, but I know he won't. It's his head and it won't get much better, that's what they say. Most of the time he doesn't seem to realize he's changed, but the other day he was in tears and he said "Don't leave me", but what can I do?'

---

wards. This is unsatisfactory as some of their needs are different from those of other psychiatric patients. However, there are few units which provide specialist rehabilitation of cognitive and other deficits for patients who also have severe behavioural problems. In less serious cases, behaviour modification may help to control a patient's outbursts. For example, the patient can be ignored when swearing and rewarded when pleasant. However, to be successful, tactics of this kind need to be employed consistently by all members of the health care team and in practice this is often difficult to achieve.

Changes in emotionality may appear in conjunction with both stroke and head injury. Several studies reviewed by Heller (1990) reported that up to 60 per cent of people with left frontal-lobe lesions met the DSM III criteria for diagnosis of depression. (DSM provides criteria for the diagnosis of psychological conditions.) In contrast, people with right hemisphere damage may be euphoric and unconcerned about the physical and psychological consequences of their brain damage. Such people may also display inappropriate affect, bursting into tears for no reason or being happy when told of a sad event such as the death of a loved one. Disruption of emotions after right hemisphere damage seems particularly marked in cases where there are lesions in the parietal and temporal lobes.

Mood disorders in brain-damaged patients are not always the direct consequence of damage to areas of the brain which mediate emotional responses. In some cases they may simply be a reaction to hospitalization and loss of physical and cognitive capacities. The assumption that little can be done about an affective disorder because it is caused by the patient's brain damage is a dangerous one. Patients viewed in this way may be deprived of the understanding and support which could do much to improve both their mental state and their prognosis during the traumatic and confusing period after a stroke or head injury.

Disturbances of attention

After suffering brain damage, patients may have problems with attending to a conversation or task for any length of time. In some cases, particularly where there is a significant degree of frontal lobe involvement, the patient may be highly distractable, having an attention or concentration span of only a few seconds. Such problems in sustaining attention often co-occur with the changes in personality and emotionality which were discussed above. Patients with difficulties in sustaining attention may become frustrated and easily fatigued when required to do anything needing extended concentration, and these problems may be particularly marked when an ordered sequence of steps must be followed. However, performance can sometimes be improved if the patient is highly motivated or if the task is structured in a way that allows frequent short breaks during its completion.

DISCUSSION POINT
How might you improve a patient's motivation to complete a task and thus help overcome concentration problems stemming from frontal lobe damage?

Difficulty in orienting attention may also be seen in some people with frontal damage (Crowne, 1983) and may be particularly marked in those with parietal lesions (Posner, 1990). People with parietal damage may fail to turn their head and eyes to pay attention to events such as a light flash or the opening of a door, which would invoke an orienting response in a person who is not brain-damaged.

When there has been unilateral damage to one cerebral hemisphere, people may show signs and symptoms of *hemineglect* (see, for example, Robertson and Marshall, 1993). This syndrome is fairly common and is usually associated with strokes. However, it may also result from traumatic head injury and other types of brain damage. The acute behavioural manifestations of hemineglect are quite dramatic as patients fail to respond to objects and events in the side of space which is opposite the damaged hemisphere. Thus, patients with right hemisphere damage and left hemineglect may not dress or groom their left sides and may eat food only from the right side of a plate, leaving food on the left untouched. When asked to copy a drawing or draw from memory they may leave out or distort left side details or misplace them to the right side of the drawing. Figure 11.4 shows a clock face completed from memory by a patient with damage to the right parietal lobe and left hemineglect.

While the visual manifestations of hemineglect may be the most obvious, symptoms can also appear in the auditory and tactual modalities.

Hemineglect can appear after damage to either hemisphere but left neglect after right hemisphere damage is widely held to be more common and more severe than right neglect after left hemisphere damage. It has, however, been argued that the incidence of right neglect is underestimated because its symptoms are less obvious than those of language disturbance, which is relatively common after left hemisphere damage but rare after right hemisphere damage. Difficulties with language become the focus of attention for those involved in caring for the patient and the more subtle symptoms of right hemineglect may be missed (Ogden, 1987).

Figure 11.4 *A clock face completed from memory by a patient with left hemineglect (see text for explanation)*

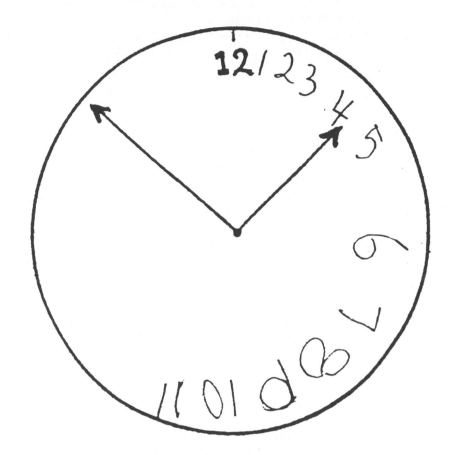

It can be demonstrated that people with hemineglect can see, hear and feel objects or events located in the neglected side of space. Thus, the mechanisms underlying their failure to respond to such stimuli are controversial and there are competing models of hemineglect (Bisiach and Vallar, 1988; Heilman and Valenstein, 1985). However, the problem seems to be at least partly attentional in nature. Recent experiments have shown that patients with hemineglect may respond to items on the neglected side if their attention is drawn to them by a cue placed on that side (e.g. Mattingley *et al.*, 1993). These findings suggest that rehabilitation of people with hemineglect can be aided by practices which encourage allocation of attention to the neglected side. For example, the nurse or therapist could position him or herself on the person's non-neglected side at the start of a conversation and then gradually move to the neglected side during the course of the interaction.

DISCUSSION POINT
The difficulties in sustaining attention and the changes in personality outlined in this and the preceding section are often profoundly distressing for both patients and their relatives. In desperation, members of a patient's family may approach *anyone* in the hospital for support and advice. If you were approached by Mrs W (Box 11.2), what would you say? What practical suggestions could you make to help her deal with her situation?

Language problems

Anomia, or difficulty in finding words when speaking, is often observed in acutely brain-damaged patients. The problem is illustrated by the interview with L. Zasetsky in Box 11.1 and is somewhat like the 'tip of the tongue' phenomenon which most people (without brain damage) also experience on occasions. Patients clearly know the word they want to use but are unable to find it at the appropriate point in a conversation. While such word-finding difficulties often resolve quite quickly after brain damage, they remain a persistent and frustrating problem for some people.

Anomia is only one of a large number of spoken language deficits or *aphasias* which may be acquired, usually as a result of left hemisphere stroke and trauma. People with such lesions may have difficulty in producing speech even if they do not have problems in actually controlling movements of the vocal musculature. In some people all speech is slow, effortful and largely devoid of grammatical structure – symptoms which, along with others, are diagnostic of *Broca's aphasia*. In other cases there may be deficits in speech comprehension and in some people production and comprehension problems co-occur. If people have problems with producing or understanding speech it might seem sensible to have them write down what they want to say and also to write down instructions for them. While in a few cases this does aid communication, many people with aphasia also have acquired *dyslexia*, which results in difficulties with reading and writing.

People with aphasia and dyslexia have been very widely studied and this work has generated a vast clinical and empirical literature. Clear and accessible accounts of the symptoms of acquired language impairment and strategies for management and rehabilitation can be found in a number of texts. Thus these topics will not receive further consideration here (for aphasia, see Goodglass, 1988; Howard and Hatfield, 1987; for acquired dyslexia, see Ellis, 1993).

Memory deficits

Disturbance of memory (see Chapter 8) is common after brain damage, particularly if it results from traumatic head injury. Patients often fail to remember the accident itself, the events that preceded it and the period immediately afterward. They may also have initial difficulties in retaining new information such as the name of the doctor who is treating them or the number of their ward. In many patients such difficulties are relatively transient. However, a subset of both stroke and head injury cases have permanent memory deficits or *amnesia*. For some brain-damaged people, persistent memory dysfunction is reflective of an overall decline in cognitive capacity. However, it may also appear in conjunction with relatively normal levels of intellect and awareness. (For discussion of procedures which differentiate memory problems from general intellectual impairment, see Parkin and Leng, 1993.) While amnesia may be apparent after stroke and head trauma, it is more commonly seen in cases of *Korsakoff's syndrome*. In these patients brain damage is usually a consequence of chronic alcohol abuse.

Amnesia seems to be associated with bilateral damage to a number of closely interconnected limbic system structures, including the hippocampus (Butters and Miliotis, 1985). Amnesia has two key features, *anterograde amnesia* and *retrograde amnesia*, which co-occur in most amnesic patients. Anterograde deficits are difficulties in remembering events that have occurred since brain damage was sustained. Retrograde deficits are problems with remembering material acquired in any period before brain damage occurred. Some patients with amnesia also *confabulate* or make up fictitious details about themselves, usually when faced with questions they cannot answer. Confabulation may reflect the patient's desire to hide his or her memory difficulties.

Anterograde amnesia seems to reflect a difficulty in transferring material from short-term memory (which can retain material for only about 30 seconds) to a more permanent long-term store (Squire and Zola-Morgan, 1991). Such problems in consolidating new information severely hinder patient care and rehabilitation. When, for example, a patient is shown a simple exercise she or he may be able to demonstrate the exercise immediately afterward. However, if questioned minutes later the patient may remember neither the exercise nor even the nurse or therapist who demonstrated it!

DISCUSSION POINT
Patients who fail to complete exercises or follow other instructions are often viewed as uncooperative and lacking in motivation to recover. How could you distinguish between failure to comply due to an attitude problem and failure due to amnesia?

Anterograde memory impairments are severe in many people with amnesia and seem to prevent acquisition of a wide range of new material. Experimental studies have, however, shown that there are some types of learning which are relatively unimpaired. These include acquisition of classically conditioned responses (Daum, Channon and Canavan, 1989; see Box 7.2, p. 137) and attainment of certain novel motor skills, for example, mirror drawing (Milner, 1965). The person may, however, retain the ability to perform the new motor task but be unable to recall learning it or performing it previously. Further discussion of implicit learning in amnesic patients is provided in Chapter 8.

Retrograde amnesia is usually far from complete. The very rare cases of total retrograde amnesia which are sometimes reported in the popular press involve people with psychological problems rather than damage to the brain (Kopelman, 1987). Brain-damaged amnesic patients usually retain their linguistic knowledge and a basic outline of their life history. However, it is often claimed that retrograde amnesia is characterized by a temporal gradient. Thus, memory for recent events (which occurred not long before the onset of amnesia) may be more impaired than memory for events which are relatively remote in time (e.g. events which occurred in a middle-aged patient's early adult years).

The notion of a temporal gradient in retrograde amnesia is controversial. It is based largely on qualitative clinical observations of patients' autobiographical memories and may be artefactual, reflecting a difference in the relative salience of events from the remote and the more recent past. Important events, which are thus remembered (e.g. marriage and the birth of children) are more likely to have occurred in the relatively remote rather than the recent past for middle-aged and elderly patients. A temporal gradient has not been demonstrated in some experimental studies where the relative salience of information from the remote and recent past has been carefully controlled. For example, Warrington and McCarthy (1988) tested an amnesic patient's memory for non-autobiographical information (the identity of famous people) from a range of time frames. The public figures, whose faces were depicted in the pictures used in the study, were matched for their salience or importance during the time period in which they became famous. The patient's memory was found to be impaired for faces from all the time frames used and there was no evidence that people from the recent past were more poorly remembered than those from the relatively remote past.

The pattern of amnesic deficits discussed above is only one of several patterns of memory disturbance which may appear after brain damage. Memory deficits associated with dementia are discussed in Chapter 24. For a comprehensive account of memory processes and memory deficits, see, for example, Squire (1987).

Recovery and rehabilitation

Cognitive and other problems resulting from stroke or head trauma usually improve somewhat during the first few months after brain damage is sustained. Improvement in function may come more slowly as the time since damage increases, but some people continue to make small gains several years after suffering a stroke or head trauma (Dombovy and Bach-y-Rita, 1988). The extent of improvement varies quite considerably from person to person and depends in part on the particular cognitive processes which are affected. For example, in many patients with hemineglect, clinically evident symptoms disappear within six months, although some deficits may still be elicited by subtle testing (Pierson-Savage et al., 1988). By contrast, the language problems of Broca's aphasia may show little improvement.

In some cases of head injury or haemorrhagic stroke initial improvement in function can be attributed to reduction of pressure when haematoma and swelling of the brain subside. The mechanisms underlying more long-term recovery of function after brain damage are not fully understood. Lost neurons are not replaced and damaged axons of cells within the central nervous system do not appear to regenerate. Empirical neuroanatomical and neurophysiological evidence suggests, however, that undamaged axons adjacent to dead neurons may develop new sprouts or become physiologically more responsive (Cotman and Nieto-Sampedro, 1982; Kaas, Merzenich and Killackey, 1983; Marshall, Drew and Neve, 1983). Nevertheless, it is likely that these changes make only a limited contribution to recovery after brain damage. Improvements in cognitive and other functions are probably the result of some form of compensation for the deficits. In some cases, such compensation may be attributed to the employment of strategies taught during rehabilitation.

The specialized topics of neuropsychological assessment and rehabilitation are quickly becoming a literature in themselves and cannot be given further consideration here. Crawford, Parker and McKinlay (1992) provide a useful discussion of assessment and there are several excellent, clinically oriented texts which describe neuropsychological rehabilitation, including Prigatano (1986). There is, however, little published research which has aimed at establishing the factors responsible for improvements in cognitive function during rehabilitation and few quantitative evaluations of the outcome of neuropsychological rehabilitation programmes. More collaborative research involving academics and those directly involved in patient care and rehabilitation is needed to maximize the benefits of such rehabilitation and to ensure that it is cost effective.

Summary

The cerebral hemispheres of the brain are each divided into four lobes which have different functions. The psychological effects of hemispheric damage depend in part on the lobes involved. Strokes and head trauma are the most common of a number of causes of damage. The effects of strokes and head trauma include changes in personality. Patients (particularly those with frontal lobe damage) may become highly irritable and engage in socially unacceptable behaviour. Concentration may also be impaired and some patients (particularly those with parietal lobe damage) may have problems with directing attention to the location of events. Damage to the left hemisphere often results in deficits in producing and understanding spoken and written language. Memory disturbances are common and often transient, but some patients have permanent memory problems. Some recovery is usual after brain damage and improvement probably reflects compensation for deficits which may be aided by rehabilitation.

Seminar questions

1. Outline practices not discussed in the chapter which may aid in the care and management of brain-damaged patients with psychological deficits. To help in

answering this question, you may wish to consult Prigatano (1986) or a similar text.

2. Using the further reading as a starting point, consider some of the empirical studies which have examined the psychological effects of brain damage. Outline other studies which could further the investigation of these effects.

3. Budgetary constraints often mean that intensive neuropsychologcial rehabilitation cannot be offered to all patients who need it. Should someone who habitually drives when drunk and sustains brain damage in a car accident have the same right to rehabilitation as someone whose damage is due to a ruptured aneurysm?

Further reading

McCarthy, R.A. and Warrington, E.K. (1990) *Cognitive Neuropsychology*. London: Academic Press. Provides a relatively up-to-date and advanced level coverage of clinical and experimental studies of the psychological effects of brain damage.

Sacks, O. (1985) *The Man who Mistook his Wife for a Hat*. London: Pan Books. Case histories of brain-damaged patients narrated in a lively style.

Springer, S.P. and Deutsch, G. (1989) *Left Brain, Right Brain*, 3rd edition. New York: W.H. Freeman. A very readable account of insights into functional brain asymmetry which have come from research with brain-damaged, split-brain and normal right- and left-handed subjects.

References

Andreasen, N.C. (1988) 'Brain imaging: Applications in psychiatry', *Science* **239**, 1381–8.

Baynes, K., Tramo, M.J. and Gazzaniga, M. S. (1992) 'Reading with a limited lexicon in the right hemisphere', *Neuropsychologia* **30**, 187–200.

Bishop, D. (1988) 'Can the right hemisphere mediate language as well as the left? A critical review of recent research', *Cognitive Neuropsychology* **5**, 353–67.

Bisiach, E. and Vallar, G. (1988) 'Hemineglect in humans', in F. Boller and J. Grafman (eds.) *Handbook of Neuropsychology*, Vol. 1. Amsterdam: Elsevier.

Bradshaw, J.L. (1989) *Hemispheric Specialization and Psychological Function*. Chichester: John Wiley.

Butters, N. and Miliotis, P. (1985) 'Amnesic disorders', in K.M. Heilman and E. Valenstein (eds.) *Clinical Neuropsychology*, 2nd edition. New York: Oxford University Press.

Caramazza, A. (1984) 'The logic of neuropsychological research and the problem of patient classification in aphasia', *Brain and Language* **21**, 9–20.

Cotman, C.W. and Nieto-Sampedro, M. (1982) 'Brain function, synapse renewal, and plasticity', *Annual Review of Psychology* **33**, 371–401.

Crawford, J., Parker, D. and McKinlay, W. (1992) *A Handbook of Neuropsychological Assessment*. Hove: Lawrence Erlbaum.

Crowne, D.P. (1983) 'The frontal eye field and attention', *Psychological Bulletin* **93**, 232–60.

Daum, I., Channon, S. and Canavan, A.G.M. (1989) 'Classical conditioning in patients with severe memory problems', *Journal of Neurology, Neurosurgery and Psychiatry* **52**, 47–51.

De Renzi, E. (1982) *Disorders of Space Exploration and Cognition.* Chichester: John Wiley.

Dombovy, M.L. and Bach-y-Rita, P. (1988) 'Clinical observations on recovery from stroke', in S.G. Waxman (ed.), *Advances in Neurology.* New York: Raven Press.

Dowling, J.E. (1992) *Neurons and Networks.* Cambridge, Mass.: Harvard University Press.

Ellis, A. W. (1993) *Reading, Writing and Dyslexia: A cognitive analysis*, 2nd edition. Hove: Lawrence Erlbaum.

Farah, M.J., Wong, A.B., Monheit, M.A. and Morrow, L.A. (1989) 'Parietal lobe mechanisms of spatial attention: Modality specific or supramodal?' *Neuropsychologia* **27**, 461–70.

Goodglass H. (1988) 'Language and aphasia', in F. Boller and J. Grafman (eds.) *Handbook of Neuropsychology*, Vol. 1. Amsterdam: Elsevier.

Heilman, K.M. and Valenstein, E. (1985) *Clinical Neuropsychology*, 2nd edition. New York: Oxford University Press.

Heller, W. (1990) 'The neuropsychology of emotion: Developmental patterns and the implications for psychopathology', in N.L. Stein, B. Leventhal and T. Trabasso (eds.) *Psychological and Biological Approaches to Emotion.* Hillsdale, NJ: Lawrence Erlbaum.

Howard, D. and Hatfield, F.M. (1987) *Aphasia Therapy: Historical and contempory issues.* Hove: Lawrence Erlbaum.

Kaas, J.H., Merzenich, M.M. and Killackey, H.P. (1983) 'The reorganization of somatosensory cortex following peripheral nerve damage in adult and developing mammals', *Annual Review of Neuroscience* **6**, 325–56.

Kopelman, M.D. (1987) 'Amnesia: Organic and psychogenic', *British Journal of Psychiatry* **150**, 428–42.

Levin, H.S., Eisenberg, H.M. and Benton, A.L. (1991) *Frontal Lobe Function and Dysfunction.* New York: Oxford University Press.

Luria, A. R. (1972) *The Man with a Shattered World: The history of a brain wound.* New York: Basic Books.

Marshall, J.C., Drew, M.C. and Neve, K.A. (1983) 'Recovery of function after mesotelencephalic dopaminergic injury in senesence', *Brain Research* **259**, 249–60.

Mattingley, J.B., Pierson, J.M., Bradshaw, J.L., Phillips, J.G. and Bradshaw, J.A. (1993) 'To see or not to see: The effects of visible and invisible cues on line bisection judgements in unilateral neglect', *Neuropsychologia* **31**, 1201–15.

Milner, B. (1965) 'Visually guided maze learning in man: Effects of bilateral hippocampal, bilateral frontal and unilateral cerebral lesions', *Neuropsychologia* **3**, 317–38.

Moore, B.C.J. (1989) *An Introduction to the Psychology of Hearing*, 3rd edition. London: Academic Press.

Ogden, J.A. (1987) 'The "neglected" left hemisphere and its contribution to visuospatial neglect', in M. Jeannerod (ed.) *Neurophysiological and Neuropsychological Aspects of Spatial Neglect.* Amsterdam: Elsevier.

Parkin, A.J. and Leng, N.R.C. (1993) *Neuropsychology of the Amnesic Syndrome.* Hove: Lawrence Erlbaum.

Penfield, W. and Jasper, J. (1954) *Epilepsy and the Functional Anatomy of the Human Brain.* Boston: Little, Brown.

Petersen, S.E., Fox, P.T., Posner, M.I., Mintun, M. and Raichle, M.E. (1988) 'Positron emission tomographic studies of the cortical anatomy of single-word processing', *Nature* **331**, 585–9.

Pierson-Savage, J.M., Bradshaw, J.L., Bradshaw, J.A. and Nettleton, N.C. (1988) 'Vibrotactile reaction times in unilateral neglect', *Brain* **111**, 1531–45.

Posner, M.I. (1990) 'Hierarchical distributed networks in the neuropsychology of selective attention', in A. Caramazza (ed.) *Cognitive Neuropsychology and Neurolinguistics.* Hillsdale, NJ: Lawrence Erlbaum.

Pribram, K.H. and Luria, A.R. (1973) *Psychophysiology of the Frontal Lobes.* New York: Academic Press.

Prigatano, G.P. (1986) *Neuropsychological Rehabilitation after Brain Injury.* Baltimore, MD: Johns Hopkins University Press.

Robertson, I.H. and Marshall, J. (1993) *Unilateral Neglect: Clinical and experimental studies.* Hove: Lawrence Erlbaum.

Schmidt, R.A. (1988) *Motor Control and Learning*, 2nd edition. Champaign, Ill.: Human Kinetics Publishers.

Springer, S.P. and Deutsch, G. (1989) *Left Brain, Right Brain*, 3rd edition. New York: W.H. Freeman.

Squire, L.R. (1987) *Memory and Brain.* New York: Oxford University Press.

Squire, L.R. and Zola-Morgan, S. (1991) 'The medial temporal lobe memory system', *Science* **253**, 1380–6.

Walsh, K.I. (1987) *Neuropsychology, a clinical approach*, 2nd edition. Edinburgh: Churchill Livingstone.

Warrington, E.K. and McCarthy, R.A. (1988) 'The fractionation of retrograde amnesia', *Brain and Cognition* **7**, 184–200.

PART III

Life processes and events

Most of us are required to deal with many of the events, habits or processes discussed in this section. Health professionals are as likely as anyone to experience these events and processes. Additionally, however, they are expected to understand the effects these have on others; for example, the way a medical procedure or hospital admission might be stressful and how this stress might influence health outcomes.

Chapter 12 examines the common addictions of drinking alcohol, smoking cigarettes and overeating. Starr and Chandler address the questions of why people indulge in these risky behaviours and why they find them so difficult to control. The role of the health professional in helping those who are addicted to change their behaviour is discussed.

The experience of pain is ubiquitous and causes great distress for those who suffer, and is therefore an important topic for many health professionals. Chapter 13 outlines the physiological mechanisms and psychological processes involved in pain perception. A resumé is provided of the current approaches employed in pain management.

In recent years, the subject of stress has received considerable attention. Chapter 14 examines models of occupational stress and considers how adequately they explain the stress experienced by health professionals. The chapter also discusses stress in patients and how this can best be alleviated. Finally, there is an examination of how technological changes might be introduced so that staff will experience minimum stress and patients will experience maximum benefit.

Chapter 15 discusses a related topic, the consequences of stress for health. Particular attention is paid to the effects of stress on the immune system, on the development of cancer and on heart disease. This leads on to a model which is proposed to explain the way that environmental demands lead to stress.

Death, of course, comes to us all eventually and the experience of loss and bereavement is inescapable if one lives long enough. Chapter 17 utilizes the attachment model to discuss the reactions of those who are dying or bereaved. The difficulties that nurses and other carers might experience when caring for those who are dying are also explored.

Following this, the psychological consequences of HIV infection are examined in Chapter 16. Although HIV infection is not a common life event, the issues surrounding HIV and AIDS bring together processes and events that have relevance to all health care professionals.

CHAPTER 12

Common addictive behaviours

BERYL S. STARR AND C.J. CHANDLER

Chapter outline

Introduction

People engage in many different behaviours which may harm their health. This chapter will consider examples of such behaviours which are relatively common and can have serious health consequences. The behaviours chosen, *drinking excessive amounts of alcohol*, *smoking nicotine cigarettes* and *overeating*, are ones that are likely to be met by a health care specialist either as a direct cause of an illness or as part of preventative health care programmes. The questions we shall ask are:

1. Why do we engage in smoking, drinking alcohol excessively and overeating?
2. Why do some people find it so difficult to control these behaviours?
3. What can be done to help individuals break potentially harmful habits?

What is meant by the term 'addictive behaviour'? Addiction is a concept often evoked in the face of compulsive behaviours. It was originally coined in the context of drug abuse and it implies that a person has become physically and psychologically dependent on a drug. *Physical dependence*, where the body has adapted to the drug, has two characteristics: (1) *tolerance*, where bigger and bigger doses are required to achieve the same effect; (2) and *withdrawal*, where the person experiences

231

> **BOX 12.1   THE THREE CRITERIA USED TO DIAGNOSE SUBSTANCE ABUSE (ROSENHAN AND SELIGMAN, 1984)**
>
> 1. The existence of a clear pattern of pathological use, such as a heavy daily use and an inability to stop or decrease using it.
> 2. Heightened problems in social or occupational functioning resulting from substance use, as when the person loses friends or jobs repeatedly because of it.
> 3. The existence of pathological use for at least one month.
>
> The criteria described were originally developed in the context of drug abuse, e.g. heroin or amphetamine addiction. It is easy to extend the criteria to cover drinking alcohol and possibly smoking and overeating. Nowadays the concept of addiction has broadened to include such things as gambling, exercise and shopping. Do you think that these criteria can be applied to such behaviours?

unpleasant symptoms if the drug is discontinued. *Psychological dependence* is where individuals continue to use the drug because of the pleasant effects that it produces – they rely on the drug to help them feel good and cope with life. And they centre many of their daily activities around its use. (See Glass (1991) for an overview of addiction behaviour.)

The diagnostic criteria for substance abuse are shown in Box 12.1. Smoking and drinking fit easily into the addiction model. It is less easy to do this with eating, since it is essential to survival. However, if *overeating* is considered, then psychological dependence and even the concept of withdrawal may be applied. Certainly, all three behaviours are strongly rewarding and, as we shall see, result in stimulation of 're-ward mechanisms' within the brain. The advantage of considering these behaviours in the same framework is that many of the psychological approaches to prevention and cure have common ground. First, the three behaviours will be described separately.

Drinking alcohol

Alcohol is a popular and widely used psychosocial drug. Why do people drink alcohol? Try asking friends that question and list the answers. In general you will find that the reasons given fall into two categories: positive reasons, e.g. 'I like the taste', 'It makes me feel happy'; and more negative reasons, in the sense that they refer to relieving unpleasant states, e.g. 'It helps to reduce tension', 'It helps me forget my problems'. One of the most noted effects of alcohol is disinhibition, where the drinker feels more relaxed and will engage in behaviour that she or he would normally censor. This, along with its euphoric effects, makes alcohol an excellent drug for 'oiling the wheels' on social occasions.

Why is drinking alcohol a positive experience? The psychopharmacology of alcohol suggests that, in spite of its molecular simplicity, its effects are complex. First, alcohol is absorbed from the gut into the bloodstream. It is rapidly broken down in the liver in the following stages: alcohol to acetaldehyde to acetate. The enzymes alcohol and acetaldehyde dehydrogenase facilitate the breakdown into acetate which is absorbed via normal nutritional mechanisms in the body. Acetaldehyde is a toxic substance causing flushing, nausea and, in extreme cases, death.

Alcohol disrupts the cell membrane function of neurones in the CNS and initiates a general suppression of nerve cell activity (Taraschi and Rubin, 1985). This action selectively diminishes the efficiency of 'higher' cognitive functions, leading to the phenomenon of disinhibition. On recovery, the nerve cell activity increases, a compensatory rebound effect which underlies the irritability and hypersensitivity associated with a hangover.

Alcohol also has specific consequences within the CNS. There is evidence that it promotes the activity of GABA (gamma amino butyric acid, an inhibitory transmitter) in a similar fashion to anxiolytic drugs such as benzodiazepines (Suzdak *et al.*, 1986). It has been proposed that GABA is important in dampening down 'behavioural inhibition systems' activity which when active produces arousal, heightened attention and feelings of anxiety (Gray, 1982). There is also evidence that alcohol consumption leads to increased activity in the mesolimbic dopamine pathway (Imperato and DiChiara, 1986). Activity in this area of the brain appears to be linked to the rewarding properties of particular stimuli. Thus alcohol has a dual effect on the CNS, stimulating reward and anti-anxiety systems, as well as producing a general reduction in the efficiency of neural activity.

BOX 12.2   **DIFFERENT CATEGORIES OF DRINKER AND THEIR APPROXIMATE NUMBER IN ENGLAND AND WALES (REPORT OF THE ROYAL COLLEGE OF PSYCHIATRISTS, 1986)**

Social drinker   Someone who drinks, on average, 2–3 units* of alcohol/day. They do not drink enough on any one occasion to become intoxicated.

Heavy drinker (approx. 3 million) Someone who regularly drinks more than 6 units/day but without obvious harm.

Problem drinker (approx. 1 million) Someone who experiences physical, psychological, social, family, occupational, financial or legal problems as a result of their drinking.

Dependent drinker (approx. 0.25 million) Someone who has a compulsion to drink, has developed an increased tolerance to alcohol (this may reduce again as the problem grows), has withdrawal symptoms if consumption is stopped and amelioration of withdrawal symptoms when drinking is recommenced. Drinking tends to take precedence over other activities.

* 1 unit of alcohol (8 g) is contained in ½ pint beer, 1 glass of table wine, 1 small glass of sherry or 1 measure of spirits. The upper limits of sensible drinking are 21 units/week for men and 14 units/week for women, including 2 or 3 days without alcohol.

Figure 12.1 *Relationship between categories of drinker*

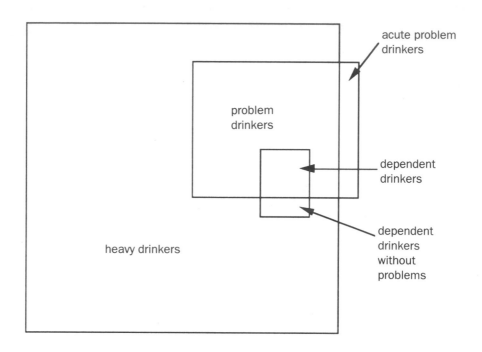

The behavioural effects of alcohol are strongly influenced by the personality of the drinker, the expectations of that person concerning the effects of alcohol, mood and the situation in which the drink is consumed. The resultant effects, whether euphoria, relaxation, anger or depression, depend on a complex interaction between the above factors. Schachter and Singer (1962), in their famous experiment on unexplained, drug-induced physiological arousal, showed that social context determined the emotion experienced by their subjects. This would appear to be true for alcohol. A moment's reflection on the different effects of alcohol drunk at a birthday party or at a funeral will serve to illustrate this point. Social/cultural ideas, rules and norms concerning drinking are absorbed at an early age (McCarty, 1985). These influence drinking behaviour and can perpetuate the notion that drinking is an appropriate and pleasant activity.

Most people drink alcohol moderately with the result that it enriches and improves their lives. But some individuals are alcohol abusers; that is, they drink in such a way that they may damage their health, personal relationships, livelihood and also other people. Alcohol abusers are sometimes categorized into heavy, problem or dependent drinkers. Definitions of these categories and their relationship are explained in Box 12.2 (see also Figure 12.1).

BOX 12.3 **SOME PROBLEMS RELATED TO ALCOHOL ABUSE**

Social	Psychological	Physical
Work problems	Suicide	Cirrhosis of the liver
Domestic violence	Depression	Cardiovascular problems
Criminal acts	Anxiety	Impotence
Drink-driving	Accidents	Digestion problems
Vandalism/hooliganism	Aggression	Cancer
Domestic disruption	Amnesia	Obesity/nutritional deficits
Inefficiency at work	Hallucinations	Foetal damage
Financial problems	Withdrawal fits	Brain damage

What causes some people to abuse alcohol? Situational factors are important since some occupations (e.g. publicans and fishermen) have higher rates of alcohol abuse. This would suggest that availability of alcohol and social isolation are potential causes. There is evidence that inherited aspects are important. The higher the degree of genetic relationship to a known abuser, the higher the probability of abuse (Goodwin, 1986). Obviously such figures are confounded by individuals sharing similar environments, but research with animals has shown that it is possible to breed strains of alcohol-drinking or alcohol-avoiding rats. Evidence relating alcohol abuse to personality traits has not been conclusive, but gender differences are well established. The ratio of males to females among adult problem drinkers is 3:1 (McCrady, 1988). In general, alcohol abusers can be found in all social classes.

What are the damaging effects of alcohol? There are several ways of approaching this question. Intoxication on just one occasion can be a dangerous state, but further problems arise as a result of regular heavy drinking. Alcohol damages the body physically, but it also has psychological effects, which in turn may have social consequences (Box 12.3). The resource cost of alcohol misuse in England and Wales in one year, including costs to industry in absenteeism and accidents, cost of legal systems and NHS expenses, has been estimated to be £1,614 million (Report of the Royal College of Psychiatrists, 1986).

One of the difficulties in coping with alcohol abuse is that alcohol is a widely used and socially acceptable drug in Western societies. It is a natural part of many different social occasions, e.g. dinner parties, business lunches, an evening with friends in the local pub and almost all kinds of celebration. It is relatively easy for some individuals to slip gradually into the habit of drinking too much. As a result many people do not realize that they have an alcohol problem and will not accept that they should cut down on their consumption. Popular excuses include 'I only drink socially' or 'I only drink beer, never spirits'. This denial can cause difficulties for a health professional trying to help clients alter their drinking behaviour (see also Chapter 6).

Smoking tobacco

Since the discovery of the Americas – and the tobacco plant – smoking tobacco has become a widespread habit adopted by all classes of society. This behaviour is still practised by countless millions despite the evidence that shows it is a serious health risk to the smoker, to those in the smoker's immediate environment and in particular to the unborn child. At worst smoking can kill, at best it will increase your life insurance premiums. The questions remain why people start smoking and why they continue when it is regarded as a threat to their health and to their pocket, and when it is increasingly seen as socially unacceptable.

Why do people start smoking? No simple answer exists in response to this question, especially as the first ever puff of a cigarette is almost invariably unpleasant. Peer pressure is undoubtedly a significant contribution. Children and adolescents aspire to adulthood and adopt available role models to imitate. If their role model smokes, then it is not surprising that they will follow in the same line. Certain personality types may be associated with a higher incidence of smoking, e.g. extroverts are more likely to smoke. Murray *et al.* (1983) have studied the factors that are linked to smoking in adolescence (see Box 12.4).

Why continue to smoke? The reasons people give are varied. It is common to hear people say that smoking is pleasant, relaxing and helps them to keep their weight down. Some individuals smoke to cope with stress (Wills, 1986). Others appear to use cigarettes to control their state of arousal, using smoking either to increase or decrease arousal (Tomkins, 1968). Research has shown that smoking aids concentration and learning (Warburton, Rusted and Muller, 1992). One pervasive reason for continuing smoking is that it is pleasant and that not smoking results in unpleasant withdrawal symptoms, e.g. craving for nicotine, irritability, frustration and anger, anxiety, difficulty in concentration, restlessness, decreased heart rate and insomnia.

What component of cigarette smoke mediates these effects? There are well over 2,000 compounds in the average cigarette. Of these 2,000, nicotine is the pharmacologically active substance. It is nicotine that makes the smoker want to continue smoking. However, the pharmacological mechanism may be enhanced by other behavioural and psychological factors. Nicotine rapidly penetrates the brain when smoked. The peak concentration of nicotine is at the end of the smoking period. After this, there is a steady decline in the nicotine level. Smokers will time the spaces between cigarettes and also the time between individual puffs to maintain a set level of nicotine within the body. This process is called titration (Schachter, 1980).

BOX 12.4 **SMOKING HABITS AND BELIEFS OF ADOLESCENTS**

Murray *et al.* (1983) studied the smoking habits and beliefs of 6,000 adolescents over two years using questionnaires. They found the following factors tended to be related to increased smoking:

- At least one parent who smoked.
- Perceived parents as lenient towards smoking.
- Siblings or friends who smoked.
- Often socialized with friends.
- Felt peer pressure to smoke.
- Held positive attitudes about smoking.
- Did not believe that smoking would harm their health.

Nicotine exerts its effect through cholinergic receptors (see Chapter 10). Similar to morphine/heroin and its endogenous counterpart the endorphins, nicotine has an endogenous receptor in the brain and periphery which is selective for nicotine and is normally responsive to the neurotransmitter acetylcholine. Nicotine receptors can be found in the periphery and in the CNS. However, it is the nicotine receptors in the brain that are responsible for the addictive and rewarding nature of smoking. Nicotine receptors in the brain can be found in the interpeduncular nucleus, medial habenulla, cerebral cortex, nuclei of the thalamus, neostriatum, ventral tegmental area, substantia nigra (pars compacta), dentate gyrus and locus coeruleus.

It has been shown that nicotine increases the activity of dopamine neurones in both mesolimbic and nigrostriatal pathways (Svensson, Grenhoff and Aston-Jones, 1986). Dopamine sites are the locations which mediate the effects of other drugs of abuse such as amphetamine and cocaine. Laboratory rats will endure electric shock in order to gain stimulation of the mesolimbic dopamine pathway. Some of the behavioural effects of nicotine are similar to those of amphetamine and cocaine, in particular the motor activation of these drugs (Wise, 1989). However, the euphoric effects of nicotine are not strong. The varied effects of nicotine have led Warburton (1988) to propose a 'functional model' of smoking behaviour, where a smoker uses nicotine as an aid to managing everyday situations. The amount an individual smokes will depend on a complex interaction between their personality and situational factors.

It is now well known that smoking has a strong link with the incidence of lung cancer (Nelson, 1984). Smoking, chewing tobacco or taking snuff is also linked to cancer of the mouth, pharynx and oesophagus. Smoking may also contribute to the development of other types of cancer (bladder, pancreas and kidney, for example) and certainly contributes to other lung diseases such as emphysema and chronic bronchitis. Smokers are more likely to die earlier from cardiovascular disease than non-smokers (Bonita *et al.*, 1986).

In spite of the widespread knowledge that smoking is dangerous, many people acquire the habit. It is probable that advertising plays a major part in introducing individuals to smoking. Once started, smoking is maintained via neurobiological, psychological and social mechanisms. Some fortunate people are able to give up without difficulty or any apparent discomfort. But these people would appear to be the exception to the rule. The majority of those who give up smoking, as indicated by the statistics, revert to smoking again (Grunberg and Bowen, 1985). People are constantly trying to give up for the umpteenth time. These people require further assistance in their efforts. An outline of methods for helping smokers fight their addiction is given later in this chapter.

Overeating

There are several kinds of behaviours associated with eating which may be injurious to health, e.g. the failure to eat a balanced diet, over- and undereating. Health professionals are likely to be faced with individuals who, for health reasons, should be encouraged or supported to change their eating behaviour. The most common problem presenting is for individuals to be overweight (exceeding weight norms for their height, gender and age group by up to 20 per cent), or obese (exceeding weight norms by more than 20 per cent). Obesity is increasingly becoming a problem in affluent Western societies (Millar and Stephens, 1987).

One of the first steps in understanding abnormal eating is to investigate the controls which normally determine how much and what we eat. Most of us eat at culturally determined mealtimes and we eat a selection of food with which we are familiar, which we enjoy and which we believe will provide a balanced diet. Sometimes, if we feel especially hungry (e.g. if we have missed a meal) we will eat uninteresting, but available food to allay hunger pangs. Should we be offered a particularly delicious food – e.g. a slice of chocolate gateau – we may eat it even if we are not hungry. If we predict that we are unlikely to have a meal for some time we will stock up with food and eat more than normal. We will also eat in response to social pressures, e.g. if your host says 'Don't you like my home-made pie?'. All these factors demonstrate that control of eating is likely to be a complex matter.

How do we know when to eat and how much to eat? Early ideas regarding control of eating, based on lesion studies, suggested that there were two 'switches' in the brain, one in the lateral hypothalamus (LH), signalling hunger, the other in the ventromedial hypothalamus (VMH), signalling satiation (the command to stop eating). It is not clear how much the LH and VMH contribute to the *normal* control of eating.

One likely factor determining eating is blood sugar level (the glucostatic hypothesis; Mayer, 1955). As blood sugar falls we feel hungry and tired; this triggers eating until blood sugar levels are back to normal. However, the level of blood glucose does not alter much under normal conditions (Le Magnen, 1981). Furthermore, animals can maintain calories by eating the correct amount of protein and fats even though blood sugar levels are slightly reduced by such a meal. Nicolaïdis (1987) has suggested that a set of neurones somewhere in the brain monitor the levels of various nutrients in the blood. This accords with experimental work which shows that animals can learn through a process of classical conditioning about the positive and negative consequences of ingesting certain substances. If rats are fed on a diet deficient in a vital nutrient such as thiamine they will ignore this diet in favour of a thiamine-rich alternative. In other words, rats can learn to associate the taste of food with its nutritive consequences. Taste aversion is the reverse of this phenomenon. Rats that are made sick after tasting a food will subsequently avoid that food (Rozin and Kalat, 1971). Patients who have suffered food poisoning, or chemotherapy-induced nausea, may 'go off' foods eaten an hour or two before the sickness. This is an example of taste aversion in humans.

We stop eating long before our bodies have had time to metabolize and convert the food to blood sugar. So how do we know when we have eaten enough food? Stomach distension and the taste of food are important factors. Deutsch, Young and Kalogeris (1978) showed that gently inflating a balloon inside a rat's stomach would stop it eating. This cannot be the whole story though, for humans fed a liquid diet through a stomach tube still feel unsatisfied (Jordan, 1969) and they will taste and chew food beyond their nutritional requirements if given the opportunity to do so. Quality of food matters, not bulk alone, since rats will eat larger quantities of a low-calorie than a high-calorie food. It seems that we are sensitive to the nutritive consequences of food and that we learn how much of particular tasting foods to eat (Blundell and Hill, 1986). One of the dangers of using artificial sweeteners is that our bodies may 'unlearn' that sweet flavour equals high calories and, in the long run, may predispose us to eat more sweet food than we need.

The duodenum may also play a role in controlling food intake. When food enters the duodenum a hormone, cholecystokinin (CCK), is released (Gibbs, Young and Smith, 1973). It is possible that CCK, which is present as a neurotransmitter in the brain, is detected by receptors in the relevant brain areas and eating is stopped. There is no evidence as yet to show how this may happen.

Eating is not only controlled by 'push' mechanisms triggered by hunger, it is also an intrinsically rewarding experience. Schwartz et al. (1989) have shown that dopamine and serotonin are released from the LH, and most probably other brain areas, when rats eat something that they like, especially if it is rich in carbohydrates. It is thought that dopamine is important in signalling the reward aspect of eating, while serotonin may be concerned with satiation.

It is evident that we have a variety of physiological mechanisms elegantly tailoring our food input to match our nutritional needs. However, it is also evident that we can override these mechanisms and eat highly palatable food even when we are satiated. This can be a useful ability for ultimate survival since we can store extra food as fat to maintain us in times of famine (bears, for example, must eat as much as they can when food is available since their food supply is only in season for relatively short periods of time (Herrero, 1985)). In affluent human societies, however, highly calorific food is available all the year round and obesity has become a serious health problem for some individuals.

Why are some people prone to obesity and others not? The answer lies in a complex interaction between genetic makeup and environmental factors. Certainly, there are inherited components to obesity. Stunkard *et al.* (1986) found that the body weight of individuals adopted as infants correlated highly with their biological rather than their adoptive parents. The relevant factor may be individual differences in metabolic rate and efficiency. A person with a highly efficient and low metabolic rate would have an enormous advantage in times of famine.

There is some evidence that so-called yo-yo dieting, a repeated cycle of reducing by dieting and then gaining weight, can make the weight problem worse by lowering the metabolic rate. Steen, Oppliger and Brownwell (1988) found that wrestlers who diet to maintain competitive weight and then binge had a metabolic rate 14 per cent lower than those who did not. Brownell *et al.* (1986) found that alternately starving and overfeeding rats resulted in an increase in metabolic efficiency and more rapid weight gain after starvation.

A further possibility is that individuals have a particular 'set point' or natural weight. Their bodies maintain their weight at this level using homeostatic mechanisms (Stunkard, 1986). A factor which may determine the set point is the number of fat cells in the body. The number seems to be determined partly by heredity and partly by nutritional experiences in childhood and adolescence. This would help explain the fact that obese children are much more likely to become obese adults. Some researchers have suggested that the set point may be altered by exercise or drugs, but there is no compelling evidence for this (Keesey, 1986).

Another concept that has been introduced is that of restrained versus unrestrained eaters. Unrestrained eaters eat what they want when they want. Restrained eaters are constantly worrying about what they eat and continually try to curb there appetite (Ruderman, 1986). Restrained eaters are likely to overeat under certain conditions, e.g. if they are at a party or if they have transgressed their diet by eating one chocolate bar, eating behaviour becomes disinhibited. The result is that restrained eaters get in the habit of periods of strict dieting followed by overindulgence. As previously described, yo-yo dieting may lead to weight gain. It is tempting to argue that obese people, for various reasons, are restrained eaters. But does obesity cause restrained eating, or does restrained eating cause obesity? The causal links are yet to be determined.

A review of the current literature by Rodin, Schank and Striegel-Moore (1989) showed that obese people do not eat significantly more than controls. (However, this needs to be interpreted with caution since overweight individuals may not accurately report what they have eaten.) Rodin *et al.* concluded that none of the psychological explanations for obesity has unequivocal empirical support, e.g. lack of impulse control, eating too quickly. Rodin *et al.* also found that depression seemed to be a result, and not a cause, of overweight. In fact, many of the differences in eating behaviours seen between obese and normal individuals may be caused by obese individuals being permanently on a diet and therefore always hungry.

Overweight and a poorly balanced diet are relatively common eating disorders. Two less common problems are anorexia nervosa (self-starvation) and bulimia (episodes of binge eating followed by purging). These are viewed as psychiatric disorders and are largely beyond the scope of the present chapter. Both seem to be precipitated by a combination of biological, cultural and psychological factors and they are most prevalent in adolescent girls. The cultural ideal of slimness in females leads most girls to think that they are too fat (Polivy and Thomsen, 1986). This in turn leads to dieting which in some individuals gets out of control, culminating in these destructive, compulsive behaviour patterns.

Being overweight is associated with elevated levels of cholesterol, coronary heart disease, high blood pressure and diabetes (Hubert, 1986). The more overweight the individual, compared to weight norms for their sex and age group, the more likely they are to suffer from these diseases. There are also social consequences, since an overweight individual may be less able or inclined to engage in leisure/social activities. The outcome of traditional methods for treating obesity have been discouraging. Most patients/clients will drop out of treatment programmes and of those who remain and successfully lose weight, most will regain it (Thompson, 1993). Possibilities for the control of eating behaviour are considered in the following section.

DISCUSSION POINT

It is evident that there are dangers inherent in overeating and also in trying to control eating. The majority of women in our society wage a constant campaign against their weight. Why do they do this? When should people be encouraged to use diets? And when should they be discouraged?

Why are these behaviours addictive?

We can see that the behaviours of smoking, drinking alcohol and overeating are similar in several ways. Why do we indulge in these behaviours and why are they so difficult to control? It would seem that all three activities directly or indirectly stimulate powerful reward mechanisms within the mesolimbic dopamine system (Wise and Rompre, 1989). At the same time, they have the effect of reducing anxiety and tension. They are also moulded and maintained by a combination of personal susceptibility, social pressure and environmental contingencies. Once established, the habits are very difficult to break and they may be labelled 'addictive behaviours'. All three habits, if indulged to excess, can be harmful to health. Some individuals are able to tackle the problem of giving up smoking or cutting down on alcohol and food intake on their own. For many, where the habit has become deeply ingrained or life-threatening, professional help is required.

Changing addictive behaviours

How can individuals be helped to give up harmful behaviours such as those described above? A first step is to persuade the individual that she or he does have a problem. We discussed the possibility of 'denial' in the section on alcohol. A further difficulty is that self-reporting is often used to gauge the extent of the behaviour in question. Individuals typically underestimate the units of alcohol drunk, the number of cigarettes smoked or the amount of food eaten in a given time period.

Some suggested strategies for changing addictive behaviours are described below. Realistically, the goal of such treatment may not be to return to normal, appetite-driven patterns of eating, social drinking or the occasional cigarette, since it may be too easy to relapse into old habits. Total abstinence may be the only practical alternative to alcohol and cigarette consumption. To some extent it is more difficult to prevent overeating since total abstinence is not a viable alternative! A permanent diet regime may be necessary to prevent overeating; but this requires constant vigilance and is difficult to maintain.

Cessation of smoking and reducing food intake will lead to the unpleasant effects of craving for cigarettes or food. Withdrawal effects from nicotine include irritability, insomnia, increased food consumption and difficulty in concentration. Diet regimes can result in hunger pangs, irritability and feelings of lassitude and weakness. For alcohol abusers, physical dependence on alcohol may have developed and stopping its consumption suddenly will result in severe withdrawal symptoms, including even death. As a result, withdrawal, 'drying out' or detoxification needs to be done under medical supervision.

Medical approaches

In some cases the distress of withdrawal can be mitigated by the use of substitutes. Nicotine gum and patches can provide the smoker with the pharmacological effects of nicotine without the carcinogenic effects of tar and smoke. However, nicotine on its own has undesirable effects on the cardiovascular system.

The pain of withdrawal from alcohol can be ameliorated by tranquillizers such as Valium. Although here an obvious problem is the possibility of substituting one addiction for another.

Drastic intervention for severely obese individuals can include supervised, low-calorie diets, jaw wiring, stapling the stomach or removing part of the small intestine to decrease the intake or the absorption of nutrients.

These strategies can be very useful in helping individuals through the first stages of the withdrawal process. Their main disadvantage is that they do not attempt to alter the underlying behaviour. None of them offers satisfactory, long-term solutions. For long-term 'cures' and to tackle psychological dependence, behavioural approaches should be employed.

Behavioural approaches

Aversion therapy
This involves pairing drinking alcohol or smoking with an unpleasant event. According to learning theory the habit has been established through the pairing of

---

BOX 12.5 CIGARETTE SMOKE AS AN AVERSIVE STIMULUS TO STOP SMOKING

Three easy to use methods of using cigarette smoke as an aversive stimulus have been shown to help individuals stop smoking (Lichenstein and Mermelstein, 1984):

1. *Smoke holding* The smoker holds the smoke for a long time in their mouth without inhaling.
2. *Focused smoking* The smoker puffs regularly and pays particular attention to negative stimuli such as unpleasant smells and burning sensations.
3. *Satiation* The smoker smokes at two or three times their normal rate for a period of time.

These procedures succeed in making the act of smoking negative rather than positive and aid smokers in stopping their habit. Rapid smoking, where the smoker puffs at a rate of 1 puff every 5 seconds, is not recommended because of the strain placed on the cardiovascular system.

---

these activities with pleasant consequences, e.g. euphoria or relaxation. Exchanging these events with drug-induced vomiting or electric shock should promote 'unlearning' of the habit. However, aversion therapy has not proved particularly useful in reversing the cravings associated with smoking and drinking (Kamarck and Lichtenstein, 1985; Miller and Hester, 1980).

An alternative approach used with problem drinking is to treat the subject with a drug such as antabuse. Antabuse allows the breakdown of alcohol to acetaldehyde, but prevents the breakdown of acetaldehyde leading to a buildup of this chemical in the body. As mentioned earlier, acetaldehyde produces a variety of aversive symptoms, including flushing and nausea. The result is to make drinking alcohol an unpleasant experience. Use of antabuse is effective for some individuals but the buildup of acetaldehyde can be dangerous, and even fatal, so the treatment requires careful supervision. Any treatment which involves exposing people to unpleasant or potentially harmful events poses ethical questions. A less drastic aversion technique which is effective for smoking is described in Box 12.5.

Self-management strategies

These approaches encourage the individual to help himself or herself, and, in principle, they can be applied to any form of 'addictive' behaviour. There are five main steps involved in self-management:

1. Self-monitoring to identify situations that elicit the behaviour, e.g. smoking often occurs after meals, overeating may happen in the evening if there is nothing else to do.
2. Avoiding situations which lead to the addictive behaviour and seeking out situations incompatible with the behaviour, e.g. socializing with non-drinkers.

3. Doing something else instead of the behaviour, e.g. chewing gum instead of smoking, exercise instead of eating.
4. Altering the act itself, e.g. sipping drinks slowly, not inhaling cigarette smoke, chewing every mouthful of food thoroughly.
5. Set up contracts of reward and punishment and goals associated with the behaviour, e.g. for every cigarette I smoke I give £1 to charity, a new item of clothing when I lose a stone in weight.

The advantage of such techniques is that they can be practised by individuals on their own. They do not require professional intervention, except perhaps in a monitoring role. They encourage self-reliance and self-esteem and they attempt to change and control the addictive behaviour directly. The self-management strategy may be supplemented with other techniques such as relaxation, hypnosis and exercise regimes.

Counselling and group support
Many individuals trying to give up addictive behaviours will benefit from counselling to gain an insight into the roots of their habit. Continuing support is also an aid to treatment programmes for encouragement, to check on progress and to prevent relapse. Group support is also useful, either from family and friends or from organized groups such as Alcoholics Anonymous or Weight Watchers. These groups offer understanding from fellow sufferers and an almost evangelical approach which can benefit those who are comfortable in an authoritarian regime. Intervention by family and friends may be harmful as well as beneficial to progress. This is likely to occur if significant others also engage in the addictive behaviour such as drinking and smoking. Furthermore, self-destructive addictive behaviours can arise in the context of patterns of stresses and strains within the family and effective treatment should include family members (see Chapter 4).

Relapse

Many of those who give up alcohol or smoking or reduce their weight relapse within one year. Grunberg and Bowen (1985) estimate the relapse rate for smokers to be about 70 per cent. Research has shown that individuals with high levels of self-efficacy are less likely to relapse (Baer, Holt and Lichtenstein, 1986). These are individuals who believe themselves to be capable of abstinence. Those with low self-efficacy believe that they have no will power and that it is impossible for them to change (see also Chapter 6 about adopting and maintaining healthy behaviours).

One of the obvious causes of relapse is that the factors that led to the establishment of the addictive behaviour in the first place are unlikely to have changed. Constant vigilance by the individual is needed, as well as acceptance of a relapse, e.g. one cigarette or one slice of chocolate cake without complete collapse of resolve. The continuing support of friends, family and professionals will help.

DISCUSSION POINT
What advice would you give to a client/patient who has lost weight as recommended, but is worried about putting it all back on again?

Prevention

'Prevention is better than cure': there are several factors which might help reduce the incidence of smoking, alcohol abuse and overeating in the general population.

Not all sections of society want to see a reduction in these common addictive behaviours. Tobacco, brewing and food manufacturing are multi-billion pound industries and are extremely profitable. As a result, advertising and sponsorship have been used to promote smoking, eating and drinking. In the past, the image presented of the smoker was of someone who was sophisticated, relaxed and in control of life. All these desirable attributes could be obtained by the purchase of a pack of cigarettes. The advertising of harmful products is regulated now and for cigarettes there is a requirement for packets to bear a prominent government health warning. Other legislation limits the availability of alcohol and tobacco to certain times, places and age groups; excise duty has increased the relative price of both alcoholic beverages and tobacco; and food packaging must state the nutrient content and calorific value of the contents.

Concern regarding the human cost of addictive behaviours has led to the development of health promotion and educational programmes, often directed at children or adolescents. There is now much better understanding by the scientific community and by the general public of the consequences of these potentially dangerous 'addictive' behaviours. It is often the role of the health professional to reinforce such messages, to persuade and help individuals to give up such habits and to encourage more healthful alternative behaviours (see Chapter 6).

Attitudes to addiction

Often there is little sympathy from families, friends and even health professionals for individuals practising addictive behaviours. In an attempt to increase sympathy and understanding, a disease model of such behaviours is sometimes advocated, e.g. alcohol abusers may be labelled as 'alcoholics' suffering from 'alcoholism' (Jellinek, 1960). Another approach has been to label chemical substances as 'addictive', i.e. addictive behaviour is a direct pharmacological property of a drug. Both these strategies are attractive to addicts since they allow the individual to attribute their behaviour to external factors beyond their control: 'I can't help smoking, I'm hooked on nicotine' or 'I was born with a craving for alcohol.' Booth-Davies (1992) suggests that such external attributions are not helpful since they lead to feelings of helplessness. He points out that most work on the motivation behind addictions depends on self-report and is therefore unreliable. He concludes that people engage in addictive behaviours because they want to, because they enjoy the effects and because they see no good reason why they should stop. In his opinion, addicts should be encouraged to take responsibility for their own actions and to take an active and constructive role in relation to health behaviour.

These views, although developed in relation to abuse of 'hard' drugs such as cocaine and heroin, may be usefully extended to the more common addictive behaviours described in this chapter. They imply that the key to controlling these behaviours is 'self-help'. This suggests an answer to the question posed in the introductory paragraph: 'What can be done to help individuals break potentially harmful habits?' The answer would be that the most effective role for the health professional in stopping addictive behaviours is to help the individual to develop self management strategies. Together with an emphasis on prevention and educational programmes, the health professional may contribute to combating common addictive behaviours which are harmful to health.

Summary

This chapter has considered three different forms of common addictive behaviour: drinking excessive amounts of alcohol, smoking tobacco and overeating. Physiological and psychological studies have shown that individuals engage in these harmful habits because they are directly and indirectly rewarding, in that they lead to pleasurable sensations as well as relieving anxiety and tension. Personality traits, learning experiences and social factors contribute to the formation and the maintenance of these habits. Once established they are very difficult to break. The most effective method of helping individuals overcome these addictive behaviours is to encourage self-management strategies.

Seminar questions

1. When should a health professional intervene to try to prevent harmful addictive behaviours? Where should the boundaries be drawn with respect to the extent of the intervention?
2. Consider different sorts of addictive behaviours, e.g. gambling, exercise, taking sleeping pills. To what extent are they determined by pharmacological mechanisms, individual susceptibility or social factors?

Further reading

Orford, J. (1992) *Excessive Appetites: A psychological view of addictions.* Chichester: John Wiley. A biological, psychological and social perspective on five forms of addictive behaviour: alcohol, food, drugs, gambling and sex.

Booth-Davies, J. (1992) *The Myth of Addiction.* Glasgow: Harwood Academic Publishers. This applies the psychological theory of attribution to drug use and questions the assumption that addiction is a pharmacological property of drugs of abuse.

References

Baer, J.S., Holt, C.S. and Lichtenstein, E. (1986) 'Self-efficacy and smoking re-examined: Construct validity and clinical utility', *Journal of Consulting and Clinical Psychology* **54**, 846–52

Blundell, J.E. and Hill, A.J. (1986) 'Behavioural pharmacology of feeding: Relevance of animal experiments for studies on man', in M.O. Carruba and J.E. Blundell (eds.) *Pharmacology of Eating Disorders.* New York: Raven Press.

Bonita, R., Scragg, R., Stewart, A., Jackson, R. and Beagle-Hole, R. (1986) 'Cigarette smoking and risk of premature stroke in men and women', *British Medical Journal* **293**, 6–8.

Booth-Davies, J. (1992) *The Myth of Addiction.* Glasgow: Harwood Academic Publishers.

Brownell, K.D., Greenwood, M.R.C., Stellar, E. and Shrager, E.E. (1986) 'The effects of repeated weight loss and regain in rats', *Physiology and Behavior* **38**, 359–464.

Deutsch, J.A., Young, W.G. and Kalogeris, T.J. (1978) 'The stomach signals satiety', *Science* **201**, 165–7.

Gibbs, J., Young, R.C. and Smith, G.P. (1973) 'Cholecystokinin decreases food intake in rats', *Journal of Comparative and Physiological Psychology* **84**, 488–95.

Glass, I. B. (1991) *International Handbook of Addiction Behaviour.* London and New York: Tavistock/Routledge.

Goodwin, D. W. (1986) 'Heredity and alcoholism', *Annals of Behavioral Medicine* **8**, 3–6.

Gray, J. A. (1982) *The Neuropsychology of Anxiety: An enquiry into the functions of the septo-hippocampal system.* Oxford: Clarendon Press.

Grunberg, N.E. and Bowen, D.J. (1985) 'Coping with the sequelae of smoking cessation', *Journal of Cardiopulmonary Rehabilitation* **5**, 285–89.

Herrero, S. (1985) *Bear Attacks: Their causes and avoidance.* Piscataway, N: Winchester.

Hubert, H. B. (1986) 'The importance of obesity in the development of coronary risk factors and disease: The epidemiologic evidence', in L. Breslow, J.E. Fielding and L.B. Lave (eds.) *Annual Review of Public Health*, Vol. 7. Palo Alto, Calif.: Annual Reviews.

Imperato, A. and DiChiara, G. (1986) 'Preferential stimulation of dopamine release in the accumbens of freely moving rats by ethanol', *Journal of Pharmacology and Experimental Therapeutics* **239**, 219–28.

Jellinek, E. (1960) *The Disease Concept of Alcoholism.* New Jersey: Hill House.

Jordan, H. A. (1969) 'Voluntary intragastric feeding', *Journal of Comparative and Physiological Psychology* **68**, 498–506.

Kamark, T.W. and Lichtenstein, E. (1985) 'Current trends in clinic-based smoking control', *Annals of Behavioral Medicine* **7**, 19–23.

Keesey, R. E. (1986) 'A set point theory of obesity', in K.D. Brownell and J.P. Foreyt (eds.) *The Physiology, Psychology and Treatment of the Eating Disorders.* New York: Basic Books.

LeMagnen, J. (1981) 'The metabolic basis of dual periodicity of feeding in rats', *Behavioral and Brain Sciences* **4**, 561–607.

Lichtenstein, E. and Mermelstein, R. J. (1984) 'Review of approaches to smoking treatment: Behavior modification strategies', In J.D. Matarazzo, S.M. Weiss, J.A. Herd, N.E. Miller and S.M. Weiss (eds.) *Behavioral Health: A handbook of health enhancement and disease prevention.* New York: John Wiley.

Mayer, J. (1955) 'Regulation of energy intake and the body weight: The glucostatic theory and the lipostatic hypothesis', *Annals of the New York Academy of Science* **63**, 15–43.

McCarty, D. (1985) 'Environmental factors in substance abuse: The microsetting', in M. Galizio and S.A. Maisto (eds.) *Determinants of Substance Abuse: Biological, psychological and environmental factors.* New York: Plenum Press.

McCrady, B.S. (1988) 'Alcoholism', in E.A. Blechman and K.D. Brownell (eds.) *Handbook of Behavioral Medicine for Women.* New York: Pergamon.

Millar, W.J. and Stephens, T. (1987) 'The prevalence of overweight and obesity in Britain, Canada and the United States', *American Journal of Public Health* **77**, 38–41.

Miller, W.R. and Hester, R.K. (1980) 'Treating the problem drinker: Modern approaches', in W.R. Miller (Ed.) *The Addictive Behaviors: Treatment of alcoholism, drug abuse, smoking and obesity.* New York: Pergamon.

Murray, M., Swan, A.V., Johnson, M.R.D. and Bewley, B.R. (1983) 'Some factors associated with increased risk of smoking by children', *Journal of Child Psychology and Psychiatry* **24**, 223–32.

Nelson, G.E. (1984) *Biological Principles with Human Perspectives.* New York: John Wiley.

Nicolaïdis, S. (1987) 'What determines food intake? The ischymetric theory', *NIPS* **2**, 104–7.

Polivy, J. and Thomsen, L. (1988) 'Dieting and other eating disorders', in E.A. Blechman and K. Brownell (eds.) *Handbook of Behavioral Medicine for Women.* New York: Pergamon.

Report of the Royal College of Psychiatrists (1986) *Alcohol our Favourite Drug.* London: Tavistock.

Rodin, J., Schank, D. and Striegel-Moore, R. (1989) 'Psychological features of obesity', *Medical Clinics of North America* **73**, 47–66.

Rosenhan, D.L. and Seligman, M.E.P. (1984) *Abnormal Psychology.* New York: Norton.

Rozin, P. and Kalat, J.W. (1971) 'Specific hungers and poison avoidance as adaptive specialisations of learning', *Psychological Review* **78**, 459–86.

Ruderman, A.J. (1986) 'Dietary restraint: A theoretical and empirical review', *Psychological Bulletin* **99**, 247–62.

Schachter, S. (1980) 'Urinary pH and the psychology of nicotine addiction', in P. D. Davidson and S.M. Davidson (eds.) *Behavioral Medicine: Changing health life styles.* New York: Bruner/Mazel.

Schachter, S. and Singer, J.E. (1962) 'Cognitive, social and physiological determinants of emotional state', *Psychological Review* **69**, 379–99.

Schwartz, D.H., McClane, S., Hernandez, L. and Hoebel, B. (1989) 'Feeding increases extracellular serotonin in the lateral hypothalamus of the rat as measured by microdialysis', *Brain Research* **479**, 349–54.

Steen, S.N., Oppliger, R.A. and Brownell, K.D. (1988) 'Metabolic effects of repeated weight loss and regain in adolescent wrestlers', *Journal of the American Medical Association* **260**, 47–50.

Stunkard, A. J. (1986) 'Regulation of body weight and its implications for the treatment of obesity', in M.O. Carruba and J.E. Blundell (eds.) *Pharmacology of Eating Disorders.* New York: Raven Press.

Stunkard, A.J., Sorensen, T.I.A., Hanis, C., Teasdale, T.W., Chakraborty, R., Schull, W.J. and Schulsinger, F. (1986) 'An adoption study of obesity', *New England Journal of Medicine* **314**, 193–8.

Suzdak, P.D., Glowa, J.R., Crawley, J.N., Schwartz, R.D. and Paul, S.M. (1986) 'A selective imidazo benzodiazepine antagonist of ethanol in the rat', *Science* **234**, 1243–7.

Svensson, T.H., Grenhoff, J. and Aston-Jones, G. (1986) 'Midbrain dopamine neurones: Nicotinic control of firing patterns', *Society for Neuroscience Abstracts* **12**, 1154.

Taraschi, T.F. and Rubin, E. (1985) 'Effects of ethanol on the chemical and structural properties of biologic membranes', *Laboratory Invest.* **52**, 120–31.

Thompson, S.B.N. (1993) *Eating Disorders: A guide for health professionals.* London: Chapman & Hall.

Tomkins, S. (1968) 'A modified model of smoking behavior', in E.F. Borgatta and R.R. Evans (eds.) *Smoking, Health and Behavior.* Chicago: Aldine.

Warburton, D.M. (1988) 'The puzzle of nicotine use', in M. Lader (ed.) *The Psychopharmacology of Addiction.* Oxford: Oxford Medical Publications.

Warburton, D.M., Rusted, J.M. and Muller, C. (1992) 'Patterns of facilitation of memory by nicotine', *Behavioural Pharmacology* **3**(4), 375–8.

Wills, T. A. (1986) 'Stress and coping in early adolescence: Relationships to substance use in urban school samples', *Health Psychology* **5**, 503–29.

Wise, R.A. (1989) 'Opiate reward: Sites and substrates', *Neuroscience and Biobehavioral Reviews* **13**, 129–33.

Wise, R.A. and Rompre, P.P. (1989) 'Brain dopamine and reward', *Annual Review of Psychology* **40**, 191–225.

CHAPTER 13

Approaches to pain control

BERYL S. STARR

Chapter outline

Introduction

This chapter explores the complexities of pain perception. It illustrates how pain is not always related to the extent of an injury and how psychological factors are important in the experience of pain. A brief account of underlying physiological mechanisms is provided and a description of the gate control theory of pain. The chapter ends with a consideration of some of the different approaches that may be employed in managing pain.

What is pain?

Most lay people regard pain as a simple, immediate, inevitable response to injury and usually describe it in such terms, e.g. a sore finger, a stomach ache. But try to recollect the last time you experienced pain. What did it feel like? What did you do? After some reflection you will appreciate that pain, as well as possessing definable sensory qualities, is in fact an extremely complex emotional and motivational event. Consider patients that you have observed and their reports of pain. Sometimes severe injuries do not immediately generate pain while pain can also be felt without any sign of tissue damage. The term pain is a broad label which covers many different sensory experiences from tingling, throbbing and itching sensations to the 'pain' of bereavement and disappointed love.

The subjective nature of pain makes it difficult to find a satisfactory scientific definition. An attempt at defining pain is offered by Merskey (1986): 'An unpleasant sensory and emotional experience associated with actual or potential tissue damage, or described in terms of such damage.' There is much to be said for this definition, although the word 'unpleasant' may not be strong enough to indicate the agony that characterizes severe pain.

Early ideas about pain regarded it as a result of stimulation of pain receptors in the skin by noxious stimuli leading to messages being relayed via pain pathways to a pain centre in the brain. If this adequately accounted for the experience of pain, then one might expect it to be relatively easily controlled by switching off this pathway by either surgical or chemical means. However, only 50 per cent of acute pain is adequately managed in hospitals (Royal College of Surgeons, 1990). A further complication is the occurrence of chronic pain. This may be conveniently defined as pain that lasts for more than six months after an injury. In spite of some successes, chronic pain can prove remarkably resistant to medical intervention. There is evidence that chronic pain is increasing, e.g. given that painful episodes are not always reported, it is estimated that about 21 per cent of adults suffer low back pain in any one fortnight (O'Connor and Goddard, 1993).

The experience of pain can be influenced by many factors and what we know of the physiology and anatomy of pain perception indicates a complex, multifaceted system. Certainly, such things as personal attributes, past experiences, context, cultural and social factors all contribute to the perception of pain. This suggests that the understanding of pain and its control would benefit from a psychological perspective.

The experience of pain

The experience of pain varies between individuals exposed to an identical physical stimulus. Furthermore, an individual may experience a similar intensity stimulus as more or less painful on different occasions. In other words, personal characteristics and situational factors influence the perception of pain.

Individual differences

The majority of people have similar sensation thresholds to such stimuli as radiant heat or electric shock (Sternbach and Tursky, 1965). This is the lowest level of a physical stimulus which induces sensations such as tingling in the subjects. However, people may have different pain thresholds, i.e. the lowest stimulus value that is reported as painful. Some individuals with 'high pain thresholds' may suffer heart attacks without being aware of any symptoms (Droste, Greenlee and Roskamm, 1986). The reasons for such individual differences are not clearly understood.

A study by Taenzer, Melzack and Jeans (1986) showed that post-operative pain was influenced by personality variables, specifically anxiety, neuroticism and extroversion. A particular pattern was identified where some patients responded emotionally and pessimistically to the experience of pain, a process known as 'catastrophizing'. A typical piece of 'catastrophizing' in response to post-operative pain might be: 'I am in terrible pain. The operation must have failed. I will never be able to work again. My life is a complete waste of time and I'm a failure. I will never get better.' Patients who tend to respond to crises by such illogical catastrophizing are likely to experience more pain. This applies to chronic pain as well as to post-operative pain. Wade *et al.* (1992) suggests that personality factors have their greatest impact on suffering and pain behaviour rather than on ratings of pain intensity and unpleasantness. This implies that personality variables are of more relevance when considering chronic pain.

Attention, suggestion and anxiety

Sudden severe pain tends to be an overwhelming sensation which demands our immediate attention. However, since a painful stimulus is only one of a variety of stimuli demanding attention, it follows that less severe or slowly rising pain may be diverted by other distracting events. If the other distracting events are themselves attention-grabbing, then they may completely swamp the pain, e.g. competitors may sustain injuries during a game, which they notice only when the excitement has died down (Melzack and Wall, 1991).

The power of suggestion to increase or decrease perception of pain has been amply demonstrated. Hall and Stride (1954) found that simply including the word pain in the experimental instructions increased subjects' tendency to report a particular stimulus as painful. In contrast, the use of placebos to control pain is surprisingly effective. Beecher (1959) reported that 35 per cent of patients experienced relief of severe pain after a placebo compared to 70 per cent of those treated with morphine. The placebo effect (see also Chapters 10 and 15) appears to be a combination of lowered anxiety with the patient's expectation of pain relief (Evans, 1985).

Individuals scoring high on trait anxiety tests tend to have an increased sensitivity to pain. From this one might justifiably conclude that anxiety is a predisposing factor in the perception of pain. In general, high anxiety levels lead to a more devastating experience of pain. Anxiety appears to be the key when considering the effects of actual or perceived control of pain. Patients who are allowed to carry out necessary painful procedures on themselves, e.g. debridement of dead skin in severe burn cases, find the pain is reduced compared to the same procedure being performed by a nurse (Melzack and Wall, 1991). Studies on 'learned helplessness' (Seligman, 1975) indicate that lack of control in a traumatic situation leads to stress, anxiety, apathy and depression.

Cultural differences, learning and experience

Some of the variability in pain thresholds, referred to earlier, may be related to cultural differences. Nepalese porters, who carry immense loads over very difficult terrain on Himalayan climbing expeditions, are less likely to report electric shocks as painful than their Western companions (Clark and Clark, 1980).

The apparent effects of cultural differences on pain perception are in the area of pain tolerance, i.e. the stimulus level at which the subject requests that the stimulation should stop. Several studies reviewed by Melzack and Wall (1991) have demonstrated such cultural differences, e.g. women of Italian origin tolerate less shock than those of Old American or Jewish descent. Bates, Edwards and Anderson (1993) have also demonstrated ethnocultural influences in the experience of chronic pain. Differences in attitudes, beliefs and emotional/psychological states associated with the different ethnic groups appeared to influence pain intensity variation.

The above examples imply that learning and early experience may have an effect on later perception of pain. For instance, the life of the Nepalese porters is likely to be dramatically different from that of Western mountaineers. Melzack (1965) demonstrated the importance of early experiences by rearing puppies in isolation. These puppies, which had presumably missed out on the normal rough and tumble of puppy life, failed to respond appropriately to painful stimuli such as a pinprick. They withdrew from the stimulus but, unlike normal dogs, did not immediately avoid the pin on subsequent exposure. Melzack and Wall (1991) suggest that children are likely to be affected by their parents' attitudes to pain and injury. Some parents will make a tremendous fuss over a minor injury to a child, while others will ignore it. It is easy to see how these early experiences might affect response to pain in adulthood.

Meaning and context

Cultural differences in pain perception also highlight the importance of the meaning and overall context of the painful event. Rituals embedded within particular cultures may result in injury which is not interpreted as painful by the participants. Early studies by Pavlov (1927) showed that if electric shock was used as a conditioned stimulus in a classical conditioning experiment, then the dogs would learn to salivate and wag their tails on receiving a shock that had previously elicited whining and signs of pain. Meaning and context may drastically alter the experience of pain for an individual (see Box 13.1).

BOX 13.1   THE EFFECT OF MEANING AS PAIN

Beecher (1959) noted that soldiers suffering severe wounds in World War II would often experience very little pain immediately after their injury. He interpreted this as being due to the meaning of the injury. The soldiers, he suggested, were in a state of euphoria having escaped from the immediate dangers of the battle front. Their relative insensitivity applied only to the pain resulting from their original injury. They would complain heartily of discomfort arising from a routine medical procedure.

DISCUSSION POINT

How might meaning affect the experience of pain for a woman in labour or a patient suffering unexplained chest pains?

Implications for understanding pain

The psychological aspects of pain perception emphasize the disassociation between the extent of any physical injury and the experience of pain. We tend to assume that it is possible to specify a physical cause for a particular pain. This is often the case for acute pain, although the factors described above will influence how the pain is perceived. Chronic pain is even more likely to be influenced by psychological aspects. For some conditions the causal agent is obscure, e.g. low back pain and migraine are two conditions which can produce severe and prolonged pain with no observable precipitating physical damage (see Loeser, 1980, for back pain; Olesen, 1986, for migraine). Because of their unknown aetiology, treatment by surgical or chemical means is often problematic. Occasionally, these conditions may improve spontaneously or they can be susceptible to psychological methods of pain control. (This will be discussed in a later section.)

In certain clinical syndromes, e.g. phantom limb pain, causalgia and neuralgia, patients experience long-term pain brought on spontaneously or by gentle stimulation. In the past, patients suffering from such pains have been thought to have psychiatric problems, since the symptoms persist and intensify long after the precipitating damage has healed (Kolb, 1954). This kind of prejudice arises from the mistaken belief that pain and injury always exist hand in hand. Recent ideas concerning pain perception and the relative success of treatments involving manipulation of sensory inputs (see later section) have argued against Kolb's interpretation. Indeed, chronic pain patients often suffer concomitant emotional disturbances and may become reclusive and depressed (Flor and Turk, 1985). This is hardly surprising in view of the debilitating consequences of severe, unremitting pain triggered by mild stimulation!

Some individuals experience severe pain with no apparent physical cause. Physicians have concluded that such patients somehow *need* pain and have labelled such cases as examples of 'psychogenic' pain. It should be borne in mind that for these patients the experience of pain is just as real as for a patient with a broken leg. Pain and suffering are a subjective experiences which do not have to be tied to tissue injury. If a patient reports and acts as if they are in pain, then they should be treated accordingly. In these cases psychological methods of pain control may be more effective.

In conclusion, the experience of pain is the result of an interplay of physical and psychological factors. Different pain experiences will involve different mixes of these two aspects. In general, chronic pain is likely to be more dissociated from any physical cause than is acute pain. At this point it may be useful for the reader to reconsider the question posed at the beginning of the chapter. Exactly what is pain? It should be evident that simple descriptions in terms of a response to tissue damage are inadequate.

Pain and the central nervous system

It is beyond the scope of this chapter to provide a detailed insight into controversial issues surrounding the biological basis of pain perception. However, it is necessary to provide a brief overview of the anatomy, physiology and pharmacology of pain pathways in order to appreciate some key aspects of pain control.

Receptors

It is generally accepted that noxious stimuli applied to the skin activate free nerve endings. These receptors, which have large overlapping receptive fields, consist of widely branching networks of fibers. It is important to note that free nerve endings are *not* pain receptors since experience of pain is influenced by information picked up from other types of receptor, and free nerve endings may be implicated in a whole range of sensations (Melzack and Wall, 1991).

Nerve fibers

Nerve fibers carrying somatic sensory information can be classified into three groups: A-beta (large myelinated); A-delta (small myelinated); C (unmyelinated). A-beta fibers conduct information rapidly, have low response thresholds and are fast adapting, i.e. they cease to respond relatively quickly after stimulation. They respond mainly to light touch. A-delta and C fibers conduct information more slowly, have high thresholds and adapt slowly. They respond to light and heavy pressure, heat, chemicals, cooling (A-delta) and warmth (C). It is tempting to postulate that A-delta and C fibers carry information about pain, but once again the relationship between fiber activity and sensation is more complex. Wall and McMahon (1985) demonstrated this using microelectric recordings from specific

BOX 13.2 **THE GATE CONTROL THEORY**

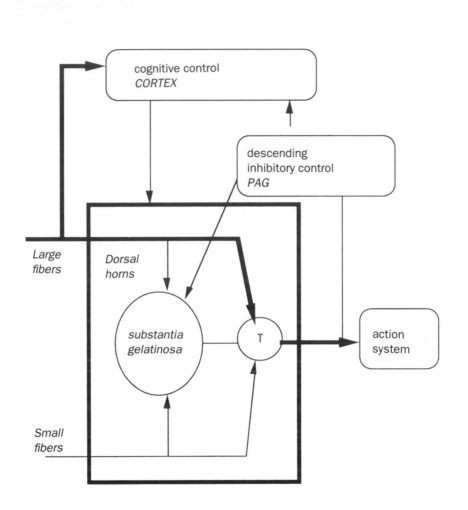

A schematic representation of the gate control theory of Melzack and Wall. Possible anatomical locations of aspects of the theory are indicated. T represents transmission cells and PAG the periaqueductal grey in the midbrain. Whether pain is experienced depends on the output of the gate in the spinal cord.

The diagram shows the three major influences on pain perception, the input from the periphery, the cognitive control from the higher cortical centres and the descending inhibitory pathway from the PAG. See text for details.

types of nerve fibers in somato sensory nerves in conscious subjects. They found a lack of correlation between activity in particular types of nerve fiber and subjects' accounts of their sensory experience.

Spinal cord

Afferent fibers from the skin terminate in the dorsal horns of the spinal cord. The dorsal horns are composed of six cell layers. The most dorsal layers, layers 1 and 2, named the substantia gelatinosa, contain short, densely packed nerve fibers, which are diffusely interconnected. The dorsal horns also receive multiple descending inputs from the brain. These descending inhibitory fibers originate in the reticular formation, the raphe nuclei and the locus coeruleus (Basbaum and Fields, 1978). The physiology of the dorsal horns suggest that much important processing regarding pain perception operates at this level. It is thought that the substantia gelatinosa is particularly significant in modulating the output of the dorsal horns and constitutes the 'gate' in Melzack and Wall's gate control theory (see Box 13.2).

Brain mechanisms

Messages concerning noxious stimulation ascend to the brain through a number of pathways. These can be roughly divided into slow, diffuse as opposed to rapidly conducting, somatically highly organized systems. The fast systems project to the somatosensory areas of the neocortex via the ventrobasal complex of the thalamus. Melzack and Wall (1965) suggest that the rapidly conducting pathways transmit information regarding noxious stimuli that influences processing *before* discriminative and motivational systems are activated. In other words, they constitute a 'feed forward' loop, which allows cognitive factors such as meaning and past experience to affect the perception of pain (see Box 13.2).

It appears that many areas of the brain are involved in processing and responding to noxious stimulation. Early notions that the somatosensory cortex or the thalamus were pain centres were refuted by the finding that lesions in these areas failed to abolish pain (Melzack and Wall, 1991). Complex circuitry involving the reticular formation and the limbic system appear to be important in the aversive properties and the behavioural avoidance which form part of pain behaviour.

A major descending pathway which modulates dorsal horn activity originates in the periaqueductal grey (PAG) in the midbrain (see Box 13.2). The transmitter substance in the cells of the PAG is enkephalin, an opiate. Some of the analgesic effects of morphine are thought to be produced through stimulation of this pathway. Two other transmitter substances, serotonin and noradrenaline, are also involved. In general, this system acts to inhibit prolonged pain rather than acting on the sudden immediate pain felt on injury (Woolf and Wall, 1986). This ties in with the beneficial effects of morphine, which operates by stimulating opiate receptors in

BOX 13.3 **SURGICAL CONTROL OF PAIN**

A patient had suffered unexplained loin and kidney pains from the age of 16. She had been shunted through several different specialists and had been prescribed a variety of extremely potent analgesic drugs to no great effect. In February 1993, she underwent an operation which involved the removal of all the nerves surrounding her kidneys. After the operation the pain worsened and became more diffuse. This case provides a clear and tragic example of how traditional methods of pain control can be woefully inadequate.

chronic, as opposed to acute, pain. The function of this system appears to be to shut down distracting pain information when the organism needs to make an efficient, coordinated response in spite of injury. (For a more detailed account, see Melzack and Wall, 1991.)

In summary, the advances in the understanding of the biological basis of pain perception show that the mechanisms are extremely complex and that they involve many areas of the CNS. It must be remembered that information concerning noxious stimulation impinges on an active and self-regulating nervous system. This information is heavily modulated, even at its input stage in the dorsal horns of the spinal cord. This supports the evidence that information about innocuous stimulation and many psychological processes can profoundly influence both the registration and the response to pain. Melzack and Wall (1965) proposed the gate control theory of pain (Box 13.2) which provides a useful framework for considering many of the phenomena of pain perception.

Pain control

There are no completely satisfactory methods of controlling pain which are effective for all patients with particular pain conditions. Traditional methods of pain control can be surprisingly unsuccessful (see Box 13.3). Often the best procedure is to attack the pain with several different techniques and adopt those which work. In this section some of the available methods of pain control will be discussed. For convenience they have been divided into invasive and non-invasive techniques. Invasive techniques include such approaches as surgery and drugs. Non-invasive techniques use physical and psychological methods of pain control. Occasionally, a single technique (e.g. sensory stimulation) maybe practised in an invasive and a non-invasive form.

Invasive techniques

Drug treatment
Although the prescription of drugs is usually under a doctor's control, nurses have a crucial role in drug treatment since they usually administer the treatment and

monitor its effects. There are many different types of painkillers available as the pharmaceutical industry competes to increase the armoury of analgesic drugs. Since this field is complex and changing rapidly, only the general classes of painkillers will be considered here (but see Chapter 10 for more information on drugs and their effects).

One class of widely used analgesics are non-steroidal anti-inflammatory drugs (NSAIDs). Aspirin is the most common of these agents. It acts by blocking the synthesis of prostaglandins, thus diminishing the local effects of injury such as inflammation and sensitization of nerve endings. These drugs are most effective against pain produced by prolonged tissue damage, e.g. pain produced by an arthritic joint or that felt after tooth extraction. One problem with aspirin is its tendency to induce gastric irritation so that it should not be used by patients with gastric disorders.

Several types of powerful analgesics have been derived from opium, the extract of poppies. These drugs (narcotics) can now be manufactured synthetically and include morphine, heroin and codeine. Narcotics may be injected, administered orally or delivered gradually by means of a mini-pump. As well as producing analgesia, narcotics have a range of undesirable side-effects including a 'drunken feeling', headache, nausea, constipation and respiratory depression (Jaffe and Martin, 1980). Recently, a technique has been developed whereby narcotics are injected into the fluid around the spinal cord (Yaksh, 1986). Here they produce analgesia, at a much lower dose and without the unpleasant, centrally mediated side-effects of the drug.

There is some hesitancy about giving morphine to control pain because tolerance to its effects may develop and there is the possibility of addiction to the euphoria generated by the drug. Melzack and Wall (1991) argue that this caution is unwarranted and unfair to suffering patients. First, they point out that addiction is unusual with morphine-treated patients. In fact, patients allowed to self-administer morphine use less than they would have been given by normal prescription regimes (Keeri-Szanto, 1979). Second, when morphine is used to control chronic pain, tolerance does not seem to develop (Twycross, 1978). Experiments in rats have shown that although tolerance to morphine occurs when it is used to control acute pain, there is little evidence of tolerance with chronic pain (Abbott, Melzack and Leber, 1982). This ties in with the evidence cited in the previous section that the opiate-initiated PAG descending control system seems to operate in cases of prolonged pain.

Sometimes patients will be reluctant to use analgesics (Ward et al., 1993). The reasons for this include, beliefs that 'good' patients do not complain about pain, fear of addiction and concern about side-effects. The combined factors of practitioner and patient anxiety about using analgesics can lead to undermedication and unnecessary suffering (Donovan, Dillion and Mcguire, 1987). Children in pain may be undermedicated for similar reasons (see Box 13.4).

DISCUSSION POINT
What are the pros and cons of using powerful narcotics to obtain pain relief?

BOX 13.4 **PAIN IN CHILDREN**

There is evidence that pain in children may be ignored, partly because of false beliefs that children, especially neonates, do not experience pain in the same way as adults and partly because young children are not able to locate a pain or describe their experience adequately. Alternative ways of evaluating pain have been developed, e.g. using pictures of facial expressions associated with varying degrees of pain. The lack of recognition of pain in children leads to unnecessary suffering and may play a role in predisposing individuals to chronic pain behaviour in adulthood (Caillet, 1993).

Low doses of antidepressants, particularly the tricyclic drugs, can help control pain (Monks and Merskey, 1984). These drugs increase the level of serotonin in the CNS, which may increase the effectiveness of inhibitory mechanisms such as the descending PAG system. Major tranquillizers are also used in pain control, either alone or in conjunction with antidepressants. Other treatments include inhalation of a nitrous oxide/oxygen mixture (Entonox), which can be particularly effective against acute bursts of pain.

Pain may also be controlled by the use of local anaesthetics which block the action of sensory nerves. Although useful for short-term analgesia, the effects wear off rapidly and all types of sensation, not just pain, are abolished from the area. Paradoxically, long-term relief in clinical pain syndromes may be obtained by a relatively short-acting injection of a local anaesthetic. Melzack and Wall (1991) suggest that the cessation of neural input allows a reorganization of firing patterns within the CNS into a more normal state.

Surgery
It has already been stated that surgical control of pain has not met with much success. This is due to the complexity of underlying pain mechanisms and the fact that chronic pain, once established, appears to migrate from being peripherally to being centrally generated. An example of the failure of surgical approaches is given in Box 13.3.

Sensory stimulation
In the previous section it was pointed out that stimulation of the A-beta peripheral nerves had the effect of inhibiting the activity of pain-signalling cells in the dorsal horns. Thus it comes as no surprise to discover that various kinds of peripheral stimulation can be effective in controlling pain. In fact, most of us unconsciously use this technique. If we bump into something hard we automatically rub the spot to relieve pain.

The list of these techniques is long and includes manipulation, massage, exercise, superficial heat (e.g. poultices), deep heat (e.g. ultrasound), cooling (e.g. ice packs) and electrotherapy (e.g. TENS). TENS (transcutaneous electric nerve stimulation) involves application of an electric current to peripheral nerves by means of electrodes placed on the skin. The patient is issued with a pocket-sized, battery-charged stimulator and can alter the frequency, intensity and duration of the electrical pulses. TENS was developed as a direct result of gate control theory and has bought pain relief that outlasts the stimulation to thousands of patients (Marchand *et al.*, 1993; Melzack and Wall, 1991). The effects of the traditional Chinese art of acupuncture may operate along similar lines, except that here the stimulation is produced by manipulating needles inserted into particular trigger points in the body.

It is not clear whether this stimulation-produced analgesia is caused by direct stimulation of dorsal horn cells leading to the closing of the gate in the substantia gelatinosa or by indirect activation of the descending inhibitory PAG system. Both factors may underlie the resulting analgesia, depending on the particular method of stimulation employed.

Non-invasive techniques

Earlier I described a variety of evidence which emphasized the contribution of various psychological factors to the perception of pain. Unsurprisingly, these can be exploited in a battery of effective techniques aimed at helping patients/clients to control their pain. Because these techniques are non-invasive it is possible for a health professional to help encourage patients/clients to use them. Some of these methods involve a behavioural approach (e.g. operant techniques), or a cognitive/behavioural approach (e.g. coping skills and cognitive behaviour therapy).

Relaxation

Anxiety has been shown to increase the severity of perceived pain both directly and indirectly. It is possible to train patients/clients in simple relaxation techniques. These lead to measurable physiological changes, which can be used as indices of relaxation (e.g. reduction in blood pressure). Also, relaxation leads to a reduction in a wide range of clinical pains (Philips, 1988). States of relaxation may be more easily achieved by the use of biofeedback. This allows patients/clients to monitor the progress of relaxation by direct access to a physiological measure such as the proportion of alpha activity in the EEG. However, it is not clear whether biofeedback is any more effective than simple relaxation training alone (Chapman, 1986).

Distraction and cognitive coping skills

A further psychological influence on pain perception is the amount of attention directed to the pain. In some cases distraction by music or noise can be an effective method of pain control (Fernandez, 1986). Miller, Hickman and Lemasters (1992) demonstrated that the use of videos of beautiful scenery with accompanying music significantly decreased pain and anxiety for burn injury patients.

It is possible to divert someone's attention away from pain by encouraging the use of cognitive coping skills. Patients/clients may be invited to imagine a pleasant place or experience incompatible with pain or to direct their attention on to some external stimulus (positive emotion induction). Alternatively, they can be encouraged to take part in some activity or possibly some self-generated mental exercises. It is sometimes useful for the individual to focus attention on the pain but in a detached and analytic manner – is it really pain or is it an itch? The health professional can actively help patients/clients to use these strategies. Some people already have their own pain coping strategies in which case they should be encouraged to employ them. Several studies have evaluated the effectiveness of coping strategies and, on the whole, they prove to be effective in controlling pain (Fernandez and Turk, 1989). Rokke and al'Absi (1992) using the Cognitive Coping Strategy Inventory showed that using strategies 'matched' to subjects' natural strategies was beneficial for managing acute pain.

Part of the success of coping strategies is that they increase an individual's perceived control over the pain. Lipchik, Milles and Covington (1993) demonstrated that patients' beliefs regarding 'locus of control' are important in pain perception. They reported the positive effect of a short therapeutic programme designed to increase perceived personal control over pain as opposed to control by 'powerful others'. Patient-controlled analgesia allows patients to determine their own medication and again increases the experience of 'control'.

In a study by Langer, Milles and Covington (1975) patients about to undergo major surgery were given precise information about the type and level of post-operative pain they should expect and then trained on coping skills such as controlled breathing, distraction and relaxation techniques. These patients experienced reduced pain, and the critical factor was found to be the perceived control over the situation provided by the coping strategies. However, these techniques need careful handling, since information on its own may increase anxiety and attention to discomfort, while coping strategies that do not work can be worse than having no means of control at all (Weisenburg et al., 1985). Certainly, the patient's belief that therapies will reduce pain is important in pain control (the placebo effect). Any strategy that increases a patient's confidence in the therapeutic procedures, the staff and their own efforts in managing pain will be beneficial.

Cognitive behaviour therapy
A further method of pain control is to employ the technique of cognitive behaviour therapy (Turk and Rudy, 1987; see Chapter 16, this volume, for a description of this approach). Briefly, the patient/client is encouraged to substitute realistic and constructive thoughts about his experience of pain as opposed to unrealistic negative thoughts. Several studies have attested to the effectiveness of this approach in relieving chronic pain (e.g. Turner and Jensen, 1993).

Operant techniques
An intriguing approach to the control of chronic pain examines the effects of reward on 'pain behaviour'. This behavioural approach to pain was developed by Fordyce (1976). It is based on the concept of operant conditioning introduced by Skinner

(1953), who believed that all behaviour was controlled by its consequences, i.e. by rewards and punishments. For behaviourists like Skinner, observable behaviour alone lends itself to objective study. Subjective experiences are regarded as unreliable and of little significance for scientific psychology. According to Fordyce, pain behaviour *is* pain and the subjective experience and reports of pain are irrelevant. Fordyce sees pain as consisting of respondent and operant components. The respondent component is the immediate response to pain. The operant component is the long-term pain behaviour, such as limping, wincing, complaining and remaining immobile, which is reinforced by such things as attention and sympathy from others, pain medication, avoiding activity and avoiding responsibility. This is not to say that the pain is not real or that the patient is malingering; they have no conscious recognition of the reward mechanisms affecting their behaviour. Furthermore, 'pain behaviour' such as inactivity may hinder the return of the CNS to a more normal state.

Treatment involves a stay in hospital of 4–8 weeks when the patient's behaviour is modified by operant conditioning techniques. Pain behaviour is ignored and behaviour incompatible with pain, such as exercise, is rewarded. Turk, Meichenbaum and Genest (1983) have shown that operant procedures successfully increase patients' activity levels and decrease the use of medication. However, not all patients appear to respond well to this approach (e.g. cancer patients with chronic/progressive pain). A review article by Rachlin (1985) discusses the case for an operant approach to pain control.

Hypnosis, counselling and psychotherapy

A combination of directed attention and suggestion may explain the phenomenon of hypnotic analgesia. It is possible to conceive of hypnosis as a state in which the subject's attention is strongly fixed on the hypnotist. In this state, and with appropriate suggestions, analgesia to all kinds of painful stimuli can be induced in a particular area of the body. Unfortunately, only a certain proportion of subjects may be deeply hypnotised (Spira and Spiegel, 1992), so its use as an analgesic tool is probably limited.

Sometimes intensive behavioural treatment may be supplemented by psychological counselling or individual psychotherapy. These approaches encourage patients to develop insight into their own pain behaviour and how this behaviour has affected their relationships. Turk, Meichenbaum and Genest (1983) have shown that programmes with an insight-oriented therapy component are effective in reducing pain. Recently, it has been recognized that the long-term effects of an accident resulting in injury, incapacitation and pain are similar to those suffered by individuals caught up in major catastrophes, i.e. post-traumatic stress syndrome. Such patients respond well to specialist counselling (Muse, 1986).

There are many advantages in using group therapy for patients suffering from chronic pain as well as the obvious increase in efficiency (Gentry and Owens, 1986). The other patients form a useful reference group and their comments are more likely to be believed than those of a pain-free therapist. They can also say things to each other that would appear cruel and unfeeling coming from a non-sufferer.

One of the criticisms of the gate control theory is that, although it provides a model for how psychological factors affect the experience of pain, it does not aid our understanding of the impact of chronic pain on all aspects of life, i.e. social, vocational, recreational and familial (Flor and Turk, 1985). An individual suffering chronic pain will place particular stresses and strains on their family. They may not be able to contribute to family income by employment, to take on household chores or feel inclined to take part in excursions and social occasions. The attitude of other family members, especially the spouse, to these problems may add further stresses and strains; they may be overprotective towards the patient or become angry and impatient. Tota-Faucette *et al.* (1993) showed that the pre-treatment family environment influenced the outcome of treatment for chronic pain patients. In some families chronic pain in one individual may act as a stabilizing factor for that family and as such there may be resistance to cure. All this suggests that for effective treatment of chronic pain, the patient should be viewed in a family-wide context.

Multiple convergent therapy

In recent years it has been recognized that there are no easy answers to the problem of pain and clinicians have tended to adopt a multiple convergent therapy approach. Several kinds of therapy may be tried and the two or three which complement each other and suit the particular patient may be retained. The efficacy of multidisciplinary programmes has been supported by a number of studies (Flor, Fydrich and Turk, 1992; Lipchik, Milles and Covington, 1993; Roberts, Steinbach and Polich, 1993).

Summary

Knowledge about the complexity of pain mechanisms has increased the repertoire of methods for pain control. However, patients undergoing medical care may still not obtain the pain relief that they deserve. Often, this is because of a medical practitioner's and the patient/client's lack of understanding about pain. Pain is expected to have an easily identifiable cause and people with certain afflictions could only be experiencing a certain amount of pain. Patients whose pain does not fit these expectations may be labelled 'troublemakers' or 'complainers'. Greater allowance needs to be made for the vagaries of pain perception and the differences that exist between individuals in their physical makeup, their personality, their cultural background and their past experiences of pain. It should be remembered that the experience of pain crosses both physical and emotional boundaries. Appropriate psychological methods of pain management have an important place in the control of pain.

Seminar questions

1. How might individual differences in the way patients/clients respond to pain affect the attitudes of health practitioners towards them? What might be the consequences of this for patient/client care?
2. A discussion on individual techniques for controlling pain. Material for this discussion may be gathered by individuals reflecting on their own experience or by conducting a small survey on friends. Questions asked could include:

   - Do you experience menstrual pain or headaches or back pain? (Any recurrent discomfort will do.)
   - If yes, how do you cope, e.g. take medication or exercise or rest?
   - How successful is your pain control technique, e.g. how long before the pain subsides?
   - When and why did you start using this technique? Consider the influence of family, friends, etc.

Further reading

Melzack, R. and Wall, P.D. (1991) *The Challenge of Pain*, 3rd edition. Harmondsworth: Penguin Books. An easy-to-read, but intellectually stimulating text on the puzzles surrounding pain. Viewed from a clinical, physiological and psychological perspective.

Sofaer, B. (1992) *Pain: A handbook for nurses.* London: Chapman & Hall. A practical text concerning day-to-day management of patients in pain.

Gibson, H.B. (1993) *Psychology, Pain and Anaesthesia.* London: Chapman & Hall. A comprehensive account of prevention, management and relief of pain, emphasizing cognitive and behavioural factors.

References

Abbott, F.V., Melzack, R. and Leber, B.F. (1982) 'Morphine analgesia and tolerance in the tail-flick and formalin tests: Dose–response relationships', *Pharmacological Biochemical Behaviour* **17**, 1213–19.

Basbaum, A.I. and Fields, H.L. (1978) 'Endogenous pain control mechanisms: Review and hypothesis', *Ann. Neurol.* **4**, 451–62.

Bates, M.S., Edwards, W.T. and Anderson, K.D. (1993) 'Ethnocultural influence on variation in chronic pain perception', *Pain* **52**, 101–12.

Beecher, H.K. (1959) *Measurement of Subjective Responses.* New York: Oxford University Press.

Caillet, R. (1993) *Pain: Mechanisms and management.* Philadelphia: F.A. Davies.

Chapman, S.L. (1986) 'A review and clinical perspective on the use of EMG and thermal biofeedback for chronic headaches', *Pain* **27**, 1–43.

Clark, W.C. and Clark, S.B. (1980) 'Pain responses in Nepalese porters', *Science* **209**, 410–12.

Donovan, M.I., Dillion, P. and Mcguire, D. (1987) 'Incidents and characteristics of pain in a sample of medical-surgical inpatients', *Pain* **30**, 69–78.

Droste, C., Greenlee, M.W. and Roskamm, H. (1986) 'A defective angina pectoris pain warning system: Experimental findings of ischemic and electrical pain test', *Pain* **26**, 199–209.

Evans, F.J. (1985) 'Expectancy, therapeutic instructions and the placebo response', in L. White, B. Turskey and G.E. Schwartz (eds.) *Placebo: Theory, research and mechanisms.* New York: Guilford Press.

Fernandez, E. (1986) 'A classification system of cognitive coping strategies for pain', *Pain* **26**, 141–51.

Fernandez, E. and Turk, D.C. (1989) 'The utility of cognitive coping strategies for altering pain perception: A meta-analysis', *Pain* **38**, 123–35.

Flor, H., Fydrich, T. and Turk, D.C. (1992) 'Efficacy of multidisciplinary pain treatment centres: A meta-analytic review', *Pain* **49**, 221–30.

Flor, H. and Turk, D.C. (1985) 'Chronic illness in an adult family member: Pain as a prototype', in D.C. Turk and R.D. Kerns (eds.) *Health, Illness and Families: A life-span perspective.* New York: John Wiley.

Fordyce, W.E. (1976) *Behavioral Methods for Chronic Pain and Illness.* St Louis: C.V. Mosby.

Gentry, W.D. and Owens, D. (1986) 'Pain groups', in A.D. Holzman and D.C. Turk (eds.) *Pain Management: A handbook of psychological treatment approaches.* New York: Pergamon.

Hall, K.R.L. and Stride, E. (1954) 'The varying response to pain in psychiatric disorders: A study in abnormal psychology', *British Journal Medical Psychology* **27**, 48–60.

Jaffe, J.H. and Martin, W.R. (1980) 'Opioid analgesics and antagonists', in A.G. Gilman, L.S. Goodman and A. Gilman (eds.) *The pharmacological basis of therapeutics.* New York: Macmillan.

Keeri-Szanto, M. (1979) 'Drugs or drums: What relieves post-operative pain?' *Pain* **6**, 217–30.

Kolb, L.C. (1954) *The Painful Phantom: Psychology, physiology and treatment.* Springfield, Ill.: C.C. Thomas.

Langer, E.J. (1975) 'The illusion of control', *Journal of Personality and Social Psychology.* **32**, 311–28.

Lipchik, G.L., Milles, K. and Covington, E.C. (1993) 'The effects of multidisciplinary pain management treatment on locus of control and pain beliefs in chronic non-terminal pain', *Clin. J. Pain* **9**(1), 49–57.

Loeser, J. D. (1980) 'Low back pain', in J.J. Bonica (ed.) *Pain.* New York: Raven Press.

Marchand, S., Chorest, J., Li, J., Chenard, J.R., Lavignolle, B. and Laurencelle, L. (1993) Is TENS purely a placebo effect? A controlled study in chronic low back pain', *Pain* **54**(1), 99–106.

Melzack, R. (1965) 'Effects of early experience on behaviour: Experimental and conceptual considerations', in P. Hoch and J. Zubin (eds) *Psychopathology of Perception.* New York: Grune & Stratton.

Melzack, R. and Wall, P.D. (1965) 'Pain mechanisms: A new theory', *Science* **150**, 971–9.

Melzack, R. and Wall, P. (1991) *The Challenge of Pain.* Harmondsworth: Penguin Books.

Merskey, H. (1986) 'Classification of chronic pain: Descriptions of chronic pain syndromes and definitions of pain terms', *Pain* (Suppl. 3), S1–S225.

Miller, A.C., Hickman, L.C. and Lemasters, G.K. (1992) 'A distraction technique for control of burn pain', *Journal Burn Care Rehabilitation* **13**(5), 576–80.

Monks, R. and Merskey, H. (1984) 'Psychotropic drugs', in P.D. Wall. and R. Melzack (eds.) *Textbook of Pain*. Edinburgh: Churchill Livingstone.

Muse, M. (1986) 'Stress-related, post-traumatic chronic pain syndrome: Behavioral treatment approach', *Pain* **25**, 389–94.

O'Connor, M. and Goddard, A.K. (1993) 'The management of intractable low back pain', in H.E. Gibson (ed.) *Psychology, Pain and Anaesthesia*. London: Chapman & Hall.

Olesen, J. (1986) 'The pathophysiology of migraine', in F.C. Rose (ed.) *Handbook of Clinical Neurology*, Vol. 48. Amsterdam: Elsevier.

Pavlov, I.P. (1927) *Conditioned Reflexes*. Oxford: Humphrey Milford.

Philips, H. C. (1988) 'Changing chronic pain experience', *Pain* **32**, 165–72.

Rachlin, H. (1985) 'Pain and behaviour', *The Behavioural and Brain Sciences* **8**, 43–83.

Roberts, A.H., Sternbach, R.A. and Polich, J. (1993) 'Behavioral management of chronic pain and excess disability: Long-term follow-up of an outpatient program', *Clinical Journal Pain* **9**(1), 41–8.

Rokke, P.D. and al'Absi, M. (1992) 'Matching pain coping strategies to the individual: A prospective validation of the cognitive coping strategy inventory', *Journal Behavioural Medicine* **15**(6), 611–25.

Royal College of Surgeons (1990) *Pain after Surgery*. Report of the Working Party of the Commission in the Provision of Surgical Services of the Royal College of Surgeons of England and the College of Anaesthetists.

Seligman, M.E.P. (1975) *Helplessness: On depression, development and death*. San Francisco: W.H. Freeman.

Skinner, B.F. (1953) *Science and Human Behaviour*. London: Macmillan.

Spira, J.L. and Spiegel, D. (1992) 'Hypnosis and related techniques in pain management', *Hospital Journal* **8**(1–2), 89–119.

Sternbach, R.A. and Tursky, B. (1965) 'Ethnic differences among housewives in psychophysical and skin potential responses to electric shock', *Psychophysiology* **1**, 241–6.

Taenzer, P.A., Melzack, R. and Jeans, M.E. (1986) 'Influence of psychological factors in postoperative pain, mood and analgesic requirements', *Pain* **24**, 331–42.

Tota-Faucette, M.E., Gil, K.M., Williams, D.A., Keefe, F.J. and Goli, V. (1993) 'Predictions of response to pain management treatment. The role of family environment and changes in cognitive processes', *Clinical Journal Pain* **9**(2), 115–23.

Turk, D.C., Meichenbaum, D. and Genest, M. (1983) *Pain and Behavioral Medicine: A cognitive behavioral perspective*. New York: Guilford Press.

Turk, D.C. and Rudy, T.E. (1987) 'Towards a comprehensive assessment of chronic pain patients', *Behaviour Research and Therapy* **25**, 237–49.

Turner, J.A. and Jensen, M.P. (1993) 'Efficacy of cognitive therapy for chronic low back pain', *Pain* **52**, 169–77.

Twycross, R.G. (1978) 'Relief in pain', in C.M. Saunders (ed.) *The Management of Terminal Disease*. London: Edward Arnold.

Wade, J.B., Dougherty, L.M., Hart, R.P., Rafii, A. and Price, D.D. (1992) 'A canonical correlation analysis of the influence of neuroticism and extroversion on chronic pain, suffering and pain behaviour', *Pain* **51**, 67–73.

Wall, P.D. and McMahon, S.B. (1985) 'Microneuronography and its relation to perceived sensation', *Pain* **21**, 209–29.

Ward, S.E., Goldberg, N., Miller-McCauley, V., Mueller, C., Nolan, A., Pawlik-Plank, D., Robbins, A., Stormoen, D. and Weissman, D.E. (1993) 'Patient-related barriers to management of cancer pain', *Pain* **52**, 319–24.

Weisenberg, M., Wolf, Y., Mittwoch, T., Mikulincer, M. and Aviram, D. (1985) 'Subject versus experimenter control in the reaction to pain', *Pain* **23**, 187–200.

Woolf, C.J. and Wall, P.D. (1986) 'A dissociation between the analgesic and antinociceptive effects of morphine', *Neuroscience Letter* **64**, 238.

Yaksh, T.L. (1986) *Spinal Afferent Processing*. New York: Plenum Press.

CHAPTER 14

Managing stress in health care

Issues for staff and patient care

FIONA JONES

Chapter outline

Introduction

'Stress' has received a great deal of coverage in recent years in the media and has been the subject of considerable psychological research. This chapter focuses on the specific stressors present for both staff and patients in the health service. It examines how such stressors can be prevented or alleviated by interventions focused on individual or organizational change. To this end the chapter draws on two, largely separate strands of research from occupational psychology and from health/clinical psychology.

Over the past few years, occupational psychologists have conducted research aimed at identifying work stressors; that is external, relatively permanent features of the work environment or the work itself (e.g. the extent to which a job provides an individual with autonomy). This has led to the development of models postulating a wide variety of job characteristics that are regarded as stressful. Such emphasis is perhaps arbitrary, since it is well known that situations which one individual will take in her stride may place an intense strain on another. Individual differences in personality, hardiness or coping mechanisms, for example, are clearly important. Nevertheless, it is possible to identify those features of the work environment which are likely to be a source of strain for many workers. A major implication of such approaches to occupational stress is that they have far-reaching implications in terms of changing the way work is designed, as well as treating stress in the individual (see also Chapter 1 for a discussion of organizational issues).

Health and clinical psychologists similarly have recognized the importance of minimizing patients' stress in health care settings. Here psychologists' interventions have primarily focused on a variety of interventions to help the individual to cope with stressful medical procedures. For example, researchers have focused on the effects of different types of information in preparation for medical and surgical procedures.

The aim of this chapter will, therefore, be to bring together research carried out by occupational psychologists into stress at work and research largely conducted by clinical or health psychologists into the effects of hospitalization. The issues are often complex and not clear cut, but the chapter will provide a review of current thinking into the major ways that contact with the health service could be made a less stressful experience for both staff and patients/clients.

Stress

Stress is a much misused term; it has been variously treated as synonymous with such concepts as 'strains', 'demands', 'stressors' and 'pressures'. The semantic confusion causes uncertainty over such basic issues as whether a certain amount of stress is 'a good thing'. (The answer is likely to be different if stress means 'pressure' rather than 'strain'.) Some researchers have suggested that the term is consequently meaningless and should be abandoned (Briner and Reynolds, 1993; Pollock, 1988). However, the usual approach, which is adopted in both this chapter and Chapter 15, is to regard it as a general term to encompass a broad area of study, which includes the study of environmental stressors, strains (which may be physical, psychological or behavioural) and moderating influences, including a range of factors to do with personality and the availability of supports. The study of stressors alone has included a wide range of different types of factor. They may be acute or chronic, with effects that are brief or long-lasting, instantly traumatic or with negative effects that build up over time. Some researchers have focused on major life events (such as divorce or bereavement) and their effects on wellbeing (Holmes and Rahe, 1967). At the other extreme, it has been suggested that minor, everyday hassles are more important in predicting ill health (DeLongis *et al.*, 1982) and that interpersonal stressors are the most upsetting of daily stressors (Bolger *et al.*, 1989). Most occupational research has taken an intermediate level of analysis, looking at relatively stable and enduring aspects of the work environment.

An individual is often subject to a wide range of diverse stressors. A hospital patient may, for example, be suffering a major acute life event, enduring the relatively chronic stressors of a poorly designed hospital environment as well as minor daily inconveniences of irritating or restless fellow patients. The effects of such stressors on the patient will be influenced by a range of factors, including personality, availability of social support and type of coping strategy used.

Stress among health care professionals

Models of occupational stress

It is clear that work stress is not a simple issue. For example, the heavy workload junior doctors experience may well be a source of stress, but the extent to which it leads to strain will depend on a number of intervening variables. The extent of resources to deal with the load, the amount of autonomy the doctor has and the amount of social support will all be important. Researchers working in the study of occupational stressors have used a number of different approaches or models to define the relationships between stressors and strains. Such models have clear implications for the way work could be designed to minimize stress. Two of these models, Warr's vitamin model and Karasek's demand-discretion model, are discussed below. (See also the catastrophe model, discussed in Chapter 15.)

Warr's vitamin model
Warr has identified a number of environmental features affecting mental health. Although the importance of these factors has primarily been studied in the context of work or unemployment, they provide a framework for studying all kinds of environment. These are as follows:

1. *Opportunity for control.* Mental health is likely to be affected by the extent to which situations offer opportunity for personal control over activities or events. Warr (1987: 4) suggests that the 'opportunity for control has two main elements: the opportunity to decide and act in one's chosen way, and the potential to predict the consequences of action.'
2. *Opportunity for skill use.* Mental health is likely to be affected by the extent to which the environment affords the opportunity to use existing skills or develop new skills.
3. *Externally generated goals.* Mental health is likely to be affected by the extent to which the environment makes demands or generates goals.
4. *Variety.* The extent to which environments offer variety will further influence mental health.
5. *Environmental clarity.* This includes:
   (a) feedback about the consequences of one's own actions;
   (b) the degree to which other people and things in the environment are predictable;

(c) the clarity of role requirements.

6. *Opportunity for interpersonal contact.* This is important in meeting needs for friendship and social support. In addition, many goals may be achieved only through group membership.

7. *Availability of money.* The availability of money is clearly a factor likely to influence mental health by causing anxiety about the individual's ability to provide for their own, or their family's basic needs. In addition, shortage of money is likely to influence the extent to which the individual may be able to gain access to sufficient levels of the other factors, such as variety or control.

8. *Physical security.* In the work context this would include such factors as job security and poor working conditions.

9. *Valued social position.* The final aspect considered important for mental health is that of having a position within a social grouping which leads to being held in esteem by others.

Warr uses the analogy of vitamins to explain the way that these work features affect mental health. Low levels of vitamins lead to poor physical health and similarly low levels of each of the listed environmental features will lead to poor mental health. As with vitamins, Warr suggests that above a certain level there is no added benefit if more of the feature is added. For example, above a certain level an increase in money or interpersonal contact will not lead to a further improvement in mental health. In the case of some vitamins (for example, Vitamins A or D), very large amounts may be harmful for health. Other vitamins (for example, C or E) can safely be consumed in large quantities. Similarly, Warr suggests that certain environmental features will be harmful if levels are very high. This is true of elements 1–6 listed above. The other three elements are not harmful at high levels. Thus, the model predicts that too much money or physical security will not be harmful, but too much control or variety may be.

Warr suggests that the presence of control is particularly important in that it is likely to give scope for determining the other eight elements. Of all the work characteristics, control has probably received the greatest amount of research. It is a key element in the next model to be described, Karasek's demand-discretion model (Karasek, 1979).

Karasek's demand-discretion model
This model is one of the most well-known and influential approaches to occupational stress. Karasek considers that the effects of job demands are moderated by job control or discretion (referred to as 'decision latitude' by Karasek). Figure 14.1 identifies the types of jobs which are thought to result from the various combinations of demands and discretion. The model predicts that a combination of high job demand and low levels of job discretion would lead to high levels of psychological and physical strain – a 'high strain' job. By contrast, low levels of demand and high levels of discretion would be 'low strain' jobs. High job demands with a high level of discretion makes for 'active jobs', which are not unduly stressful because they allow

Figure 14.1 *Karasek's (1979) job strain model*

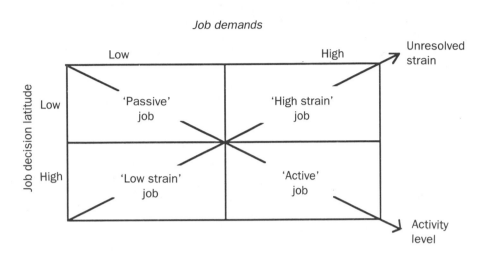

the individual to develop protective behaviours. Jobs with low demands and low discretion, on the other hand, tend to be passive, resulting in reduced activity and learned helplessness. Thus while active and passive jobs are intermediate in terms of strain outcomes, a passive job would lead to higher levels of strain than an active job.

This approach helps to explain why high levels of strain are often found in the lower levels in organizational hierarchies in studies of a range of organizations including the British civil service (Marmot *et al.*, 1991). While there are clearly stressors associated with senior positions, these are likely to be mitigated by greater control and ability to delegate. (See also Chapter 15 for a discussion of the effects of demand and discretion on physical health.)

Studies of professional groups

There are a large range of widely diverse professional groups within the health service and a large literature has developed which looks at the stressors in different groups. A number of studies have suggested that health workers experience more stress than comparable samples of non-health workers (Payne and Firth-Cozens, 1987; Rees and Cooper, 1992). It is clear from Warr's summary of occupational stressors that many health professionals are likely to suffer from organizational stressors that are common to many other jobs (lack of clarity and conflicting roles, overload, lack of control), but often suffer additional stressors that are intrinsic to the nature of the job; for example providing terminal care, counselling bereaved parents or dealing with disturbed and violent patients. Payne and Firth-Cozens (1987) have suggested that an additional problem for health service workers is that their stress may have a direct effect on the recipients of the service, such that communication with patients may deteriorate. This is confirmed by a study by Motowidlo, Packard and Manning (1986), which found that nurses reporting higher levels of subjective stress were rated by their supervisors as poorer on interpersonal aspects of their work performance, such as interpersonal effectiveness and tolerance. Clearly, stress is an important issue in maintaining a high standard of patient care.

A review of the literature on stress in health professionals is beyond the scope of this chapter. Nursing alone consists of a wide range of different types of role which have been subjected to individual study. For example, a study by Parkes (1982) compared stressors and strains of student nurses during assignment to medical and surgical wards. She found that medical wards caused higher levels of depression and lower levels of job satisfaction among the students. Surgical wards offered work which was rated higher on a number of key characteristics such as control or job discretion, opportunity for use of skills and acquisition of new skills. Work on medical wards was more emotionally demanding with lower levels of social supports. Other relevant studies are described elsewhere in this book. In Chapter 3, Horton discusses an early study by Menzies (1970), which gives a psychodynamic account of the role conflicts experienced by nurses. A study by Vachon (1987) on the occupational stress of caring for people who are dying is discussed in Chapter 17. Burnout and coping in those who care for people with HIV is discussed in Chapter 16.

Junior doctors have also been the focus of a number of studies (see Firth-Cozens, 1989). Suicide rates, alcoholism and depression have been found to be high in the medical profession and particularly among junior doctors. The long hours of work are a particular problem, but the responsibilities of dealing with death and dying and the possibility of making mistakes are among a number of other important work stressors.

It should, however, also be pointed out that there are a number of positive aspects about many jobs within the health service which might also be expected to lead to high levels of satisfaction. The work is valued by society and some of Warr's 'vitamins' are likely to be present (for example, variety, skill utilization and intellectual challenge) which are likely to compensate for other potential stressors (Payne and Firth-Cozens, 1987). Nevertheless, the numerous studies indicate that work stress in the health service is a significant problem.

DISCUSSION POINT

Look again at Karasek's model. Which cell best describes your work experiences to date? Do some work roles within the health service have less job strain associated with them than others? If so, why do you think this is?

Managing stress at work

It has been suggested that there are three stages at which it is possible to provide interventions to help reduce or eliminate occupational stress (Ivancevich *et al.*,

1990). The first type of intervention focuses on the stressors and aims to modify the environment. This may involve changes in the work organization; for example, jobs may need to be redesigned to reduce stressors or increase workers' control. The second aims to change the individual's cognitions (for example, through stress management training courses). And the third aims to reduce stress by treating the individual (for example, by counselling).

Focusing on the organization: job design

The models of stress discussed in this chapter and Chapter 15 have clear implications for the design of jobs within the health service, in terms of increasing levels of certain work features (or 'vitamins') such as control. For example, a study of a large sample of white-collar workers in Sweden looked at the relationship between job reorganization and health. They found that where individuals had influence in the reorganization process and where they obtained increased task control as a result, they had lower levels of a wide range of physical and psychological symptoms (Karasek, 1990). It is reasonable, on the basis of research into occupational stress, to conclude that highly demanding jobs may be made less stressful by increasing the individual's control or the supports available to them. Research studies investigating a range of health service occupations have made recommendations for organizational change along these lines (see e.g. Fletcher, Jones and McGregor-Cheers, 1991). However, there is a lack of studies evaluating the effects of such changes on mental health within the health service.

One recent area of organizational concern within the health service is the influence of budget cuts, a feature of modern work which has not been given much consideration in stress research. However, Jick (1987) has suggested that the traditional models of stress research could be applied in such new areas. Budget cuts typically lead to a number of perceived stressors (perceived job insecurity, high level of work overload, underutilization of skills, conflict, time pressures, etc.). These are factors which correspond to Warr's vitamins and Fletcher's demands, supports and constraints (see Chapter 15). Such effects could be counteracted by increasing levels of certain vitamins or supports. Examples suggested by Jick include (1) keeping staff well informed by meetings and fact sheets, thus providing environmental clarity (increasing the predictability of events), and (2) the encouragement of participation to stimulate innovative methods which require fewer resources.

Focusing on the individual: training and counselling

While occupational psychology research would suggest the importance of designing work so that many sources of stress are minimized, the main approaches taken by employers over the past few years have been either to train the individual to cope with stress by means of stress management courses or to treat the individual by means of counselling schemes. Similarly, there has been a disproportionate emphasis in the research literature on individual interventions and outcomes. It is ethically questionable to train employees to tolerate poorly designed organisations (Ganster *et al.*, 1982). However, stressful work demands are inherent in the nature of the work for many health service professionals. While attention to job design within the health service is important, it is undoubtedly easier to reduce stress in factory work than in health care. A two-pronged approach, focusing both on the organization and the individual, is likely to be most effective. The two individual approaches to stress most widely used are the provision of stress management courses and counselling schemes.

Stress management training

Sending employees on stress management training courses is a measure frequently adopted by employers. A typical course might include a diverse range of techniques, including training about work stressors, relaxation (or meditation) techniques, assertiveness and time management. A key element is likely to be the use of cognitive-behavioural techniques, based on the view that stress is often caused by negative 'self-talks'. Training would focus on replacing these with more positive internal dialogues. Attempts to evaluate such interventions have tended to show relatively limited changes in the wellbeing of participants. This may be due in part to the fact that many of those sent on courses may not have been suffering from stress in the first place. A classic study by Ganster *et al.* (1982) provided a very thorough evaluation of a stress management programme in an American Social Services agency. The researchers found that after sixteen hours of training, there were small reductions in depression, anxiety and adrenaline secretion in participants compared with a control group. These changes were maintained four months later. However, the authors comment that many commercially available training programmes offer courses that last no more than half a day and so are unlikely to produce noticeable improvements. There has, as yet, been insufficient research to identify which of the diverse elements are particularly effective.

Many of the techniques taught in stress management courses are also widely available in an ever-increasing number of self-help manuals, some of which are geared for particular work groups. (See the suggestions for Further Reading at the end of this chapter.)

Counselling schemes

Over the past few years there has been a growth in the number of organizations providing counselling services for their employees. These may take the form of either in-house confidential counselling services, as provided by some large organizations such as the Post Office (Sadu, Cooper and Allison, 1989); or counselling services provided by independent companies offering employee advice service, which are increasingly being used by British companies. Typically, the latter offer advice and counselling for a wide range of problems, from minor consumer or legal issues to more serious psychological problems. While public sector employers have generally

---

BOX 14.1   A STAFF COUNSELLING SCHEME WITHIN THE HEALTH SERVICE

In recent years there has been a growing trend for large companies to provide Employee Assistance Programmes (EAPs). Such schemes are provided by a number of companies specializing in the provision of counselling services. Typically, these will offer a wide range of confidential advice, ranging from simple information services to counselling for personal and work-related problems, advice on legal and financial problems and trauma counselling. Each employee will be given a card giving telephone contact numbers. Following an initial contact by an employee, arrangements for face-to-face meetings can be arranged if necessary. Alternatively, employees may be referred to a range of specialists; for example, those offering legal advice. Schemes such as these offer employees access to a much wider range of services than can normally be employed within a single organization. Companies typically receive information about how many calls were made and the nature of the calls, but no information about who made them. This enables the companies to tackle organizational problems that cause stress to their employees.

The initial growth of EAPs has been within the private sector, where providing support to employees is increasingly considered to be cost-effective. Similar schemes are now being developed within the health service. For example, Employee Advisory Resource Ltd (EAR), of Uxbridge, Middlesex, has been contracted to provide an EAP for the staff of New Possibilities NHS Trust in Colchester, which provides services for people with learning difficulties. They have found that about 20 per cent of their employees contact the service each year, a similar rate to commercial organizations. Typically, approximately 20 per cent of problems were work-related and 80 per cent were personal.

---

been slower to recognize the benefits of providing counselling support for staff, these are beginning to become available within the health service (see Box 14.1).

A number of studies have attempted to examine the effectiveness of counselling or therapy for work stress. An evaluation of the Post Office scheme showed improvements in psychological wellbeing and sickness absence after counselling (Sadu, Cooper and Allison, 1989). A study by Firth and Shapiro (1986) found large reductions in symptoms after sixteen hours' therapy for work-related distress. Two different types of therapy showed similar results, though one of these, 'prescriptive therapy', utilizing cognitive-behavioural approaches similar to those often used in stress management training, showed particularly promising results. Studies have tried to determine what elements in therapeutic interventions are most effective. Often, findings show that widely different types of therapy have tended to produce very similar results (Stiles, Shapiro and Elliot, 1986). It seems that little headway has been made towards determining exactly what it is about counselling that works. However, Firth-Cozens' study suggests that sixteen hours spent treating distressed individuals may be a more useful and cost-effective way of achieving stress management than an equivalent amount of time providing stress management training for individuals who are not experiencing stress.

DISCUSSION POINT
Think of a particular job within the health service (for example, hospital porter, district nurse, nurse on a medical ward). From the available stress literature, what aspects of the job would you expect to be particularly stressful and what could be done to improve the situation in terms of job redesign and provision of help to manage stress?

Stress among patients and clients

All individuals will come into contact with the health services at different stages in their lives. Frequently, contacts with the health service are major events in an individual's life (accidents, serious illness, surgery or childbirth). These may involve losses from which the individual may grieve (e.g. loss of health, loss of family contacts, loss of independence; see Chapters 16 and 17). Many other more trivial medical procedures may be intensely stressful to patients because of their unfamiliar, invasive or painful nature.

Similarly, illness may cause changes in many of Warr's environmental characteristics, and these may cause additional stress. For example, serious illness is likely to lead to a loss of autonomy, with others taking control over aspects of an individual's life. It is likely to prevent skill use, to reduce the opportunities for goal-directed behaviour and to lead to less variety in the activities an individual can undertake. The environment and future events are likely to become uncertain and unpredictable. There may be less opportunity for interpersonal contact. In extreme cases, loss of money, status and physical security may follow. Such stressors will be intensified in the case of the hospital patient, who will have greatly diminished control and contact with their families. Such environmental stressors will also be additional to the intrinsic stress associated with the illness itself (e.g. loss of function or pain).

In addition to the effects of stressful medical treatments on psychological wellbeing, the mounting evidence concerning the impact of stress on physical wellbeing (see, for example, Fletcher's discussion of stress and immune system functioning in Chapter 15), suggests that it is important to minimize stress among patients. Some research has also indicated that pre-operative anxiety is associated with poor recovery and increased pain, though results are inconsistent and conflicting (see Kincey and Saltmore, 1990: Chapter 16 discusses such stresses associated with HIV infection).

Managing stress among patients and clients

Psychologists' primary contribution has been the development of interventions for patients/clients, which have aimed to reduce stress by altering the way a patient perceives the environment. This may be by the provision of information or assistance in developing appropriate coping strategies. While these may not change objective features of the external environment in terms of Warr's environmental vitamins, they may have the effect of making the environment more controllable by making treatment predictable; allowing the patient to make informed choices where possible; and encouraging the patient to engage in active coping strategies.

A particular focus of research has been the evaluation of stress management procedures for unpleasant medical procedures. Four particular types of approach have been commonly investigated:

1. Information provision.
2. Relaxation.
3. Cognitive behavioural approaches.
4. Modelling.

The evidence for their effectiveness has been reviewed by Ludwick-Rosenthal and Neufeld (1988) and Kendall and Epps (1990) and is summarized below.

Information provision

Many studies have focused on the effects of providing information about medical treatments. Two main types of information have been considered: (1) procedural, which gives factual information about the sequence of events that the patient is likely to experience; and (2) sensory information about the sorts of feelings and sensations that the patient is likely to experience. Results of such studies have been complex, contradictory and have not resulted in clear guidelines for the practitioner.

Studies that take account of individual differences in personality or coping style help to account for some of the inconsistent effects. For example, Kendall and Epps (1990) suggest that there is a continuum of coping styles from 'avoidant' to 'non-avoidant'. Those with avoidant styles, sometimes known as 'blunters' or 'repressors', may deal with stressful situations by denying the information or distancing themselves from it. Those with a non-avoidant style, sometimes known as 'monitors' or 'sensitizers', cope by seeking information and preparing plans of action. Kendall and Epps suggest that information should be given in a manner consistent with the preferred coping style of the patient. Thus non-avoiders may benefit from specific procedural and sensory information. Avoiders may prefer more general information.

Relaxation approaches

A number of studies have taught patients such techniques as progressive relaxation, in which they concentrate on tensing and relaxing different groups of muscles in turn. The intention of such interventions is to replace the anxious response with a response that is incompatible with anxiety. Relaxation techniques have been found to be effective for a wide variety of situations from childbirth to chemotherapy, and are frequently used in conjunction with other approaches (e.g. cognitive-behavioural approaches). Studies of anticipatory nausea in chemotherapy patients have shown that receiving training in progressive muscle relaxation combined with therapist-guided imagery results in better performance on a range of physiological measures of anxiety as well as the reporting of less nausea (Burish and Lyles, 1981; Lyles *et al.*, 1982).

Cognitive-behavioural approaches

An example of this approach is stress inoculation training (Meichenbaum, 1977). This is similar to the kind of intervention provided by many occupational stress management training courses described above. In phase 1 of the training, patients are taught the rationale of the method and given an understanding of the effects of cognition on behaviour. In phase 2 they are taught a number of cognitive be-havioural techniques (for example, replacing anxiety-provoking 'self-talks' with new and more positive ways of talking to yourself about stressful situations), and in phase 3 they rehearse these techniques. The majority of studies have shown benefits of these types of approaches (e.g. Kaplan, Atkins and Lenhard, 1982; Kendall *et al.*, 1979).

Modelling

This approach stems from the work of Bandura (1969). It is based on the view that exposure to a model (for example, on a video) who is coping successfully with a particular experience can teach the patient to utilize similar appropriate coping strategies. In one study patients undergoing gastrointestinal endoscopy were shown a film of individuals undergoing similar treatment (Shipley *et al.*, 1978). A control group were shown an unrelated video. Subjects exposed to the model had signifi-cantly lower levels of anxiety during the medical procedure. Overall, studies re-viewed by Ludwick-Rosenthal and Neufeld (1988) provide strong support for modelling interventions.

Ludwick-Rosenthal and Neufeld (1988) conclude that there is some evidence that all the above interventions can reduce patient stress during aversive medical procedures. While modelling and cognitive-behavioural approaches have generally demonstrated more positive effects, this may be at least partly due to the fact that these interventions are likely to include elements of information-giving or relaxa-tion. As with studies investigating the effects of occupational stress management interventions, there has been insufficient research to identify which of the particular elements are most useful. The best current advice to practitioners would be to provide a broad range of support, taking into account the needs, wishes and pre-ferred coping styles of the individual patient.

BOX 14.2   **IN-HOSPITAL COUNSELLING FOR MALE MYOCARDIAL INFARCTION PATIENTS AND THEIR WIVES, LEICESTER GENERAL HOSPITAL CORONARY CARE UNIT (CCU) (THOMPSON, 1990; THOMPSON AND MEDDIS, 1990a, 1990b)**

Coronary patients suffer from considerable emotional strain during the acute phase of the illness. A recent study at Leicester General Hospital evaluated the effects of a programme of in-hospital counselling provided by a coronary care nurse.

Sixty male patients who had been admitted to a CCU following their first myocardial infarction were randomly assigned either to a treatment group in which they received four additional 30-minute sessions of counselling during their first five days in hospital, or a control group in which they received routine medical and nursing care only. The counselling sessions included education about the nature, impact and management of heart attacks, and counselling focused on the patients' reactions and feelings. The aims of the programme included alleviating uncertainty and fear by providing information, providing psychological support and involving the patients in decision-making aspects of care. It further aimed to enable the patients to discover positive coping mechanisms rather than the negative reactions of anxiety and depression and to engender a realistic but optimistic outlook. Wives were included in the counselling sessions.

The study found that, although patients in both groups had similar levels of initial anxiety and depression, after the counselling sessions the treatment group reported significantly lower levels than the control group. This effect remained six months after discharge from hospital. Anxiety levels were also reduced for spouses who received counselling – an effect that also lasted the six months of the study. This suggests that a simple, inexpensive intervention, taking only two hours over a one-week period, can have significant impacts in reducing stress, and that the inclusion of spouses is likely to be an important factor.

While the above approaches have focused on medical interventions, it is recognized that surgical interventions are likely to be particularly stressful (Volicer, Isenberg and Burns, 1977). Surgery in many cases has more long-term effects than the types of procedure discussed above. Nevertheless, similar approaches have been found to be useful in dealing with stress. Wells *et al.* (1986) found that stress inoculation training reduced anxiety and pain and improved post-operative adjustment. Generally, approaches aimed at reducing anxiety (for example, relaxation and emotional support) have been more effective than those aimed at education only (Mumford, Schlesinger and Glass, 1982).

A major challenge for the future – the influence of technological change in the health service

The many changes within the NHS in recent years will clearly have an impact on both staff and patients/clients. Such changes have the potential to be stressful, but may be introduced in ways which either maximize or minimize damage. The impact of organizational change is discussed elsewhere (see Chapter 1). A specific change which has been studied by psychologists is the impact of modern technology. There have clearly been major advances in medical technology in recent years. Some of the most sophisticated equipment currently used by nurses is that employed for patient monitoring in intensive care units (ICUs).

Fitter (1987) suggests that there are a number of dangers inherent in the introduction of such technology. For nurses, there is the danger that if they come to rely on such technology, their role may become more passive and this could lead to deskilling and the loss of conventional nursing skills, which may be particularly dangerous if machines fail. In reviewing a range of studies, he suggests that there are a number of stress factors directly related to the use of new technology:

1. Enhanced cognitive demands, owing to the complexity of equipment.
2. Poor design and equipment failures which, for example, may lead to the stress of frequent false alarms.
3. Lack of adequate training.
4. Ethical problems; for example, it may be distressing to nurses that life can be sustained despite its poor quality.

For patients, there is the danger that they will find themselves not only in an unfamiliar and alarming high-tech environment, but also that they will be distanced from nursing staff. This will compound the inevitable stress associated with admission to an ICU and may impair recovery. Studies have revealed that while patients were generally positive about the service, the environment of the ICU was stressful and could invoke anxiety, although in part this depended on the amount of compensating support provided by nursing staff.

Fitter (1987: 227) suggests that a recurring theme is the lack of involvement that nurses have in the introduction of new technology even where they are its main users: 'Many of the nurses commented that they felt the technology could be of greater benefit to patient care and less stressful to them, if they were involved in its development and plans for its use.' Similar issues emerge in studies in manufacturing industries, where it has been found that new technology can be introduced in ways that deskill workers, reduce job satisfaction, reduce job performance and increase stress, or in ways that utilize a new range of skills, enhance performance, enhance job satisfaction and reduce stress (Buchanan and Boddy, 1983; Wall *et al.*, 1990). New technology needs to be designed and introduced in ways that meet the requirements of the nurses and patients, rather than nurses and patients having to adapt to the requirements of the technology. For this to happen, there has to be management commitment to nurse involvement in the development and implementation of technological change. In addition, the impact of these and other changes in the health service on the psychological wellbeing of both staff and patients/clients will require monitoring in future years.

DISCUSSION POINT
1. Think of a patient/client (if possible a patient /client you have encountered) undergoing a major operation; for example heart surgery or a hysterectomy. List

aspects of their experience which might be particularly stressful. What could be done to minimize the stress?

2. Think of a patient /client or carer in the community whom you consider to be showing signs of stress. Discuss how they could be helped by health professionals, either by changing the environmental stressors (with reference to Warr's vitamin model), or by employing the stress management strategies listed above.

Summary

Warr's model suggests that a low stress environment (whether at work or elsewhere) should have opportunities for control, skill use and goal attainment. It should have variety, clarity and opportunity for interpersonal contact. There should be adequate money, physical security and social position. Illness may threaten the existence of these basic factors. Contact with the health services has the potential either to exacerbate or minimize stress. This chapter has reviewed some recent approaches to reducing patients' stress by increasing perceived environmental control through techniques designed to increase predictability and active coping.

Staff under pressure will not only suffer themselves, but will be less able to meet the needs of their patients. Stress in a changing health service may be reduced by the use of methods similar to those used with patients, by increasing the control experienced by staff, by providing information and increased involvement in decision making. The emphasis in psychological research so far has been to view stress as an individual problem to be treated by individual stress management interventions. There is, however, a need for a greater focus on organizational factors and approaches to organizational change which may minimize stress for both staff and patients.

Seminar questions

1. What is stress? How can it be defined? Is it a useful concept?
2. Why might organizational change be stressful? How can it be handled to minimize stress?

Further reading

Payne, R. and Firth-Cozens, J. (eds.) (1987) *Stress in Health Professionals.* Chichester: John Wiley. This book contains chapters discussing the problems of stress in a wide range of medical professions, including physicians, surgeons, psychiatric nurses and technicians.

Johnston, M. and Wallace, L. (eds.) (1990) *Stress and Medical Procedures*. Oxford: Oxford University Press. This book provides detailed coverage of issues surrounding the stress associated with diagnosis and a range of treatments (including medical, surgical, obstetric and paediatric treatments).

Steptoe, A. and Appels, A. (eds.) (1989) *Stress, Personal Control and Health.* Chichester: John Wiley. This book discusses issues of control in both occupational and clinical settings.

A wide range of useful self-help guides for dealing with occupational stress is available; for example:

Arroba, T. and James, K. (1987) *Pressure at Work, A Survival Guide.* Maidenhead: McGraw-Hill.

Burnard, P. (1991) *Coping with Stress in the Health Professions: A practical guide.* London: Chapman & Hall.

References

Bandura, A. (1969) *Principles of Behavior Modification.* New York: Holt, Rinehart & Winston.

Bolger, N., DeLongis, A., Kessler, R.C. and Schilling, E.A. (1989) 'Effects of daily stress on negative mood', *Journal of Personality and Social Psychology* **57**(5), 808–18.

Briner, R.B. and Reynolds, S. (1993) 'Bad theory and bad practice in occupational stress', *SAPU memo 1405.* Sheffield University.

Buchanan, D.A. and Boddy, D. (1983) 'Advanced technology and the quality of working life: The effects of computerized controls on biscuit-making operators', *Journal of Occupational Psychology* **56**, 109–19.

Burish, T.G. and Lyles, J.N. (1981) 'Effectiveness of relaxation training in reducing adverse reactions to cancer chemotherapy', *Journal of Behavioral Medicine* **4**, 65–78.

DeLongis, A., Coyne, J.C., Dakof, G., Folkman, S. and Lazarus, R.S. (1982) 'Relationships of daily hassles, uplifts, and major life events to health status', *Health Psychology* **1**(2), 119–36.

Firth, J. and Shapiro, D.A. (1986) 'An evaluation of psychotherapy for job-related distress', *Journal of Occupational Psychology* **59**, 111–19.

Firth-Cozens, J. (1989) 'Stress in medical undergraduates and house officers', *Journal of Hospital Medicine* **41**, 161–3.

Fitter, M. (1987) 'The impact of new technology on nurses and patients', in R. Payne and J. Firth-Cozens (eds.) *Stress in Health Professionals.* Chichester: John Wiley.

Fletcher, B.(C)., Jones, F. and McGregor-Cheers, J. (1991) 'The stressors and strains of health visiting: Demands, supports, constraints and psychological health', *Journal of Advanced Nursing* **16**, 1078–89.

Ganster, D., Mayes, B.T., Sime, W.E. and Tharp, G.D. (1982) 'Managing organizational stress: A field experiment', *Journal of Applied Psychology* **67**(5), 533–42.

Holmes, T.H. and Rahe, R.H. (1967) 'The social readjustment rating scale', *Journal of Psychosomatic Research* **11**, 213–18.

Ivancevich, J.M., Matteson, M.T., Freedman, S.M. and Phillips, J.S. (1990) 'Worksite stress management interventions', *American Psychologist* **45**(2), 252–61.

Jick, T.D. (1987) 'Managing and coping with budget-cut stress in hospitals', in R. Payne and J. Firth-Cozens (eds.) *Stress in Health Professionals.* Chichester: John Wiley.

Kaplan, R.M., Atkins, C.J. and Lenhard, L. (1982) 'Coping with a stressful sigmoidoscopy: Evaluation of cognitive and relaxation preparations', *Journal of Behavioral Medicine* **5**, 67–82.

Karasek, R.A. (1979) 'Job demands, job decision latitude and mental strain: Implications for job design', *Administrative Science Quarterly* **24**, 285–308.

Karasek, R.A. (1990) 'Lower health risk with increased job control among white collar workers', *Journal of Organizational Behavior* **11**, 171–85.

Kendall, P.C. and Epps, J. (1990) 'Medical treatments', in M. Johnston and L. Wallace (eds.) *Stress and Medical Procedures*. Oxford: Oxford University Press.

Kendall, P.C., Williams, L., Pechacek, T.F., Graham, L.E., Shisslak, C. and Herzoff, N. (1979) 'Cognitive-behavioral and patient education interventions in cardiac catheterization procedures: The Palo Alto Medical Psychology Project', *Journal of Consulting and Clinical Psychology* **47**, 49–58.

Kincey, J. and Saltmore, S. (1990) 'Surgical treatments', in M. Johnston and L. Wallace (eds.) *Stress and Medical Procedures*. Oxford: Oxford University Press.

Ludwick-Rosenthal, R. and Neufeld, R.W.J. (1988) 'Stress management during noxious medical procedures: An evaluative review of outcome studies', *Psychological Bulletin* **104**(3), 326–42.

Lyles, J.N., Burish, T.G., Krozely, M.G. and Oldham, R.K. (1982) 'Efficacy of relaxation training and guided imagery in reducing the aversiveness of cancer chemotherapy', *Journal of Consulting and Clinical Psychology* **50**, 509–24.

Marmot, M.G., Smith, G.M., Stansfield, S., Patel, C., North, F., Head, J., White, I., Brunner, E. and Feeney, A. (1991) 'Health inequalities among British civil servants: The Whitehall II study', *The Lancet* **337**, 1387–93.

Meichenbaum, D. (1977) *Cognitive-behavior Modification*. New York: Plenum Press.

Menzies, I. E. P. (1970) *The Functioning of Social Systems as a Defence against Anxiety*. London: Tavistock Institute of Human Relations.

Motowidlo, S.J., Packard, J.S. and Manning, M.R. (1986) 'Occupational stress: Its causes and consequences for job performance', *Journal of Applied Psychology* **71**(4), 618–29.

Mumford, E., Schlesinger, H.J. and Glass, G.V. (1982) 'The effects of psychological intervention on recovery from surgery and heart attacks: An analysis of the literature', *American Journal of Public Health* **72**, 141–51.

Parkes, K.R. (1982) 'Occupational stress amongst student nurses: A natural experiment', *Journal of Applied Psychology* **67**, 789–96.

Payne, R. and Firth-Cozens, J. (1987) *Stress in Health Professionals*. Chichester: John Wiley.

Pollock, K. (1988) 'On the nature of social stress: Production of a modern mythology', *Social Science and Medicine* **26**(3), 381–92.

Rees, D. and Cooper, C.L. (1992) 'Occupational stress in health service workers in the UK', *Stress Medicine* **8**, 79–90.

Sadu, G., Cooper, C. and Allison, T. (1989) 'A Post Office initiative to stamp out stress', *Personnel Management* (August), 40–5.

Shipley, R.H., Butt, J.H., Horwitz, B. and Farbry, J.E. (1978) 'Preparation for a stressful medical procedure: Effect of stimulus pre-exposure and coping style', *Journal of Consulting and Clinical Psychology* **46**, 499–507.

Stiles, W.B., Shapiro, D.A. and Elliot, R. (1986) 'Are all psychotherapies equivalent?' *American Psychologist* **41**(2), 165–80.

Thompson, D.R. (1990) *Counselling the Coronary Patient and Partner*. London: Scutari Press.

Thompson, D.R. and Meddis, R. (1990a) 'A prospective evaluation of in-hospital counselling for first-time myocardial infarction men', *Journal of Psychosomatic Research* **34**(3), 237–48.

Thompson, D.R. and Meddis, R. (1990b) 'Wives responses to counselling early after myocardial infarction', *Journal of Psychosomatic Research* **34**(3), 249–58.

Vachon, M.L.S. (1987) *Occupational Stress in the Care of the Critically Ill, the Dying and the Bereaved*. Washington: Hemisphere.

Volicer, B.J., Isenberg, M. and Burns, M. (1977) 'Medical-surgical differences in hospital stress factors', *Journal of Human Stress* (June), 3–13.

Wall, T.D., Clegg, C.W., Davies, R.T., Kemp, N.J. and Mueller, W.S. (1987) 'Advanced manufacturing technology and work simplification: An empirical study', *Journal of Occupational Psychology* **8**, 233–50.

Wall, T.D., Corbett, J.M., Martin, R., Clegg, C.W. and Jackson, P. (1990) 'Advanced manufacturing technology, work design and performance: A change study', *Journal of Applied Psychology* **75**, 691–7.

Warr, P.B. (1987) 'Job characteristics and mental health', in P.B. Warr (eds.) *Psychology at Work*. Harmondsworth: Penguin Books.

Wells, J.K., Howard, G.S., Nowlin, W.F. and Vargas, M.J. (1986) 'Presurgical anxiety and postsurgical pain and adjustment: Effects of a stress inoculation procedure', *Journal of Consulting and Clinical Psychology* **54**(6), 831–5.

CHAPTER 15

The consequences of stress

BEN (C.) FLETCHER

Chapter outline

Introduction

This chapter outlines the role of psychological factors in organic disease and its precursors. It presents a conceptualization of what is meant by stress which is both predictive and pragmatic. This conceptualization does not require that 'stress' be felt in order to have negative effects. The purpose of the chapter is not to discuss the stress of nursing and caring, nor the stress of coping with illness (see Chapter 14). Rather, it is to show the importance of psychological factors in the functioning of the immune system and the role of stress in cancer, heart disease and life expectancy.

It will probably come as no surprise to the reader to say that stress plays an important role in physical illness and does not just make people feel low, depressed or tired. I have already stated:

> Stress kills. It is responsible for more industrial disease than any other aspect of work. It compromises the immune system, plays a highly important role in the onset of major diseases, and results in premature death. It also makes people feel anxious and depressed, lowers their job and life satisfaction, makes for bad decisions, a poor organizational climate, increases alcohol and cigarette

consumption, increases health service costs, leads to accidents, and reduces efficiency. This is only the tip of the iceberg. (Fletcher, 1990)

However, the extent of the influence of stress in illness is a very controversial topic with many commentators sceptical about how strong the research evidence is for a causal link (e.g. Steptoe, 1993).

Stressors and strains

Stress is an ambiguous word which has been defined in many ways. For this reason it is necessary to distinguish between 'stressors' and 'strains'. *Stressors* may be environmental or psychosocial factors within the person (e.g. personality) which cause the individual to suffer strain. This *strain* is the consequence of being exposed to stressors of sufficient magnitude or duration. Strain may be manifested in many ways, including psychological ill-health and elevation of biological risk factors (e.g. blood pressure, hormonal changes, immune deficiency). Stressors may be major enough to have a relatively immediate and observable effect on the person (e.g. the death of a close friend or moving jobs). They may, however, be less obvious to the person and even go unnoticed. Stressors may not even be considered to be harmful by the person exposed to them. This is why stress is so often considered a 'silent killer': stressors which persist for some length of time may have a cumulative and insidious effect on the person's wellbeing.

DISCUSSION POINT
What signs of stress usually pass unnoticed in colleagues or patients?

There are many ways of measuring stress (biological, epidemiological and psychological) and it is now clear that modelling the stress process is essential if progress is to be made. It is common in psychology to measure stress with the use of the self-report, anonymous questionnaires. These range from simple, but valid, measures of strain in terms of psychological health (e.g. Goldberg's (1972) General Health Questionnaire; or Crown and Crisp's (1979) Experiential Index) to broad-ranging tools based on sophisticated theory which measure both stressors and strains within a specific context (e.g. Fletcher's (1991b, 1991c) *The Cultural Audit: An individual and organisational tool*). The benefit of theoretically driven tools is that they overcome some of the problems inherent in self-report measures because they do not rely simply on the subjective evaluations of the respondents. Unfortunately, many models of stress are restricted to the examination of a narrow range of phenomena or define stress too narrowly. For example, Selye's (1976) early pioneering General Adaptation Model defined stress in terms of physiological effects (primarily secretions of steroids from the adrenal cortex or catecholamines from the adrenal medulla), chronic elevations of which could compromise a person's wellbeing. Another influential approach has been championed by Lazarus (1993). This emphasizes the role of cognitive and emotional mediation: the strain effects of an external factor are largely determined by how the person appraises (and, therefore, copes with) the stressor.

This chapter presents the reader with evidence which suggests that psychological factors in the environment as well as aspects of personality can cause physical disease. This does not imply that if a person is exposed to these factors, or if they have a particular type of personality, they will invariably suffer from illness. Stress should be treated as a risk factor in disease in the same way that other 'causal' agents are treated, such as smoking behaviour.

It is likely that stress exacerbates the negative effects of other traditional risk factors in disease and can, therefore, be a trigger for onset, as well as having independent effects in causing disease. Karmack and Jennings (1991) in their review conclude that although it has not been shown conclusively that stressors independently cause heart attacks, there is abundant evidence that the physiological precursors of sudden death (e.g. vasoconstriction, platelet aggregation, plaque rupture, thrombosis, arrhythmias) are exacerbated by psychological challenge. If further research confirms such findings, it is likely that psychologically oriented treatments, used in combination with traditional ones, will be effective and that psychological therapies will be real prophylactics against major killers such as cancer and heart disease (Eysenck and Grossarth-Maticek, 1991).

The fact that many potential stressors go unnoticed and that stress is not necessarily perceived also suggests that other psychological factors should be considered when discussing these issues. Some are very important in the medical context, especially for treatment. For example, the powerful effects of placebo treatments, and the consequential requirements of medical science to use double-blind clinical trials, are themselves indications of the potentially large contribution of psychological factors. It is commonly supposed that around 30–50 per cent of any patient sample will be placebo responders (i.e. they will show symptom relief even though the 'treatment' has no physiological action) and that the power of the placebo increases with the seniority of the person administering it, confidence in the treatment and the sophistication of the equipment and procedures used (see Chapter 10; and Richardson, 1989). With psychiatric disorders placebo treatments seem very effective. The placebo effect may also be responsible for a large part of the benefits observed using alternative medicine. The power of the effects should not be underestimated: up to 85 per cent of patients suffering from angina pectoris have been shown to obtain clinical symptom relief from a sham operation (Dimond, Kittle and Cockett, 1960). Unfortunately, it is likely that stress problems are not as self-limiting (i.e. improve without treatment) as many physical dysfunctions that are presented to the doctor or nurse.

How many suffer from stress and who are they?

Broadly speaking, at any one point in time, around 10 per cent of an ostensibly 'healthy' workforce are likely to be suffering from some major disabling psychological strain (such as clinically relevant levels of depression or free-floating anxiety), with a further 25 per cent or so having more minor, but significant, problems

(Fletcher, 1991a). In a large random sample of British adults 14 per cent of men and 19 per cent of women reported having experienced unpleasant emotional strain for at least half of the (week)day before the interview, with work being identified as the most important cause (Warr and Payne, 1982). The problems were not confined to the day before the interview (what might be called 'acute strain') since 15 per cent of men and 20 per cent of women had suffered the strain for more than one month. In a major study of heart disease, the Framingham Heart Study, 48 per cent of those aged 45 years or over described themselves as being 'often troubled by feelings of tenseness, tightness, restlessness, or inability to relax', and 37 per cent as being 'usually pressed for time' (Haynes et al., 1978).

Examinations of particular occupational groups in the caring professions reveal high levels of strain in some jobs. For example, in one study, over 21 per cent of student nurses scored at least as high as one would expect of people being treated for anxiety or depression (Parkes, 1982). A similar level was found in social workers (Jones, Fletcher and Ibbetson, 1991), but not in health visitors (Fletcher, Jones and MacGregor-Cheers, 1991). These studies also show much higher levels of strain than those found in women who work in industry. This strain also appears to be causally related to work factors in so far as it is associated with various psycho-logical aspects of the work environment. Rose, Mullan and Fletcher (1994) also suggest that direct care staff in small group homes and hospital settings, who had higher strain levels than those staff in larger community homes, did so because of their higher staff:client ratios and higher levels of work-related interactions with residents.

The higher workers are on the occupational ladder, the less likely they are to suffer from psychological and physical ill health and the longer they live (e.g. Fletcher, 1991a; Stansfield and Marmot, 1992). This is shown in the Whitehall study, a large, longitudinal investigation of disease risk and grade of employment in the civil service. Self-perceived health status and actual angina pectoris, cardiac isc-haemia and chronic bronchitis symptoms were all worse in those with lower status jobs. There were also clear differences between the grades in a range of physiologi-cal risk factors as well as poor health behaviours and family history. These grade differences were partly predicted by job monotony, low job discretion and poorer social supports (Marmot et al., 1991).

The link between stress and disease

Stressors, strains and the immune system

There is a growing body of evidence to link a person's state of mind or mood with lowered efficiency of the body's immune system (Weisse, 1992). In a recent review of studies linking depression and immunity, Herbert and Cohen (1993) found that depression was associated with large alterations in immunocompetence including natural killer cell activity (involved in cancer surveillance) as well as more general indicators of function such as white blood cell counts and lymphocyte proliferation to mitogen challenge. They also observed that the immune system changes were greater for older and hospitalized patients. The explanation given was not in terms of neuroendocrinal mechanisms but through health-related behaviours: depression causes changes in sleep patterns, poorer diet, lowered exercise and increases in smoking and alcohol, all of which have been shown to alter immune responses. This explanation suggests that health practices could be the key to maintaining immuno-competence in such people (see Chapters 5 and 6). Other reviewers examining the link between stress and infectious pathology/diseases have shown that there is marked association between stress and illness behaviour such as use of medical care services (Cohen and Williamson, 1991).

For many viral invasions of the body such as colds and 'flu only a small propor-tion of those infected develop clinical symptoms. The explanation lies in psycho-logical factors (including stress) that mediate between pathogen/antigen and resulting clinical disease symptoms. The role of personality differences in suscep-tibility to infection has also been researched. It is now recognized that the im-mune system and the cardiovascular system are conditionable (i.e. they learn) and must be considered as integral *behavioural* systems. The importance of this is that it shows one way in which stress may influence the disease process. In a famous study by Ader and Cohen (1975), rats were given a drink of sodium saccharin at the same time as they were injected with a powerful immune system suppressant. After a further three days some of the animals were given a second drink of the sodium saccharin. This was found to have a powerful immunosuppressive effect by itself, apparently as a consequence of the association between the drink and the previously administered injection; thus the immune system had learned a relationship. More recent studies have shown that this is a very wide-ranging effect on many aspects of immunocompetence which is likely to be of consider-able clinical significance (Ader and Cohen, 1993). If we consider that humans are much more susceptible than rats to psychological influences, the effects of stress and other psychological factors on the human immune system is likely to be very large indeed. One demonstration of this is given by Smith and McDaniel (1983). They gave students the TB scratch test once a month for six months on one arm and a saline scratch on the other. The TB scratch test is given to ascertain whether or not the person already has the antibodies in their blood to fight tuberculin infection. If they have, a red lump develops later at the site of the TB scratch (known as the Mantoux reaction). Nothing develops where the saline scratch is given. The investigators used only students who showed this delayed Mantoux reaction. However, without telling the students, on the sixth month some TB and saline scratches were given on the opposite arm to that used previously. What the researchers found was that expectancy had a very significant effect on the size of the Mantoux lump: it was almost non-existent when the students were expecting it to appear on the other arm.

Other studies on humans have shown that bereavement, long vigils, surgery, examination taking and loneliness can all have a marked effect on immune system functioning (see Fletcher, 1991a). For example, students who are lonely have poorer immune system responses than those who are not; separated or divorced women have fewer natural killer cells than married women and the more divorced women were attached to their husbands the less able was their immune system to fight infections (Kennedy, Kiecolt-Glaser and Glaser, 1988). In a longitudinal study of genital herpes simplex recurrence, Kemeny *et al.* (1989) have shown that life stressors do have an influence over T-lymphocyte levels and that such factors as state of mind are predictive of recurrence rates.

Stress and cancer

Cancer is the leading cause of death of men and women of working age in Britain. Evidence that stress plays a role in cancer development includes a considerable amount of animal research showing that quite mild stressors can affect tumour development and growth. This is especially true for such factors as the unpredictability of the stressor and lack of control over it. Stress hormones, such as corticosterone, can also produce a marked enhancement of tumour growth (see Fletcher, 1991a).

There are obviously scientific problems in examining the role of stress in human cancer especially since there are over 100 types of cancer with different causal mechanisms, some of which take 20–30 years to develop. The weight of evidence is, however, increasingly strong. For example, one large study (Shaffer, Duszynski and Thomas, 1982) suggests that students who subsequently developed cancers, especially the major ones, perceived themselves as less close to their parents. Impaired father–son relationships demonstrated the strongest links with cancer, with cancer patients scoring substantially lower on closeness than healthy men.

Felt hopelessness and depression may also be related to cancer risk. Schmale and Iker (1971) report a psychological investigation of women attending hospital after having positive cervical smears. They were given cone biopsies to determine whether the abnormalities were cancerous or not, but prior to the outcome of the biopsies they were classified according to the degree to which they exhibited felt hopelessness in response to life events that had occurred in the preceding six months. From this information alone the researchers were able to categorize correctly over 75 per cent of the women in terms of whether or not malignant cells were present. More recently, the Courtauld study has shown that, for women with breast cancer, recurrence-free survival after fifteen years is nearly three times lower in women who respond to their diagnosis with feelings of stoic acceptance or hopelessness, compared to those who exhibited a fighting spirit or a denial of their cancer. This difference is independent of such factors as age, menopausal status, clinical stage, type of operation, tumour size and post-operative radiotherapy (Greer, 1991).

Other aspects of personality have also been linked to cancer risk (see Fletcher, 1991a). Two cancer-prone personality characteristics are:

1. Repression of emotions, rational or non-emotional reactions, or remaining isolated from emotionally important objects such as people.
2. Ambivalent or inconsistent reactions, such as having different feelings or behaving in different ways to the same situation on different occasions.

Some researchers now argue that aetiological models of cancer must incorporate psychological and psychophysiological factors. Lambley (1993), for example, has formulated a model of cervical cancer which gives a central place to such factors and implies that psychologically-based treatments could play a much greater part than they have in the past. This is confirmed by other studies, which show that the survival rates of cancer patients can be considerably improved through the use of behavioural interventions. An example of this is Eysenck and Grossarth-Maticek's (1991) work, which shows that terminally ill cancer patients have enhanced survival times if they undergo creative novation therapy (CNT; see Box 15.1). In one study the CNT group lived for an extra two years longer than the 3.1 years of the control sample. In another study of 100 women with mammary cancer and visceral

---

BOX 15.1 CORE ELEMENTS OF CREATIVE NOVATION THERAPY (ADAPTED FROM GROSSARTH-MATICEK AND EYSENCK, 1991)

The basis of CNT is represented by the following ideas, which form the crux of personal behavioural change:

- People can alter their behaviour to achieve an independent and healthy personality.
- Behaviours can have consequences that are unpleasant, negative and harmful.
- People can do one of three things in the face of unpleasant circumstances:
    1. Change behaviour.
    2. Withdraw or avoid circumstances which make one unhappy.
    3. Change mental attitudes and values.
- To change behaviour or attitudes one must:
    1. Observe oneself carefully and identify:
        (a) the conditions which produce unpleasantness.
        (b) what can be done to change the conditions.
        (c) what new behaviours could be used in these conditions.
    2. Imagine new and alternative behaviours and try them out in mind and action.
    3. Remember that your own needs are important and do not always give precedence to others' needs.
- Trial and error will need to be employed because success will take time and experience of failure as well as success.
- A person should aim to produce autonomous, self-activated behaviour to lead a happy life.
- Replace behaviours that produce unhappiness with those that produce happiness.
- Support and help of others will be useful and important.
- Contentment through changed behaviours is achievable.

metastasis, CNT was as effective as traditional chemotherapy treatments at enhancing survival and when used in conjunction with chemotherapy, doubled the survival times compared to chemotherapy alone. The essential aim of the treatment is the acquisition of new autonomous behaviours to replace potentially damaging old habits.

In the original longitudinal studies of CNT, it was found that initially disease-free people aged 30–69 years who had received CNT for only a short duration (typically for 20 or so hours over a few months) were less than half as likely to have developed cancer or heart disease as control groups without CNT. In many cases, the prophylactic benefits were considerably greater and were also obtained in group therapy sessions. For example, in a seven-year follow-up study using group therapy, 7.5 per cent of the CNT group died from cancer compared to 47.4 per cent of the control group. Furthermore, the benefits were as strong when bibliotherapy was employed (i.e. written explanation of the therapy to be followed rather than individual therapy sessions).

This work has not been without its critics (e.g. Pelosi and Appleby, 1992). However, when the same criteria of scientific rigour are applied to these studies as is usual in medical and psychological science, the findings remain impressive (see Eysenck, 1992, for a response to critics). In my view, the primary limitation of CNT is that it deals only with consciously identifiable stressors and ignores the 'hidden' stressors which are likely to be at least as damaging to health and well-being.

DISCUSSION POINT
What is creative novation therapy and how could its central tenets be employed by health professionals?

Stress and heart disease

Coronary heart disease is a generic term which is used to describe conditions including coronary atherosclerosis and myocardial infarction. Such diseases are a primary cause of death. There is a vast amount of research showing that psychological factors act as stressors affecting the cardiovascular system. For example, it has been shown in coronary patients that mental stress in the form of public speaking, reading to an audience, doing maths and other cognitive tasks can produce abnormalities in heart wall functioning, without any accompanying chest pain (i.e. silent ischaemias), as great in magnitude as that caused by treadmill exercise (Rozanski et al., 1988). In studies which have measured traditional biological and psychosocial variables (albeit very crude ones, such as personality and religious affiliations) the psychosocial variables are at least as good as the biological variables in predicting heart disease, and usually better (Fletcher, 1991a).

The social environment in which the person lives can have a marked effect on resistance to disease. Meaningful and therefore relatively long-term social contacts act as social supports which reduce the effects of stress and therefore have a protective effect. For example, the particularly strong patriarchal Catholic Italian-

Americans, who have a very cohesive and strong social structure with clearly defined social roles, were shown to have less than half the rate of heart attacks than inhabitants of a nearby town which was socially heterogeneous. Similarly, in a study of the effects of social networks in California, Berkman and Syme (1979) have shown that those with few social ties were more than twice as likely to have died from heart disease and cancer as those with more extensive networks. Marriage, it seems, also has a protective effect. Fletcher and Jones (1993) have argued that the higher rates of heart disease apparent in blue collar workers may also be partly associated with a low degree of social support.

A major topic of research into CHD has been the role of personality, following the pioneering work of Friedman and Rosenman (1974), who coined the phrase 'coronary prone behaviour', or type A personality, which is characterized by: extreme competitiveness, constant striving for achievement, high job involvement, aggressiveness and hostility in interactions, haste, impatience, explosiveness of speech, tense facial expression, feeling of being under pressure of time and high responsibility, and constantly having to do more and more. Type B people show the absence of such characteristics.

Approximately 50 per cent of people can be categorized as type As, with half of them showing the more extreme forms of the behaviour. It is not an 'executive' behaviour or one confined to people in selling professions, since it is as common among blue-collar workers. Type A behaviour has been associated with an increased risk of heart disease. In a follow-up study of over 3,000 men initially free of CHD, those aged 39–49 years with type A personalities were 6.5 times more likely to have developed CHD within 2½ years as their counterparts with type B personalities. In follow-ups the magnitude of the difference had reduced but, even when all traditional risk factors for heart disease had been statistically controlled (e.g. parental history of heart disease, blood pressure, cholesterol and triglyceride levels), the overall excess risk of being type A was about two-fold.

However, a more recent 22-year follow-up of the same sample of people has cast doubt on the long-term predictability of the type A personality in CHD (Ragland and Brand, 1988). Other recent research also suggests that the effects of personality on CHD is more complicated than previously thought. It seems that other negative emotions are also likely to play a role. Booth-Kewley and Friedman (1987) in a review paper concluded that: 'Overall the picture of the coronary prone personality emerging . . . seems to be one of a person with one or more negative emotions: perhaps someone who is depressed, aggressively competitive, easily frustrated, anxious, angry or some combination.'

There has been considerable and related debate over how useful the type A/B concept is for predicting CHD (e.g. Friedman and Booth-Kewley, 1988; Ivancevich and Matteson, 1988; Matthews, 1988; Ray, 1991) and some clinicians have suggested that such aspects as grief, hostility, social isolation, fear and work demands are of greater significance than type A (e.g. Conduit, 1992). A more recent conceptualization of the coronary prone personality type has emerged from the large prospective studies of Grossarth-Maticek and co-workers (e.g. Eysenck, 1988;

Eysenck and Grossarth-Maticek, 1991; Grossarth-Maticek, Bastiaans and Kanazir, 1985). According to this view, CHD-prone people are not successful at putting their life into perspective and they become dependent on things that cause them emotional problems. They find certain people or conditions upsetting, but these are also highly important to them. Instead of distancing themselves from these situations they continue to strive towards them, often knowing this is not sensible, and experience problems as a result of dependence on stress-inducing conditions or people. Such individuals are much more likely to get premature CHD than other personality types (and less likely to get cancer than 'cancer-prone' personalities).

Whatever the contribution of type A personality in CHD, there are clear physiological differences between As and Bs in their response to stress, even when the person is not actually conscious. In a study of patients undergoing surgery, type A men showed greater blood pressure changes while they were anaesthetized during coronary bypass surgery (as much as 30 mmHg higher than type Bs) and were much more likely to have complications during the surgery which could be attributed to enhanced sympathetic nervous system activity (Krantz *et al.*, 1982). This is not to deny the potential benefits of behavioural therapy since type As have been shown to devote more of their own or 'discretionary' time to work (a potential stress) (Byrne and Reinhart, 1989) and are more likely to experience life events which need to be coped with because they initiate them (Jarvikoski and Harkapaa, 1988).

DISCUSSION POINTS
Why is it useful to use the term 'psychological factors' instead of just the word 'stress'?
What does it mean to say that psychological factors cause disease?

A wider view of stress

Transmitting work stress and health

The very significant role that work stressors play in disease is shown further by my own research on occupational mortality (e.g. Fletcher, 1983, 1988, 1991a, 1992; Jones and Fletcher, 1993a). This work was originally based on an analysis of occupational mortality data and the demonstration that a married woman's life expectancy and very specific disease risk was predictable from the husband's occupation. Some examples from among the 550 or so occupations studied are shown in Table 15.1 for broad categories of cause of death (the findings are as strong if one looks at specific causes). The statistics shown are Standardized Mortality Ratios (SMRs) where 100 is the average and higher figures reflect increased risk. You will notice that there is both occupational and disease specificity: similar jobs have different risk rates which are also different for different diseases, but that the disease concordance for men and married women is very strong. For example, photographers (and women married to them) have lower than average mortality from respiratory diseases, but higher than average for external causes such as accidents, poisonings and death from violence.

Table 15.1 *Examples from each social class of disease–specific occupational mortality (SMRs) for men and women married to men in those occupations[a]*

	Cancer		Heart disease		Respiratory		External[b]	
	Men	Women	Men	Women	Men	Women	Men	Women
Social Class 1								
Judges	82	114			53	28		
Govt assistant secs+	115	147					88	64
Medics & Dentists					26	25	115	151
Social Class 2								
Authors, Journalists			79	68			120	155
Musicians	110	94			166	161		
Social Class 3 (non-manual)								
Photographers					58	64	133	143
Site managers/foremen	57	65					32	33
Police sergeants	163	164					71	81
Policemen	109	106			61	75		
Social Class 3 (manual)								
Chefs	126	131					169	190
Foremen (machinery)	161	175			88	81		
Social Class 4								
Winders, Reelers	16	47			130	164		
Textile processors			122	162			51	81
Deck hands, Boatmen, etc.			232	269			499	315
Stevedores, Warehousemen					134	138	89	87
Social Class 5 Labourers:								
Coke ovens & gas workers	119	100			191	171		
Textiles	187	84	225	248				
Coal miners					359	429	279	234

Notes
a. For clarity, only two sets of SMRs are included for any occupation.
b. Accidents, poisoning, violence, etc.

Source: Fletcher (1988); and abstracted from OPCS (1986).

One reason for suggesting that work stress is transmitted from husband to wife is that a whole array of more obvious explanations were carefully ruled out (including couples sharing the same social conditions or class; transmission of toxic substances; elevation in the death rate of women following the death of their spouse due to a bereavement; partners doing broadly similar work; people with similar risk profiles marrying each other; data inaccuracies with SMRs, etc.).

More recently, our research has investigated actual stress transmission in married dual-career couples and has included the daily completion of extended in-depth questionnaires by participating couples. It does appear that couples do fluctuate together in mood and health symptoms and that what transmission takes place is from the man to his partner and not vice versa, even in dual-career households (Jones and Fletcher, 1993b and c). I have proposed that 'non-heeded' or unconsciously perceived factors within the workplace may be responsible for the transmission of specific disease risk and the observed disease concordance in married couples (Fletcher, 1992). This posits a central role for a person's 'cognitive architecture' (or way of thinking) in health and explicitly suggests that the work a person does affects their cognitive structures which are in turn transmitted to partners. It also puts a very important emphasis on unconscious or non-heeded influences and implies that future stress research should concentrate more on such cognitive processes than on *feelings* of pressure and stress.

DISCUSSION POINT
Think about and list ways that stress might actually be transmitted from one person to another.

Stress and the catastrophe model

More general models of stress are covered in Chapter 14. Models are essential in this field because they provide a way of predicting the 'who, when, why and how' of strain. They are useful, for example, in predicting why it is that some jobs are associated with higher levels of strain and why there are subtle differences between jobs in their strain levels even though they may look superficially similar. Models have also reinforced the idea that we are not likely to be successful at isolating the psychological causes of ill-health by introspection. Stress is clearly not to be equated with feeling under demand or under pressure.

Central to my *catastrophe model* is the idea that strain results when there is a lack of balance in the demands and constraints placed on a person in relation to the supports that are available to them (Fletcher, 1991a). The dimensions of the model are:

■ *Demands.* This is the degree to which the environment contains stimuli which peremptorily require attention and response. The stimuli may be technical, intellectual, social or financial. Demands are the things that have to be done. Table 15.2 presents some common job demands.

Table 15.2 *Work Stressors as Demands or Supports/Constraints*

Work demands	Work Supports/Constraints
Job pressure	Being clear about role
Having too much to do	Job discretion, autonomy or control
Having too little to do	Quality of relationships with:
Being responsible for people	Boss
Responsibility for things (equipment)	Colleagues
Demands from others	Subordinates
Conflicting demands/roles	Union membership
Over/under-promotion	Role ambiguity
Keeping up with others/organizations	Variety level/skill utilization
Organizational climate	Social perception of job
Office politics	Participation in decisions
Organizational structure	Payment/reward system
Organizational/job changes	Quality of equipment
Major decisions	Physical working conditions
Expectancies of others/organization	How work is planned/managed

- *Supports.* This is the degree to which there are resources which are relevant to meeting the demands of the individual or the group. These supports may be technical, intellectual, social, financial, etc. For example, being part of a happy cohesive workforce or having a supportive spouse may reduce the impact of demands.
- *Constraints* are those aspects of the environment which prevent a person or group from coping with demands. For example, the lack of relevant resources to do a job well. Such constraints can act to prevent people maximizing the benefits of supports, as well as affect how they can cope with the demands. Table 15.2 shows some common work supports/constraints.

According to the catastrophe model, strain results from a lack of balance between the demands, supports and constraints. Thus, high job demands may not be stressful if the job (or the non-work environment) also provides good levels of support and low constraints. In fact, high demands can be beneficial in the right circumstances. They provide stimulation and utilize the worker's abilities – underutilization of abilities and boredom are among the most potent stressors and usually occur in work environments where supports are low and constraints high. This is common of jobs in the lower social classes, which generally have the highest strain levels. Karasek (e.g. Karasek, Russell and Theorell, 1982; Karasek, 1990) has done a considerable amount of work to show that one support, namely job discretion, can moderate the effects of job demands on the cardiovascular system (see the next section). In situations of high demand, adrenalin levels are increased, with consequent changes in blood pressure and blood lipid values. It seems, however, that low discretion or lack of control is also associated with higher levels of the stress hormone cortisol. Karasek suggests that the worst combination for the cardiovascular system is when demands are high and are not offset by controllability. He has applied this to the long-term prediction of heart disease rates in both the United States and Sweden. It was found that having low job discretion significantly increased the risk of heart attacks, over and above the effects of job demands. This relationship between job demands and job discretion has also been successful in predicting pill consumption, depression rates, felt exhaustion, absence from work, life and job satisfaction (Karasek, 1979). Nevertheless, it is clear from other research that social factors, especially related to social support, are much more likely to affect strain levels (e.g. Fletcher and Jones, 1993).

One obvious practical implication of the model is that highly demanding jobs can be made less stressful without reducing the level of the demands: instead, the level of supports can be increased or the constraints reduced. The model has implications for redesigning work to reduce the amount of strain in an organization while at the same time boosting efficiency and this has been tested with nurses, health visitors and social workers (Fletcher *et al.*, 1991; Jones, Fletcher and Ibbotson, 1991; Rose, Mullan and Fletcher, 1993).

DISCUSSION POINT

In your workplace how could constraints be reduced and supports increased in order to reduce stress without lowering demands?

The model proposes that 'catastrophe' may occur with a very small change in the environmental or personal conditions. Central to the model is the idea of a threshold level of strain potential, above which a person would show or develop clinical symptoms. The strain potential is the aggregate of all demands, supports and constraints, and people may also have different threshold levels. These may be exceeded as a result of significant life events or a particularly poor circumstance, causing clinical manifestations such as elevated blood pressure, anxiety or stress hormone secretion. For most people, however, it is the sum of minor, sub-threshold stressors that determines strain levels. This implies that people are unlikely to know what is the cause of their strain, because they have no conscious access to this information. The model is called the catastrophe model, however, because it also predicts that above the threshold level certain of the demand, support and constraint factors will be perceived differently. For example, coffee breaks or social interaction with colleagues suddenly become stressful to the person who is not coping with job demands.

This model has a number of important practical implications for dealing with stress issues. It predicts that (1) the stressed person will perceive the world differently; (2) a distinction has to be drawn between the primary causes of strain and the factors which are only secondarily associated with it; (3) people cannot be presumed to know what the causes of stress are; and (4) one cannot simple 'cure' the person by removing the true causes (or increasing relevant supports) because the catastrophe will have resulted in changed perceptions which will need to be tackled themselves.

Summary

This chapter has considered what is meant by the term 'stress' and suggested that a whole array of psychological factors are likely to play a role in the onset of disease. Only some of these factors would normally be associated with increased pressure or environmental demand, which is why the use of the term 'stress' can be misleading and unhelpful. Of particular importance is the fact that many 'stressors' are unlikely to be noticed by people although they will still affect them. Psychological therapies are likely to be of use in the prevention of major diseases but their potential requires greater conceptual clarity and development of predictive models of stress which emphasise cognitive and behavioural, rather than affective, processes.

Seminar questions

1. What is meant by the term stress?
2. Identify the ways that health care professionals can reduce the effects of stressors on those in their care.
3. Discuss the role of psychological factors in causing illness and disease.

Further reading

Fletcher, B. (1991) *Work, Stress, Disease, and Life Expectancy.* Chichester: John Wiley. The most comprehensive single source which covers all the issues raised here.

Carroll, D. (1992) *Health Psychology: Stress, behaviour and disease.* Brighton: The Falmer Press. This looks at topics including pain, AIDS, exercise and treatment adherence, as well as issues covered in Fletcher (1991).

Gatchel, R.J., Baum, A. and Krantz, D.S. (1989) *An Introduction to Health Psychology*, 2nd edition. New York: Random House. An American text with a reasonable general coverage.

References

Ader, R. and Cohen, N. (1975) 'Behaviourally conditioned immunosuppression', *Psychosomatic Medicine* **37**, 333–40.

Ader, R. and Cohen, N. (1993) 'Psychoneuroimmunology: Conditioning and stress', *Annual Review of Psychology* **44**, 53–85.

Berkman, L.F. and Syme, S.L. (1979) 'Social networks, lost resistance, and mortality: A nine-year follow-up study of Alameda County residents', *American Journal of Epidemiology* **109**(2), 186–204.

Booth-Kewley, S. and Friedman, H.S. 'Psychological predictors of heart disease: A quantitative review', *Psychological Bulletin* **101**, 343–62.

Byrne, D.G. and Reinhart, M.I. (1989) 'Work characteristics, occupational achievement and the type A behaviour pattern', *Journal of Occupational Psychology* **62**, 123–34.

Cohen, S. and Williamson, G.M. (1991) 'Stress and infectious disease in humans', *Psychological Bulletin* **109**(1), 5–24.

Conduit, E.H. (1992) 'If A–B does not predict heart disease, why bother with it? A clinician's view', *British Journal of Medical Psychology* **65**(3), 289–96.

Crown, S. and Crisp, A.H. (1979) *Manual of the Crown–Crisp Experiential Index.* London: Hodder & Stoughton.

Dimond, E.G., Kittle, C.F. and Cockett, J.E. (1960) 'Comparison of internal mammary artery ligation and sham operation for angina pectoris', *American Journal of Cardiology* **4**, 483–6.

Eysenck, H.J. (1988) 'Personality, stress and cancer: Predicition and prophylaxis', *British Journal of Medical Psychology* **61**, 57–75.

Eysenck, H.J. (1992) 'Psychosocial factors, cancer and ischaemic heart disease', *British Medical Journal* **305**, 457–9.

Eysenck, H.J. and Grossarth-Maticek, R. (1991) 'Creative novation therapy as a prophylactic treatment for cancer and coronary heart disease: Part II – effects of treatment', *Behaviour Research and Therapy* **29**, 17–31.

Fletcher, B. (C) (1983) 'Marital relationships as a cause of death: An analysis of occupational mortality and the hidden consequences of marriage – some UK data', *Human Relations* **36**(2), 123–34.

Fletcher, B. (C) (1988) 'Occupation, marriage and disease-specific mortality concordance', *Social Science and Medicine* **27**(6), 615–22.

Fletcher, B. (C) (1990) *Clergy under Stress.* London: Mowbrays.

Fletcher, B. (C) (1991a) *Work, Stress, Disease, and Life Expectancy.* Chichester: John Wiley.

Fletcher, B. (C) (1991b) *The Cultural Audit: An individual and organisational investigation.* Cambridge: PSI. (First edition 1989).

Fletcher, B. (C) (1991c) *The Micro-cultural Audit: An individual and organisational tool.* Cambridge: PSI.

Fletcher, B. (C) (1992) *Cognitive Architecture and Disease Risk.* Second public lecture, British Psychological Society, Annual Conference, Blackpool.

Fletcher, B. (C) and Jones, F. (1993) 'The role of occupational demands and decision lattitude in casual blood pressure, psychological health and satisfaction', *Journal of Organisational Behaviour* **14**, 319–30.

Fletcher, B., (C), Jones, F. and McGregor-Cheers, J. (1991) 'The stressors and strains of health visiting: Demands, supports, constraints and psychological health', *Journal of Advanced Nursing* **16**, 1078–89.

Friedman, M. and Rosenman, R.H. (1974) *Type A Behaviour and Your Heart.* New York: Knopf.

Friedman, H.S. and Booth-Kewley, F. (1988) 'Validity of the type A construct: A reprise. *Psychological Bulletin* **104**(3), 381–4.

Goldberg, A. (1972) 'The detection of psychiatric illness by questionnaire', *Maudsley Monograph No. 21.* Oxford: Oxford University Press.

Greer, S. (1991) 'Psychological response to cancer and survival', *Psychological Medicine* **21**, 43–9.

Grossarth-Maticek, R. and Eysenck, H.J. (1991) 'Creative novation therapy as a prophylactic treatment for cancer and coronary heart disease: Part I – description of treatment', *Behaviour Research and Therapy* **29**, 1–16.

Grossarth-Maticek, R., Bastiaans, J. and Kanazir, D.T. (1985) 'Psychosocial factors as strong predictors of mortality from cancer, ischaemic heart disease and stroke: The Yugoslav prospective study', *Journal of Psychosomatic Research* **29**, 167–76.

Haynes, S.G., Feinleib, M., Levine, S., Scotch, N. and Kannel, W.B. (1978) 'The relationship of psychosocial factors to coronary heart disease in the Framingham Study: II. Prevalence of coronary heart disease', *American Journal of Epidemiology* **107**(5), 384–402.

Herbert, T.B. and Cohen, S. (1993) 'Depression and immunity: A meta-analytic review', *Psychological Bulletin* **113**(3), 472–86.

Ivancevich, J.M. and Mattesson, M.T. (1988) 'Type A behaviour and the healthy', *British Journal of Medical Psychology* **61**, 37–56.

Jarvikoski, A. and Harkapaa, K. (1988) 'Type A behaviour and life events', *British Journal of Medical Psychology* **61**, 353–63.

Jones, F. and Fletcher, B. (C) (1993a) 'Disease concordances amongst marital partners: Not "way of life" or mortality data artifact', *Social Science and Medicine* **12**(3), 1525–33.

Jones, F. and Fletcher, B. (C) (1993b) 'An empirical study of occupational stress transmission in working couples', *Human Relations* **46**(7), 881–903.

Jones, F. and Fletcher, B. (C) (1993c) 'A theory of occupational stress transmission.' Paper presented to the 7th European Health Psychology Conference, Brussels, September.

Jones, F., Fletcher, B. (C) and Ibbetson, K. (1991) 'Stressors and strains amongst social workers: Demands, supports, constraints and psychological health', *British Journal of Social Work* **21**, 443–69.

Karasek, R.A. (1979) 'Job demands, job decision lattitude and mental strain: Implications for job design', *Administrative Science Quarterly* **24**, 285–308.

Karasck, R.A. (1990) 'Lower health risk with incresed job control among white collar workers', *Journal of Organisational Behaviour* **11**, 171–85.

Karasek, R.A., Russell, R.S. and Theorell, T. (1982) 'Physiology of stress and regeneration in job-related cardiovascular illness', *Journal of Human Stress* **8**(1), 29–42.

Karmack, T. and Jennings, J.R. (1991) 'Biobehavioural factors in sudden cardiac death', *Psychological Bulletin* **109**(1), 42–75.

Kemeny, M.E., Cohen, F., Zegans, L.S. and Conant, M.A. (1989) 'Psychological and immunological predictors of genital herpes recurrence', *Psychosomatic Medicine* **51**, 195–208.

Kennedy, S., Kiecolt-Glaser, J.K. and Glaser, R. (1988) 'Immunological consequences of acute and chronic stressors : Mediating role of interpersonal relationships', *British Journal of Medical Psychology* **61**(1), 77–87.

Krantz, D.S., Arabian, J.M., Davia, J.E. and Parker, J.S. (1982) 'Type A behaviour and coronary bypass surgery: Intraoperative blood prcssure and perioperative complications', *Psychosomatic Medicine* **44**(3), 273–84.

Lambley, P. (1993) 'The role of psychological processes in the aetiology and treatment of cervical cancer: A biopsychological perspective', *British Journal of Medical Psychology* **66**, 43–60.

Lazarus, R.S. (1993) 'From psychological stress to the emotions: A history of changing outlooks', *Annual Review of Psychology* **44**, 1–21.

Marmot, M.G., Smith, G.D., Stansfield, S., Patel, C., North, F., Head, J., White, I., Brunner, E. and Feeney, A. (1991) 'Health inequalities among British civil servants: The Whitehall II study', *The Lancet* **337**, 1387–93.

Matthews, K.A. (1988) 'Coronary heart disease and type A behaviors: Update on and alternative to the Booth-Kewley and Friedman (1987) quantitative review', *Psychological Bulletin* **104**, 373–80.

OPCS (1986) *Occupational Mortality 1979–80, 1982–3.* Decennial supplement, Part II. Microfiche tables, Series D5, no. 6. London: HMSO.

Parkes, K.R. (1982) 'Occupational stress among student nurses: A natural experiment', *Journal of Applied Psychology* **67**(b), 789–96.

Pelosi, A.J. and Appleby, L. (1992) 'Psychological influences on cancer and ischaemic heart disease', *British Medical Journal* **303**, 1295–8.

Raglan, D.R. and Brand, R.J. (1988) 'Coronary heart disease mortality in the Western Collaborative Group Study: Follow-up experience of 22 years', *American Journal of Epiemiology* **127**(3), 462–75.

Ray, J.J. (1991) 'If "A–B" does not predict heart disease, why bother with it? A comment on Ivancevich & Mattesson', *British Journal of Medical Psychology* **64**(1), 85–90.

Richardson, P. (1989) 'Placebos: Their effectiveness and modes of action', in A.K. Broome (ed.) *Health Psychology: Processes and applications.* London and New York: Chapman & Hall.

Rose, J., Mullan, E. and Fletcher, B. (C) (1994) 'An examination of the relationship between staff behaviour and stress levels in residential care', *Mental Handicap*, in press.

Rozanski, A., Bairey, C.N., Krantz, D.S., Friedman, M.D., Resser, K.J., Morell, M., Hilton-Chalfen, S., Hestrin, L., Bietendorf, J. and Berman, D.S. (1988) 'Mental stress and the induction of silent myocardial ischemia in patients with coronary artery disease', *The New England Journal of Medicine* **318**(16), 1005–11.

Schmale, A.H. and Iker, H.P. (1971) 'Hopelessness as a predictor of cervical cancer', *Social Science & Medicine* **5**, 95–100.

Selye, H. (1976) *The Stress of Life.* New York: McGraw-Hill.

Shaffer, J., Duszynski, K.R. and Thomas, C.B. (1982) 'Family attitudes in youth as a possible precursor of cancer among physicians: A search for explanatory mechanisms', *Journal of Behavioural Medicine* **5**, 143–64.

Smith, G.R. and McDaniel, S. M. (1983) 'Psychologically mediated effect on the delayed hypersensitivity reaction to tuberculin in humans, *Psychosomatic Medicine* **45**, 65–70.

Stansfield, S.A. and Marmot, M.G. (1992) 'Social class and minor psychiatric disorder in British civil servants: A validated screening survey using the GHQ', *Psychological Medicine* **22**, 739–49.

Steptoe, A. (1993) 'Stress and disease book reviews', *British Journal of Psychology* **84**, 102–3.

Warr, P.B. and Payne, R.L. (1982) 'Experiences of strain and pleasure among British adults', *Social Science and Medicine* **16**, 1691–7.

Weisse, C.S. (1992) 'Depression and immunocompetence: A review of the literature', *Psychological Bulletin* **111**(3), 475–89.

CHAPTER 16

Psychological implications of HIV infection

BARBARA HEDGE

Chapter outline

Introduction

Initial reports of Acquired Immune Deficiency Syndrome (AIDS) from Los Angeles, San Francisco and New York in the early 1980s described an acute illness in gay men which was usually fatal (Shilts, 1987). By 1982 cases of AIDS were also being seen in people with haemophilia, blood transfusion recipients, injecting drug users and infants, and it became apparent that AIDS was more than the 'gay plague' the media was beginning to report. In 1983 an infectious agent, the human immunodeficiency virus (HIV) was identified as the cause of AIDS and it has now become clear that infection with HIV is life-long, resulting in a chronic condition in which the asymptomatic phase may last many years, but which almost always leads to life-threatening illnesses and death.

Caring for those infected with HIV involves more than just the medical interventions aimed at preserving the immune system or fighting disease. Such procedures are able to help individuals live longer and survive repeated bouts of illness. However, the uncertainty attached to the course of disease and its poor prognosis frequently cause intense emotional reactions, even in those who are clinically well and asymptomatic. Good care addresses an individual's quality of life as well as its length; it aims to help people live with HIV infection rather than simply wait to die from it. In an attempt to meet this goal, health care for those with HIV disease is best provided by a multidisciplinary team, with doctors, nurses, psychologists, psychiatrists, dietitians, pharmacists, social workers and a variety of counsellors all bringing their skills to patients' care. As the number of people infected by HIV continues to rise, it is essential for all health carers to have some knowledge of the psychological and social implications of HIV disease.

This chapter is principally concerned with the psychological manifestations of HIV disease. But as many of these are related to the clinical course of infection, a background knowledge of the natural history of infection and disease progression is first necessary. The meanings attached to HIV infection and issues surrounding HIV testing are discussed next. Emotional distress associated with HIV infection is described and ways in which psychological interventions can improve quality of life are considered. Finally, some thought is given to the psychological effects that prolonged caring for people with HIV disease can have on carers.

The natural history of infection and disease

The human immunodeficiency viruses (HIV-1 and HIV-2) are part of a family of retroviruses which infect cells of the immune system. Particularly affected are the CD4 cells, which play a key role in orchestrating the immune system's response to infection, and the monocyte-macrophage cells in the brain. Infection of the latter can lead to cognitive impairment. Antibodies are produced in an attempt to destroy the virus, but this response appears insufficient. As a result, individuals remain infected and potentially infectious for life.

Most of the tests for HIV infection look for the presence of antibodies. As the antibodies take some time to develop there is a 'window period' during which individuals may be infected but will not test 'antibody positive'. It is therefore normal practice to test 12 weeks after a possible exposure to HIV.

Transmission of infection occurs through the exchange of infected body fluids such as blood, blood products, semen, cervical secretions and breast milk. Thus it is sexual practices such as penetrative sex between men, or between men and women, and needle or syringe sharing while injecting drugs which constitute the most risky behaviours for transmission of HIV rather than a person's sexual orientation, race or personality. HIV can also pass from mother to child across the placenta during pregnancy, at the time of delivery and after delivery via breast milk (Peckham and Newell, 1990).

Although a transient, flu-like illness may accompany the initial antibody response, many individuals remain asymptomatic for some years. As the virus replicates and destroys the immune system a variety of symptoms such as swollen lymph glands, night sweats, fatigue and diarrhoea can be experienced. A diagnosis of AIDS is made when certain opportunistic infections, tumours or encephalopathy are observed. A commonly used marker of immunosuppression is a count of CD4 cells. There is a trend for a decreasing CD4 count to be associated with increasing clinical symptoms of illness, with individuals becoming increasingly vulnerable to particular opportunistic infections and cancers. However, this measure is not sufficiently reliable to be predictive of an individual's clinical disease pattern. Current research suggests that approximately 50 per cent of people with HIV infection will have progressed to AIDS within 8–10 years of infection (Rutherford *et al.*, 1990), with poorer rates of survival in adults being associated with an older age at time of infection and a lack of antiviral treatment before diagnosis of AIDS (Graham *et al.*, 1992).

Neuropsychological complications of disease

The neuropsychological effects of HIV disease are many and varied (Grant, 1990) and can result from either the direct effect of HIV on the central nervous system or from secondary complications of immune deficiency. Neuropsychological status at various stages of HIV disease is controversial, particularly concerning the asymptomatic patient. Some investigators (eg Grant *et al.*, 1987) suggest that brain impairment due to HIV is detectable in many individuals otherwise asymptomatic, while others report no neuropsychological deficits in the asymptomatic patient (McArthur, 1987; Perry and Marrotta, 1987; WHO, 1988).

The pattern of cognitive deficits which emerges in late stage disease shows impairment consistent with some features of subcortical dementia including decline in motor speed, concentration, problem-solving and visuospatial abilities (Navia, 1990).

Reactions to a positive test result

For medical reasons alone a positive HIV test can give a person many difficult issues to come to terms with and is comparable with the diagnosis of other potentially fatal illnesses. However, people with HIV infection have to face additional problems, such as the stigma and discrimination attached to gay sex and drug use. King (1989a) reported the experiences of 192 people with HIV infection. Over 25

Table 16.1 *Reactions to HIV infection*

Fears	Symptoms
Death	Shock and denial
Pain	Anxiety
Loss of control	Depression
The future	Suicide ideation and behaviours
Sex	Guilt
Identity	Anger and frustration
Relationships	Sexual dysfunction
	Obsessive disorders

per cent had experienced stigmatizing or discriminatory actions related to their serostatus especially if they had a physical manifestation of the disease. Because the individuals were sensitive to public fear and disapproval, more than 50 per cent had not told their GP and only 35 per cent had told families of their infection.

Pre- and post-test counselling

In order to prepare people for receiving a positive test result and minimize associated distress, the former Department of Health and Social Security recommend that pre- and post-test counselling be available for all those considering having an HIV antibody test (DHSS, 1985). As shown in Table 16.1, negative reactions to a positive HIV antibody test result are commonly experienced, with patients voicing many fears and often showing symptoms of psychological distress.

There are two major aims for HIV counselling. The first is to help individuals maintain behaviours which will minimize the chance of them transmitting HIV if already infected or of them acquiring the virus if uninfected. The second is to maximize the quality of life of those infected. Pinching (1994) argues that these aims are intricately related and that public health issues are generally best served by attention to the needs of individuals. This suggests that pre- and post-test counselling aimed at supporting the individual will also benefit society in general.

Counselling involves more than simply giving information. Although an accurate understanding of the facts is essential, the role of counselling is to assist individuals in relating the relevant information to their own risks, needs, social support and coping skills, and from this assessment to make their own decisions. Counsellors, therefore, need to provide accurate, up-to-date information about HIV infection and to guide people through the problem-solving process. This involves:

- Fact-finding.
- Exploration of options.
- Decision-making.
- Living with the consequences.

BOX 16.1   **THE IMPACT OF WRITTEN LEAFLETS**

Leaflets and posters are frequently used to disseminate information widely. However, it cannot be assumed that because leaflets are provided, people are informed. Much public health information is not read because it is either not looked at when its physical packaging does not make it appear interesting (Poulton, 1969), or when the language used is too difficult to be understood (Ley and Spelman, 1967).

Sherr and Hedge (1990) analyzed three leaflets targeted at pregnant women which discussed the vertical spread of HIV. They analyzed the presentation, accuracy, errors, biases and readability of the leaflets, and assessed the impact they had on women through a group discussion. Only the most attractive leaflet would have been picked up (and then only in the privacy of a consulting room). Leaflets contained errors, omissions, confusing messages and misleading suggestions. Less than 40 per cent of the population understood some of the most important passages and all the leaflets raised more questions than they answered. Women were pleased to receive the information but wanted an opportunity to discuss the issues raised with a professional.

These findings suggest that although written information can provide a useful adjunct to counselling, it cannot not replace it.

- practical assistance.
- continuing support.

Thus the use of leaflets to provide information may be important, but can be only part of the counselling process (see Box 16.1).

Pre-test counselling

In order to make an informed decision as to whether an HIV antibody test is wanted or needed it is necessary that the test is clearly understood. A common misunderstanding is that the test determines whether a person has AIDS rather than detects the underlying infection with HIV. Additionally, people are often unaware of the window period following infection. Table 16.2 documents the essential issues which need to be addressed before testing. As people are frequently in shock when told they are HIV positive, as much information as possible should be given before testing. If they test negative the aim is for them to remain uninfected. Because such individuals may not take up the offer of post-test counselling, safer sex needs to be discussed before the HIV test.

Post-test counselling

It is always difficult to break bad news (Perakyla and Bor, 1990), but postponement does not ease the situation and can increase recipients' stress as they try to guess the

Table 16.2   *Issues to be covered during pre- and post-test counselling sessions*

Pre-test Counselling	Post-test Counselling
■ Explain what the test means and what it does not tell.	■ Focus on the reason for the session.
■ Alert to possible ramifications of a positive test result.	■ Give clear, simple, unambiguous information.
■ Assess personal risk.	■ Clarify what an HIV antibody positive test result means.

■ Prepare for a positive test result:
  – Advantages of knowing HIV serostatus.
  – Disadvantages of knowing HIV serostatus.
  – Who to tell and why to be circumspect.
	■ Expect emotional reactions: shock, denial, anxiety, anger.
	■ Address patient's immediate concerns.
	■ Identify issues of immediate importance: who to and who not to tell; who to use for support; safer sex and injecting practices.

■ Develop coping strategies. ■ Identify social support. ■ Educate in safer sex and safer injecting practices. ■ Explain confidentiality of test result.	■ Provide a lifeline, e.g. a 24-hour helpline telephone number and written information about HIV, giving details of services available. ■ Give a further appointment within a few days.

result from the demeanour and approach of the counsellor. When a person comes for the results of an HIV test it is essential to clarify the reason for this meeting immediately and to focus on the results of the blood test (Table 16.2). Even when a positive test result is expected, shock and distress are frequently experienced once HIV infection is confirmed. It is well documented that few facts are retained even a few minutes after medical consultations (Ley and Spelman, 1967), especially in times of shock. This suggests that when giving an HIV-positive test result only the most important information should be given, using clear, unambiguous language.

Patients' immediate concerns are frequently the prognosis and the likely pattern of disease. Although medical interventions are increasingly successful in reducing the effects of opportunistic infections, there remain many uncertainties in disease progression. It is important that counselling addresses the difficulties of living with uncertainty rather than attempts to provide unrealistically precise answers or un-substantiated reassurance. The former approach gives patients the opportunity to develop the necessary coping skills and not to feel further distress should their health deteriorate.

Every patient has the right to confidentiality and the stigma attached to HIV disease increases the need for confidential information to remain within the HIV care team. Ethical problems can arise when a patient refuses to tell a person who is at continuing risk of exposure (such as a sexual partner where unsafe sex is being practised). Experience shows that breaking confidentiality usually does not solve the problem as patients take their care elsewhere and are unlikely to disclose such information a second time. When confidentiality is respected there is less reason for difficulties to be hidden and for problems to remain unresolved (Pinching, 1994).

DISCUSSION POINT

Sometimes the dilemmas encountered can be extremely complex. For example, a patient told nursing staff that he intended to tell his wife of his HIV status after being discharged from hospital. The couple had been having regular, unprotected sexual intercourse and had a 4-year-old son. Unfortunately, the man's condition deteriorated and he died before he told her. Do you think his wife should be told of her husband's HIV infection or should confidentiality be maintained?

Summary

Access to counselling needs to be made available for individuals considering an HIV test in order to minimize the distress attached to a positive test result. Pre-test counselling aims to ensure that individuals are fully informed about the meaning of a positive test result and its implications, and are prepared to cope should their result be positive.

Post-test counselling provides an opportunity for patients who test positive to explore ways in which their quality of life can be enhanced while living with HIV infection and for further discussion of the prevention of further spread of infection.

The need for confidentiality is of prime importance in the testing for HIV, to maintain people's trust, to respect their rights and to prevent discrimination against them.

Psychological reactions to HIV disease

Even when pre- and post-test counselling has been made available, the continuing impact of HIV disease on a person's life can be great. This section discusses possible causes of psychological symptoms such as multiple stressors and considers issues related to suicide. The potential effect of stress on immune functioning is then outlined. Finally, adaptive coping strategies and the 'buffer' which can be provided by social support are considered.

Psychological symptomatology

Many studies have reported psychological symptomatology in persons with HIV. Tross *et al.* (1987) found the rate of psychiatric disorder in gay men with HIV disease to be 2–4 times that in the general population. King (1989b) reported 31 per cent of HIV-positive patients attending a London hospital to show psychiatric symptoms, and Catalan *et al.* (1992a) reported higher levels of mood disturbance in HIV-infected individuals with haemophilia than in seronegatives. A number of attempts (Atkinson *et al.*, 1988; Catalan *et al.*, 1992b; Chuang *et al.*, 1989) have been made to establish whether a relationship exists between psychological morbidity and the stage of infection. No consensus has yet been reached, with some authors (e.g. Gala *et al.*, 1993; Ostrow *et al.*, 1986) reporting few differences between HIV-negative and asymptomatic HIV-positive gay men; Hedge, Sherr and Green (1991) finding psychological symptomatology to be independent of stage of disease, Perry *et al.* (1990a) reporting the time of testing to be stressful and Williams *et al.* (1991) noting that the onset of symptoms or an AIDS diagnosis is associated with increased psychological distress. A definitive answer to this question is difficult to obtain because of the many confounding factors. For example, Gala *et al.* (1993), who found similarities in psychiatric morbidity between asymptomatic positive and comparable seronegative individuals seeking an HIV test, suggest that these findings may reflect raised levels of psychological morbidity in the HIV-negative group as the test itself can be stress-inducing.

Suicide ideation and behaviour

Reports by Marzuk *et al.* (1988) of a 36-fold increase in relative risk of suicide in men with AIDS in New York, and by Gala *et al.* (1992) of an increase in suicides among HIV-positive deaths, especially in those with histories of attempted suicide, are consistent with data linking cancer with an increased risk of suicide (Fox *et al.*, 1982). The methodological problems encountered in assessing the incidence of suicide in any population are enormous; many authors (e.g. Pugh, O'Donnell and Catalan, 1993) highlight misclassification and under-reporting of probable cases.

Although the time of testing has been linked with increased thoughts of suicide (Perry, Jacobsberg and Fishman, 1990a), the potential suicide risk of people with HIV infection is high at all times, as many stressors which are associated with an increased suicide risk (e.g. life events, depression, social isolation and cumulative stress) have been documented in those with HIV disease (Brown, 1979; Paykel, Prusoff and Myers, 1975; Schneider *et al.*, 1991; Slater and Depue, 1981).

Stress, coping skills and social support

A number of models have been proposed to explain how psychological and physical dysfunction are related to induced stress. For example, Lazarus and Folkman (1984) conceptualize coping as 'constantly changing cognitive and behavioural efforts to manage external and/or internal demands that are appraised as taxing or exceeding the resources of the person' and that stress occurs when the perceived biological, psychological and social resources available are not sufficient to meet the demands of the situation. It is well documented that stress, or non-coping, is frequently accompanied by various emotional reactions such as fear, anxiety, depression and anger.

Lazarus and Folkman's model suggests that the costs and benefits of possible coping behaviours are evaluated and the coping behaviour adopted is that perceived as most beneficial. There is evidence that an appraisal of the threat presented by a stressor could be 'buffered' by the availability and extent of social support systems (Cohen and Wills, 1985), the individual's perceived control over the situation (Rotter, 1966) and the coping style employed (Lazarus and Folkman, 1984).

According to this model, the way people deal with HIV disease will depend on their understanding and interpretation of the event, the stresses experienced, the coping options they perceive as available and on mediating factors such as the perceived availability of social support and the coping strategies they finally adopt.

A number of studies provide support for this model. For example, Namir (1986) described social support as being important to people with AIDS for the provision of emotional support, illness-related support and physical contact. Hedge *et al.* (1993) found that while objective measures, such as a CD4 count, were of little predictive value in identifying psychological morbidity, a self-rating of good social support contributed to a profile of psychological wellbeing. Neither the number of friends nor family involvement was predictive of psychological symptomatology, but the presence of a regular partner or a perceived stable group of close friends was associated with lower levels of psychological distress. About a third of the sample had no partner and another 17 per cent reported no close friends. Thus, it can be seen that the psychological effects of having little or no significant support is clearly an issue for many individuals.

The role of precipitating factors in reactions to stress was investigated by Hedge *et al.* (1992), who examined individuals presenting to an HIV psychology service in crisis. The most frequently reported preceding events were: personal illness (39 per cent), bereavement (30 per cent), fears concerning disclosure of HIV status (23 per cent), issues surrounding testing (17 per cent), dilemmas concerning medication (17 per cent) and child-related difficulties (both caring for children with HIV disease and explaining to children about HIV or death in the family) (10 per cent). Eighty-nine per cent of crises were preceded by two or more major events or dilemmas. These data suggest that it is a cumulative stress level which leads to an inability to cope and emphasize the need to respond to the consequences of multiple problems as well as to specific events. There is also evidence (Catalan *et al.*, 1992b; Hedge *et al.*, 1993; Namir *et al.*, 1987) that strategies used to cope with HIV disease affect the psychological distress levels experienced. Adaptive skills included the seeking of emotional support, active coping strategies and the maintenance of a high level of self-esteem.

Stress and the immune system

A key question is whether behaviour and mental health functioning are co-factors in the progression to symptomatic disease. Kemeny *et al.* (1990) linked depression with a steeper drop in CD4 cells, while Perry, Jacobsberg and Fishman (1990b) found that the association between anxiety following the death of a partner and the CD4 count was only transitory. Solomon and Temoshok (1987) reported a better immune profile to be associated with a sense of control over life. But Temoshok (1988) found a positive relationship between psychological distress and total white cell count – an effect in the opposite direction from that expected. Such discrepancies could be attributable to the numerous confounding factors and methodological problems (see Green and Hedge, 1991) that beset this area of study and the issue remains a major challenge.

Summary

Psychological distress in response to HIV infection has been documented at all stages of disease. Although most studies have reported on homosexual men there is evidence that mood disturbance is widespread. Distress can be precipitated by events such as physical illness or bereavement. The cumulative stress experienced seems to be important. Suicide can be a risk as many predisposing factors are present in the lives of those who are HIV-positive. Identification of 'buffers' such as active coping skills and social support gives suggestions for possible psychological interventions aimed at minimizing stress. It is not yet established whether stress affects the rate of progression to symptomatic disease.

Psychosocial intervention strategies

Given the high levels of psychological distress experienced by individuals with HIV disease we need to consider ways of minimizing the effects of stressors. In this section I shall explore a cognitive-behavioural model, describe some intervention studies and consider some specific issues and dilemmas.

Cognitive-behavioural model

There is a substantial body of evidence which suggests that therapy based on Beck's cognitive-behavioural model of treatment (Beck, 1976) can benefit those with psychological symptomatology. This model rests on three assumptions:

1. Thoughts determine emotions and behaviour.
2. Unrealistic and negative thoughts result in emotional disorder.
3. Decreasing unrealistic and negative thoughts and increasing realistic, positive thoughts can reduce emotional symptomatology.

A common misapprehension is that cognitive-behaviour therapy simply encourages positive thinking. In fact, it comprises a number of techniques which address

Table 16.3   *Cognitive-behavioural intervention*

Cognitive-behavioural techniques include:

- Relaxation training and breathing exercises.
- Activity scheduling.
- Thought stopping.
- Reality testing.
- Decatastrophization.
- Cognitive reframing.
- Problem-solving.
- Development of long-term and intermediate goals.

dysfunctional cognitions and behaviours within a structured therapy session (Table 16.3). For example, because many realities for those with HIV infection are negative, the technique of 'decatastrophization' is used. This is a process which attempts to separate the reality from the accompanying global negative feelings and allows the person to explore coping alternatives. A thought such as 'I'll never be well enough to return to work' may be realistic when expressed by an individual with HIV disease. If the corollary is 'So I'll never be happy again', then a depressive thought could result, whereas the follow-up thought, 'So I'll have plenty of time for reading' can be part of a positive, coping strategy. Thus, decatastrophization can play a major component in preventing a severe depressive or anxiety response. (See Chapter 13 for links between this and pain.)

The problem-solving approach aims to support individuals in making informed decisions about their present difficulties and to equip them with the general skills and strategies necessary for dealing with future problems (Hawton and Kirk, 1989; Selwyn and Antoniello, 1993). Box 16.2 gives an example of how this approach was successful in a patient with depression.

Intervention studies

Although there are many reports of high levels of psychological distress and psychiatric symptomatology in people with HIV infection, there is only a limited literature on intervention studies. George (1988) examined patients with HIV disease 6–12 months after individual, cognitive-behavioural interventions. She found a significant reduction in distress and sustained improvements in levels of anxiety and depression. Similarly, Hedge, James and Green (1990) reported increases in self-esteem and decreases in anxiety and depression following an intervention aimed at increasing coping skills. A number of group interventions have been successful in reducing distress, improving coping skills and improving quality of life (Fawzy, Namir and Wolcott, 1989; Lamping *et al.*, 1993; Moulton *et al.*, 1990). Hedge and

---

BOX 16.2   MICHAEL

Michael, a 29-year-old, HIV-positive, gay man, an actor and playwright, was admitted to the inpatient HIV unit with symptoms of diarrhoea. He had a low CD4 count but did not have an AIDS diagnosis. A pathogen was isolated, treatment commenced and the diarrhoea began to resolve. However, Michael was observed to be in low spirits; he rarely left his room, talked to other patients or spent time writing. He was referred to the clinical psychologist. Assessment established that Michael was having difficulty remaining continent of faeces. Embarrassed and concerned that he might be incontinent, he remained in his room and discouraged others from spending time with him. His thoughts focused on never regaining continence, being unable to work again and being unable to leave his house once discharged from hospital. He was clinically depressed.

By keeping a diary (behavioural intervention) it was established that Michael had at least 3 hours between bowel movements and could thus leave his room with some confidence between episodes. Michael initially left his room with some anxiety. However, by timing himself he was able to spend time talking to other patients and staff.

His dysfunctional cognitions were challenged: should incontinence remain, was staying in his room the only option? Would incontinence necessarily prevent him working? Were there alternative ways of achieving what he wanted from life? He considered the possible options and decided that should the uncontrollable diarrhoea remain and prevent him from acting, he would continue to write plays. His mood improved and he generated a number of ways in which he would cope with an episode of incontinence. Michael went home for the weekend and coped with the incontinence. His mood improved and he left hospital a week later. The general principles of the problem-solving approach were explained during follow-up outpatient sessions and Michael's mood remained high as he increasingly returned to his former way of life.

Since this intervention Michael has had a play accepted by a London theatre company and has appeared in a number of films and television series.

Glover (1990) showed that an educational group not only provided information but also relieved distress and enhanced mutual support.

Specific issues and dilemmas

Although most psychological interventions are directed at increasing the coping skills of individuals with HIV disease some issues and dilemmas require specific attention (Hedge, Sherr and Green, 1991).

Grief and bereavement
Models of the grieving process (see Chapter 17), which consider adaptive responses to bereavement, suggest a number of beneficial coping strategies. However, the reaction of an individual to a particular death will be affected by the circumstances

in which it occurs. Bereavement in the context of HIV presents some unique features. For example, those who die are usually young and the highest rate of mortality is in the age range 20–40 years. Furthermore, death is the last of many losses, as HIV-infection may have already brought the loss of relationships, sex, employment, control, a future, hope and health. In addition, those bereaved by HIV frequently are themselves HIV-positive. If bereavement or its psychological sequelae have an adverse effect on the immune system, then it could prove hazardous to health. Folkman *et al.* (1992) have described the patterns of distress experienced by caregivers during illness and death. They found that prior to the death of a partner, HIV-positive caregivers were less distressed than those not infected, while after the death the infected partners showed more distress. A possible explanation is that those who are HIV-positive view the experience as a model of their own death. First, they empathize with the patient; afterwards they realize they will face a similar experience alone, as their own infection makes it less likely that they will find a new partner. Lennon, Martin and Dean (1990) report the intensity of grief during bereavement to be related to the involvement in caretaking during end-stage disease and to the adequacy of practical and emotional support given to the caregiver during this time. Consequently, the counselling needs of bereaved people can vary widely.

Another facet of AIDS-related bereavement, the social loss, was described by Dean, Hall and Martin (1988), who reported multiple bereavement in a large cohort of gay men in San Francisco. Ninety-five per cent of the sample reported HIV-related loss, with an average of 6.2 HIV-related deaths each. With increasing numbers of AIDS-related deaths, McKusack (1991) reported increasing distress involving:

- psychological and emotional numbness,
- shrinking away from friends and resources,
- symptoms of complicated bereavement (inordinate guilt, calcified anger, rage, indifference),
- depression.

He described a cycle of negative impact: deaths led to a decrease in the available social support which resulted in higher levels of depression in those with HIV disease, which had the effect of less self-care, which increased the likelihood of mortality, etc. To combat the effects of multiple bereavement, McKusack suggested the adoption of a community-wide coping programme to enable people to stay involved rather than distance themselves from the problem, and to find some form of social support which promotes discharge of anxieties and renewal of vigour. The use of public ritual to mourn losses (Tafoya, 1992) can enable a community to reaffirm its capability to overcome these feelings of loss and to remain empowered.

Childbearing issues

The rates of transmission of HIV from mother to child vary widely, with higher rates seen in the developing world. The European Collaborative Study (1992) reported a vertical transmission rate of 14.4 per cent compared with a rate of 39 per cent in Zambia and Zaire (Hira *et al.*, 1989; Ryder *et al.*, 1988). The decision to become pregnant or to continue with a pregnancy may be difficult to make. The possible negative consequences of child bearing are:

- an infected, possibly sick child,
- a child who dies,
- guilty parents,
- parents who are too sick to care for the child,
- parents who die leaving an orphan,
- an adverse affect on the pregnant woman's health.

For these reasons termination of pregnancy is available for women who are HIV-positive. Not all women decide to remain childless; for some, childlessness would be an additional loss to bear and for others bearing a child avoids negative cultural reactions directed towards childless men and women. Although most of the literature on child bearing focuses on women, the desire to parent is seen in both men and women, heterosexual and gay (Sherr and Hedge, 1989). And despite the fact that many care workers have firm views about the desirability of childbearing in HIV-infected patients, the right to decide must remain that of the patient.

DISCUSSION POINT
Where resources are limited, e.g. in the provision of infertility treatment, some patients are refused treatment on a number of grounds, such as age and marital status. To what extent would you recommend treatment for infertility to an HIV-positive couple when natural conception had failed to occur?

Medication issues

Antiviral medications are now available which have shown some degree of effectiveness against HIV (Williams, 1993). Although these medications and those directed at opportunistic infections and tumours may be beneficial, some have disagreeable side-effects. As new drugs are developed, patients are increasingly offered the opportunity to participate in clinical trials.

Hedge *et al.* (1991) found that being offered antiviral therapy became a negative marker of health status and was frequently accompanied by high levels of stress. Requests to participate in a drug trial also produced emotive responses. Distress may be minimized if patient control is enhanced by the provision of accurate information about the drug or test procedure, and by the facilitation of informed decision making.

Management of neurological problems

HIV-related brain disorder can be the result of various causes. These include (1) the direct effect of HIV on the central nervous system; (2) secondary complications of immune deficiency such as opportunistic infections and tumours; and (3) nutritional deficiencies, drug toxicity, electrolyte imbalance, hypoxia, impaired liver or kidney function. In many cases improvement of cognitive function is found when the cause is treated. Especially in the later stages of HIV disease, cognitive and behavioural changes may also be seen which cannot be reversed. In some instances cognitive dysfunction is a result of major depression, or mood disturbance and an organic dysfunction coexist. Consequently, the differentiation of functional from organic illness can be difficult. The identification by neuropsychological testing of cognitive functions which have remained intact and those which show deficits can be useful in guiding the management of the patient.

Care of those who are severely impaired can be onerous. Provision of social and emotional support for the carers, family and friends is of great importance (Ostrow, Grant and Atkinson, 1988). If residential care is not available or is not desired by the family and caregivers, attendance at day centres and intermittent respite care can help to maintain an individual in the community.

Summary

Intervention strategies that address dysfunctional cognitions and behaviours have been found useful in reducing psychological symptomatology in people with HIV disease. Of major importance are interventions aimed at enhancing adaptive coping skills and enabling people to identify and use social support. Particular input is needed by those who are bereaved, those with decisions concerning childbearing and with dilemmas over medication. The management of individuals with neurological problems can be considerable and support may also be required by the carers.

Burnout and coping in health carers

This last section considers the issue of caring for the carers by discussing the phenomenon of burnout and the strategies to minimize it. Hortsman and McKusick (1986) reported health care workers to experience enormous stress when caring for people with HIV disease. Dealing with profound physical and mental deterioration in patients led to feelings of helplessness, frustration and inadequacy at being unable to cure. Carers showed symptoms of anxiety, depression, overwork, fatigue, stress, fear of death and decreased interest in sex. Such occupational stress has been documented in a variety of health care professionals, particularly in those caring for people who have terminal illnesses (Vachon, 1987).

Burnout

The term 'burnout' is used to characterize a syndrome which can develop when stresses are not recognized and addressed (Maslach, 1982). Maslach and Jackson (1981) defined burnout as a combination of emotional exhaustion, depersonalization and a reduced sense of personal accomplishment.

Table 16.4   *Factors associated with stress in health care professionals working with people with HIV disease*

Factors associated with stress	Association	Study
Age	Negative	Bennett, Michie and Kippax, 1991
Experience	None	Bennett, Michie and Kippax, 1991
Intense patient contact	Positive	Hortsman and McKusack, 1986
Total time in HIV/AIDS unit	Positive	Bennett, Michie and Kippax, 1991
	Negative	Hortsman and McKusack, 1986
Grief	None	Bennett, Kelaher and Ross, 1992
Sex of worker	None	Ross and Seeger, 1988
	None	Bennett, Michie and Kippax, 1991
Identification with patient	Positive	Bennett, Kelaher and Ross, 1992
Hospital-specific	Positive	Bennett, Michie and Kippax, 1991
Patient-related stress	Positive	Bennett and Kelaher, 1993
Patient characteristics (youth/age/ sexuality)	Positive	Bennett, 1992
Organizational stressors	Positive	Scott and Jaffe, 1989
External coping resources (alcohol, food, social support, activities)	Positive	Bennett, Kelaher and Ross, 1992
Internal coping resources (knowledge, skills, attitudes, values)	Negative	Bennett, Kelaher and Ross, 1992
Staff disagreement over patient treatment	Positive Positive	Ross and Seeger, 1988; Martin, 1990
Stigma of working with HIV disease	Positive Positive	Hortsman and McKusick, 1986 Vachon and Dennis, 1989
Involvement with patient	Positive	Flaskerud 1987; Buhrich 1989

Table 16.4 shows factors which have been identified as increasing the levels of stress staff experienced while working with people with HIV disease. The question of whether AIDS presents unique burdens to health care staff is not easily answered (see also Barbour, 1994 and Chapters 14 and 17). Many of the factors contributing to stress are experienced by care workers in other fields such as oncology and cystic fibrosis. However, Bennett *et al.* (1991) found that the greater patient dependency in HIV units necessitated the need for greater contact between the nurse and patient and increased the emotional intensity of the work. Bennett, Kelaher and Ross (1992) investigated factors which could be associated with burnout. They found grief not to be predictive of burnout, but that greater work-related grief was experienced when carers identified closely with patients. Burnout

was associated with an absence of internal coping strategies and with a reliance on external coping. Older, more experienced carers were less likely to experience burnout.

Strategies to minimize burnout

To minimize burnout, strategies are needed which focus on the individual's coping skills and on the organization's attempt to minimize stressors (see also Chapter 1). In line with the findings that intensity of work rather than overall length of time working on an HIV unit contributed to stress levels (Bennett, Michie and Kippax, 1991; Hortsman and McKusick, 1986) time-out techniques, e.g. rotating with staff in the genito-urinary medicine clinic, could be adopted. To utilize the coping strategies of those who are older and who have more experience, increasing the opportunities for informal sharing of problems might be beneficial. Alternatively, the provision of staff support groups could facilitate exchange of information and coping strategies between experienced and inexperienced staff.

When patients are seen for a long time by a relatively small group of care staff close emotional involvement with patients frequently occurs. Specific training in strategies aimed at expressing warmth and empathy while maintaining professional boundaries has been suggested to reduce emotional stress (Bennett, Michie and Kippax, 1991).

To facilitate carers in the above, organizational change may be required (Macks and Abrams, 1992). This may include:

- assessment of job requirements and available resources,
- task planning,
- staff development, education and training,
- enhancing communication systems,
- provision of formal support,
- enhancing informal communications and appreciation mechanisms,
- reviewing job structure and workload.

Attention to the organization or to individual coping strategies without attention to the other is likely to be ineffectual as stress is a product of both.

Summary

Although it is not possible to remove the prime stressors – sick patients and their needs – there are ways to lessen the stresses attached to caring for people with HIV disease. Caring for carers requires resources, but this may prove more cost-effective than the increased sickness rate and high turnover of staff associated with burnout.

Summary

The emotional reactions to infection with HIV are well documented. HIV is associated with multiple stressors, including physical illness, bereavement and medication dilemmas. The cumulative stress experienced is associated with an individual's ability to cope and the perceived available social support. Further work on the interaction between stressors and the functioning of the immune system is clearly needed.

There are many questions still to be answered concerning the effect that psychological intervention has on long-term coping behaviours; however, there is evidence that strategies which develop coping skills and which enable people to mobilize social support are beneficial in the short term. In relation to this, it is important to recognize the effect which bereavement from HIV-related deaths is having on communities, traditionally those who have provided social support.

The magnitude of the epidemic, with no end in sight, has resulted in high levels of stress for carers. To minimize the impact of this stress, it appears necessary to address the coping skills of carers and to make supportive managerial and organisational changes.

Seminar questions

1. If you were asked to care for patients with HIV disease what would your concerns be? Explore your thoughts and feelings concerning HIV infection, emotional distress, homosexuality and injecting drug use.
2. When do you think that issues concerning death and dying should be raised with a patient? Discuss how this might best be done.
3. Plan a psychological support service for people with HIV disease for a local clinic. What are the practical difficulties you are likely to encounter? How could you overcome them?

Further readings

Hawton, K., Salkovskis, P. M., Kirk, J. and Clark, D.M. (eds.) (1989) *Cognitive Behavioural Therapy for Psychiatric Problems: A practical guide*. Oxford: Oxford University Press. An easily understood, comprehensive account of cognitive-behavioural techniques. The chapters on problem-solving, anxiety and depression are particularly recommended.

McKusick, L. (ed.) (1986) *What to Do about AIDS*. Berkeley, Calif.: University of California Press. Although written early in the AIDS epidemic this easily readable book gives useful insights into the issues and problems experienced by those with HIV disease and identifies some useful interventions.

Miller, R. and Bor, R. (1989) *AIDS: A guide to clinical counselling*. London: Science Press. A practical guide to counselling in the HIV field. A useful introduction which provides snippets of hypothetical interviews.

References

Atkinson, J.H. Grant, I., Kennedy, C.J., Richman, D.D., Spector, S.A. and McCutchan J. A. (1988) 'Prevalence of psychiatric disorders among men infected with HIV', *Archives of General Psychiatry* **45**, 859–64.

Barbour, R.S. (1994) 'The impact of working with HIV/AIDS: a review of the literature', *Social Science Medicine*, **39**, 221–32.

Beck, A.T. (1976) *Cognitive Therapy and the Emotional Disorders*. New York: International Universities Press.

Bennett L. (1992) 'The experience of nurses working with hospitalised AIDS patients', *Australian Journal of Social Issues* **27**, 125–43.

Bennett, L. and Kelaher, M. (1993) 'Longitudinal determinants of patient care-related stress in HIV/AIDS health professionals', *IX International Conference on AIDS*. Berlin.

Bennett, L., Kelaher, M. and Ross, M. (1992a) 'Links between burnout and bereavement in HIV/AIDS professionals', *Quality of Life Satellite Symposium: VIII International Conference on AIDS*. Amsterdam.

Bennett, L., Michie, P. and Kippax, S. (1991) 'Qualitative analysis of burnout and its associated factors in AIDS nursing', *AIDS Care* **3**, 181–92.

Brown, G. W. (1979) 'The social etiology of depression: London studies', in R.A. Depue (ed.) *The Psychobiology of the Depressive Disorders: Implications for the effects of stress*. San Diego: Academic Press.

Buhrich, N. (1989) 'Psychiatric aspects of HIV infection', *Australian Conference on Medical and Scientific Aspects of AIDS and HIV infection*.

Catalan, J., Klimes, I., Bond, A., Day, A., Garrod, A. and Rizza, C. (1992a) 'The psychosocial impact of HIV infection in men with haemophilia: Controlled investigation and factors associated with psychiatric morbidity', *Journal of Psychosomatic Research* **36**, 409–16.

Catalan, J., Klimes, I., Day, A., Garrod, A. Bond, A. and Gallwey J. (1992b) 'The psychosocial impact of HIV infection in gay men', *British Journal of Psychiatry* **161**, 774–8.

Chuang, H.T., Devins, G. M., Hunsley, J. and Gill, M. J. (1989) 'Psychosocial distress and well-being among gay and bisexual men with Human Immunodeficiency Syndrome', *American Journal of Psychiatry* **146**, 876–80.

Cohen, S. and Willis, T.A. (1985) 'Stress, social support and the buffering hypothesis', *Psychological Bulletin* **98**, 310–57.

Dean, L., Hall, W.E. and Martin, J.L. (1988) 'Chronic and intermittent AIDS related bereavement in a panel of homosexual men in New York', *City Journal of Palliative Care* **4**, 54–7.

DHSS (1985) 'Information for doctors concerning the introduction of the HTLV III antibody test', *AIDS Booklet 2*.London: DHSS.

European Collaborative Study (1992) 'Risk factors for mother-to-child transmission of HIV-1', *Lancet* **339**, 1007–12.

Fawzy, F.I., Namir, S. and Wolcott, D.L. (1989) 'Structured group intervention model for AIDS patients', *Psychiatric Medicine* **7**, 35–45.

Flaskerud, J.H. (1987) 'Psychosocial aspects of AIDS', *Journal of Psychosocial Nursing* **25**, 9–16.

Folkman, S., Chesney, M., Boccellari, A., Cooke, M., Collette, L. (1992) 'Death of partner affects moods of HIV+ and HIV– caregiving gay men differently', *VIII International Conference on AIDS.* Amsterdam.

Fox, B.H., Stanek, E.J., Boyd, S.C. and Flanney, J.T. (1982) 'Suicide rates among cancer patients', *Connecticut Journal of Chronic Diseases* **35**, 85–100.

Gala, C., Pergami, A., Catalan, J., Durbano, F., Musicco, M., Riccio, M., Baldeweg, T. and Invernizzi, G. (1992) 'Risk of deliberate self-harm and factors associated with suicidal behaviour among asymptomatic individuals with Human Immunodeficiency Virus infection', *Acta Psychiatrica Scandinavica* **86**, 70–5.

Gala, C., Pergami, A., Catalan, J., Durbano, F., Musicco, M., Riccio, M., Baldeweg, T. and Invernizzi, G. (1993) 'The psychosocial impact of HIV infection in gay men, drug users and heterosexuals', *British Journal of Psychiatry* **163**, 651–9.

George, H. (1988) 'AIDS: Factors identified as helpful by patients', *IV International Conference on AIDS.* Stockholm.

Graham, N.M.H., Zeger, S.L., Lawence, P. *et al.* (1992) 'The effects on survival of early treatment of human immunodeficiency virus infection', *New England Journal of Medicine* **326**, 1037–42.

Grant, I. (1990) 'The neuropsychology of human immunodeficiency virus', *Seminars in Neurology* **10**, 267–74.

Grant. I., Atkinson, J. H., Hesselink, J. R., Kennedy, C. J., Richman, D.D., Spector, S. A. and McCutchen, J.A. (1987) 'Evidence for early central nervous system involvement in the acquired immune deficiency syndrome (AIDS) and other human immunodeficiency virus (HIV) infections', *Annals of Internal Medicine* **107**, 828–36.

Green, J. and Hedge, B. (1991) 'Counselling and stress in HIV infection and AIDS', in C. Cooper and M. Watson (eds.) *Cancer and Stress: Psychological, biological and coping strategies.* Chichester: John Wiley.

Hawton, K. and Kirk, J. (1989) 'Problem solving', in K. Hawton, P. H. Salkovskis, J. Kirk and D. M. Clark (eds.) *Cognitive Behavioral Therapy for Psychiatric Problems: A Practical Guide.* Oxford: Oxford University Press.

Hedge, B. and Glover, L.F. (1990) 'Group intervention with HIV seropositive patients and their partners', *AIDS Care* **2**, 147–54.

Hedge, B., James S. and Green, J. (1990) 'Evaluation of focused cognitive-behavioural intervention with HIV seropositive individuals', *VI International Conference on AIDS.* San Francisco.

Hedge, B., Sherr, L. and Green, J. (1991) 'To take or not to take antivirals? Psychological sequelae of the decision-making process', *VII International Conference on AIDS.* Florence.

Hedge, B., Slaughter, J., Flynn, R. and Green, J. (1993) 'Coping with HIV disease: Successful attributes and strategies', *IX International Conference on AIDS.* Berlin.

Hedge, B. *et al.* (1992) 'Psychological crises in HIV infection', *VIII International AIDS Conference.* Amsterdam.

Hira, S.K., Kamanga, J., Bhat, G.J. *et al.* (1989) 'Perinatal transmission of HIV-1 in Zambia', *British Medical Journal* **299**, 1250–52.

Hortsman, W. and McKusick, L. (1986) 'The impact of AIDS on the physician', in L. McKusack (ed.) *What to Do about AIDS.* Berkeley, Calif.: University of California Press.

Kemeny, M.E., Duran, R., Taylor, S.E., Weiner, H., Visscher, B. and Fahey, J.L. (1990) 'Chronic depression predicts CD4 decline over a five year period', *VI International Conference on AIDS*. San Francisco.

King, M.B. (1989a) 'Prejudice and AIDS: The views and experiences of people with HIV infection', *AIDS Care* **1**, 137–52.

King, M.B. (1989b) 'Psychosocial status of 192 out-patients with HIV infection and AIDS', *British Journal of Psychiatry* **154**, 237–42.

Lamping, D., Abrahamowicz, M., Gilmore, N., Edgar, L., Grover, S., Tsoukas, C., Falutz, J., Lalonde, R., Hamel, M. and Darsigny, R. (1993) 'A randomized controlled trial to evaluate a psychosocial intervention to improve quality of life in HIV infection', *IX International Conference on AIDS*. Berlin.

Lazarus, R.S. and Folkman, S. (1984) *Stress, Appraisal and Coping*. New York: Springer.

Lennon, M.C., Martin, J.L. and Dean, L. (1990) 'The influence of social support on AIDS related grief reaction among gay men', *Social Science and Medicine* **31**, 477–84.

Ley, P. and Spelman, M.S. (1967) *Communicating with the Patient*. London: Staples Press.

Macks, J. and Abrams, D. (1992) 'Burnout among HIV/AIDS health care providers', in P. Volberding and M. Jacobson (eds.) *AIDS Clinical Review*, New York: Marcel Decker.

Martin, D. A. (1990) 'Effects of ethical dilemmas on stress felt by nurses providing care to AIDS patients', *Critical Care Nursing Quarterly* **12**, 53–62.

Marzuk, P., Tierney, H., Tardiff, K., Gross, E., Morgan, E., Hsu, M. and Mann, J. (1988) 'Increased risk of suicide in patients with AIDS', *Journal of the American Medical Association* **259**, 1333–7.

Maslach, C. (1982) *Burnout: The cost of caring*. Englewood Cliffs, NJ: Prentice Hall.

Maslach, C. and Jackson, S.E. (1981) 'The measurement of experienced burnout', *Journal of Occupational Behaviour* **2**, 99–113.

McArthur, J.C. (1987) 'Neurologic manifestations of AIDS', *Medicine* **66**, 407–37.

McKusack, L. (1991) 'Multiple loss accounts for worsening distress in a community heavily hit by AIDS', *VII International Conference on AIDS*. Florence.

Moulton, J., Gorbuz, G., Sweet, D., Martin, R. and Dilley, J. (1990) 'Outcome evaluation of eight-week educational support groups, validating the model using control group comparisons', *VI International Conference on AIDS*. San Francisco.

Namir, S. (1986) 'Treatment issues concerning persons with AIDS', in L. McKusick (ed.) *What to Do about AIDS*. Berkeley, Calif.: University of California Press.

Namir, S., Wolcott, D.L., Fawzy, F.I. and Alumbaugh, M.J. (1987) 'Coping with AIDS: Psychological and health implications', *Journal of Applied Social Psychology* **17**, 309–28.

Navia, B.A,. (1990) 'The AIDS dementia complex', in J.L. Cummings (ed.) *Subcortical Dementia*. New York: Oxford University Press.

Ostrow, D.G., Joseph, J., Monjan, A., Kessler, R., Emmons, C., Phair, J., Fox, R., Kingsley, L., Dudley, J., Chmeil, J.S. and Van Raden, M. (1986) 'Psychosocial aspects of AIDS risk', *Psychopharmacological Bulletin* **22**, 678–83.

Ostrow, D.M., Grant, I. and Atkinson, H. (1988) 'Assessment and management of the AIDS patient with neuropsychiatric disturbances', *Journal of Clinical Psychiatry* **49**, 14–22.

Paykel, E.S., Prusoff, B.A. and Myers, J.K. (1975) 'Suicide attempts and recent life events', *Archives of General Psychiatry* **32**, 327–33.

Peckham, C. and Newell, M.L. (1990) 'HIV-1 infection in mothers and babies', *AIDS Care* **2**, 205–12.

Perry, S., Jacobsberg, L.B., Fishman, B. Weiler, P.H., Gold, J.W.M. and Frances, A.J. (1990) 'Psychological responses to serological testing for HIV', *AIDS* **4**, 145–52.

Perry, S., Jacobsberg, L. and Fishman, B. (1990a) 'Suicide ideation and HIV testing', *Journal of the American Medical Association* **263**, 679–82.

Perry, S., Jacobsberg, L.B. and Fishman, B. (1990b) 'Relationship between CD4 lymphocytes and psychosocial variables among HIV seropositive adults', *VI International Conference on AIDS*. San Francisco.

Perry, S. and Marrotta, R.F. (1987) 'AIDS dementia: A review of the literature', *Alzheimer Disease and Associated Disorders* **1**, 221–35.

Perakyla, A. and Bor, R. (1990) 'Interactional problems of addressing "dreaded' issues in HIV-counselling', *AIDS Care* **2**, 325–38.

Pinching, A.J. (1994) 'AIDS: Health care ethics and society', in R. Gillon (ed.) *Principles of Health Care Ethics*. Chichester: Wiley.

Poulton, E. (1969) 'How efficient is print?' *New Society* **349**, 869–71.

Pugh, K., O'Donnell, I. and Catalan, J. (1993) 'Suicide and HIV disease', *AIDS Care* **5**, 391–9.

Ross, M. and Seeger, V. (1988) 'Determinants of reported burnout in health professionals associated with the care of patients with AIDS', *AIDS* **2**, 395–7.

Rotter, J.B. (1966) 'Generalized expectancies for internal versus external control of reinforcement', *Psychological Monographs* **80**, 1–28.

Rutherford, G. W., Lifson, A. L., Hessol, N. A. *et al.* (1990) 'Course of HIV-1 infections in a cohort of homosexual and bisexual men. An 11-year follow-up study', *British Medical Journal* **301**, 1183–88.

Ryder, R.W., Nsa, W., Hassig, S.E. *et al.* (1988) 'Perinatal transmission of the human immunodeficiency virus type 1 to infants of seropositive women in Zaire', *New England Journal of Medicine* **320**, 1637–42.

Schneider, S.G., Taylor, S.E. Kemeny, M.E. and Dudley, J. (1991) 'Factors influencing suicide intent in gay and bisexual suicide ideators: Differing models for men with and without Human Immunodeficiency Virus', *Journal of Personality and Social Psychology* **61**, 776–88.

Scott, C.D. and Jaffe, D.T. (1989) 'Managing occupational stress associated with HIV infection', *Occupational Medicine*, 4, 85–93.

Schneider, S.G., Taylor, S.E. and Kemery, M.E. (1991) 'AIDS related factors predictive of suicidal ideation of low and high intent among gay and bisexual men', *Suicide and Life Threatening Behaviour* **21**, 313–228.

Selwyn, P. and Antoniello, P. (1993) 'Reproductive decision-making among women with HIV infection', in M.A. Johnson and F.A. Johnstone (eds.) *HIV Infection in Women*. Edinburgh: Churchill Livingstone.

Sherr, L. and Hedge, B. (1989) 'On becoming a mother: Counselling implications for mothers and fathers', *WHO Conference*. Paris: WHO.

Sherr, L. and Hedge, B. (1990) 'The impact and use of written leaflets as a counselling alternative in mass antenatal HIV screening', *AIDS Care* **2**, 235–45.

Shilts, R. (1987) *And the Band Played on*. London: Penguin Books.

Slater, J. and Depue, R.A. (1981) 'The contribution of environmental events and social support to serious suicide attempts in primary depressive disorder', *Journal Abnormal Psychology* **90**, 275–85.

Solomon, G.F. and Temoshok, L. (1987) 'A psychoneuroimmunologic perspective in research on AIDS: Questions, preliminary findings, and suggestions', *Journal of Applied Social Psychology* **17**, 285–307.

Tafoya, T. (1992) 'Ritual solutions to loss', *VIII International Conference on AIDS*. Amsterdam.

Temoshok, L. (1988) 'Psychoimmunology and AIDS', in T.P. Bridge (ed.) *Psychological, Neuropsychiatric and Substance Abuse Aspects of AIDS*. New York: Raven Press.

Tross, S., Hitsch, D., Rabkin, B., Berry, C. and Holland, J.C.B. (1987) 'Determinants of current psychiatric disorder in AIDS spectrum patients', *III International Conference on AIDS*. Washington.

Vachon, M. (1987) *Occupational Stress in the Care of the Critically Ill, the Dying and the Bereaved*. New York: Hemisphere Publishing.

Vachon, L.S. and Dennis, J. (1989) 'HIV, stress and the health care professional', in J.W. Dilley C. Pies and M. Helquist (eds.) *Face to Face: A guide to AIDS counselling*. San Francisco: AIDS Health Project of UCSF, Celestial Arts Distributing.

WHO (1988) *World Health Organisation Global Programme on AIDS: Report of the consultation on the neuropsychiatric aspects of HIV infection*. Geneva: WHO.

Williams, I. (1993) 'Antiviral therapy', in M.A. Johnson and F.D. Johnstone (eds.) *HIV Infection in Women*. Edinburgh: Churchill Livingstone.

Williams, J. *et al.* (1991) 'Multidisciplinary baseline assessment of homosexual men with HIV infection', *Archive of General Psychiatry* **48**, 124–30.

CHAPTER 17

Dying and bereavement

PAUL MARCH

Chapter outline

Introduction

Most nurses are confronted with the reality of death with a regularity that lay people would find shocking. This was emphasized by Menzies-Lyth in 1959 (Menzies-Lyth, 1988), who found that a number of inefficient and uncaring nursing practices were, in part, attempts by nurses to protect themselves from the pain and fear that resulted from contact with death. For example, she found unnecessary systems of checking and counter-checking, requirements on nurses to display a 'stiff upper lip', nurses referring to patients as 'the liver in bed 9' and other, similar practices.

Until recently, a death on the ward was a violent reminder of the failings of nursing and medicine (Hare and Pratt, 1989). But major developments, such as the growth of the hospice movement, indicate that the emphasis is changing from curing to caring. Nursing appears to be redefining itself to include the wholehearted care of dying and bereaved people. It is important for nurses to be sensitive to the emotional reactions of dying and bereaved people and to be aware of the difficulties of caring for them. This chapter considers these two areas.

Reactions of dying and bereaved people

A number of perspectives have been used to help understand the psychological reactions of dying and bereaved people. Littlewood (1992) summarizes seven models:

1. Illness and disease models (e.g. Lindemann, 1944).
2. Biological models (e.g. Engel, 1962).
3. Psychodynamic models (e.g. Pincus, 1976).
4. Attachment models (Bowlby, 1980).
5. Personal construct and cognitive models (Parkes, 1972).
6. Stress models, such as Caplan's (1964) model of crisis intervention.
7. Phenomenological and existential models (e.g. Smith, 1976).

All these models present mourning as an active and evolving process. Indeed, it is unusual in psychology to find such a remarkable level of agreement over the descriptions and explanations of likely reactions. So, for the sake of clarity, only one model will be presented here. This model stems from the work of Bowlby on attachment (1969, 1980). It has been used to understand the reactions of both dying and bereaved people. A summary of the theory is given below; it is also considered in Chapter 18.

The attachment model

In attachment theory a person's relationship with his/her first and primary caregiver provides a template for future relationships. A person who experiences this first relationship as loving and secure will tend to perceive future relationships in the same way. That person has basic trust in the world and in those around (Erickson 1950, 1982) and has the capacity to give and receive love. When someone whom the person loves dies, he/she is left with the contradiction of being attached to someone who is no longer there. Mourning is the process of correcting this contradiction and of overcoming the loss. The studies outlined below will demonstrate that dying people also suffer losses and have similar reactions to those who are bereaved. Consequently, I shall consider the reactions of dying and bereaved people together. Most people who are dying have people around them who are mourning their death. The feelings and behaviour of dying and bereaved people are a function of the relationship between them and should not therefore be considered in isolation from each other. Indeed, one of the guiding principles of

Table 17.1   *Three models of the process of grieving*

Bowlby	Parkes	Kubler-Ross
	Alarm	Denial
	Searching	
Protest	Anger – protest	Anger
		Bargaining
Despair	Apathy – despair	Depression
Reintegration	New identity	Acceptance

the new hospice movement is 'The unit of care is the family' (Parkes, 1986; see also Chapter 4).

How does the attachment model help us to understand the reactions to loss? Table 17.1 shows three different versions of the model. Bowlby's model is a general description of the reactions to the loss of an attachment figure. Parkes' model is derived mainly from two longitudinal interview studies of widows and widowers (Parkes, 1972; Parkes and Weiss, 1983). The Kubler-Ross model is derived from interviews with over 200 terminally ill patients (Kubler-Ross 1973). The stages outlined by the models bear close similarities to each other despite the fact that their authors collected their evidence, at least initially, independently and data were collected from quite different populations (see Table 17.1).

Before outlining these stages criticisms of this approach are briefly considered. Corr (1993) argues that a stage model, in which a person proceeds in a linear fashion from one stage to the next, has not been supported by subsequent research. He argues that such a model is a generalization from the experience of some individuals and that these models lack the flexibility necessary to describe the range of individual reactions. Thus, there are dangers when stage models are interpreted in a rigid and prescriptive way, but both Parkes and Kubler-Ross, as well as others (e.g. Worden, 1991), have made explicit that they are not making such a claim. Another problem is that different cultures prescribe different grieving rituals and the extent to which the findings of Parkes and Kubler-Ross apply to non-Western cultures is not clear (see Box 17.1 and Seminar Question 1). However, the research into bereaved and dying people suggests that when you look at a *group* of such people a predictable pattern emerges. Further, it is possible to use this pattern to understand the experiences of bereaved and dying individuals by using this perspectives as a framework while at the same time recognizing that there is a huge variety in the ways individuals react. So, when talking with a bereaved or dying person it is only proper that their experience should be in the foreground of the conversation, with the context at the back. (See Seminar Question 2.)

There are other, more general issues about the sequence of events described by the model. For bereaved people who have more warning of an impending death, their process of mourning may be shorter or less complicated because they have mourned the death in advance – so-called 'anticipatory bereavement'. Although

---

BOX 17.1 GRIEF IN OTHER CULTURES

Attachment theory attempts to explain the reactions of dying and bereaved people in terms of the personal meaning of loss. However, there are also cultural influences which may determine whether and how grief is experienced or expressed. For example, in a review of anthropological studies of grief, Stroebe and Stroebe (1987) suggest that the length of a grief reaction is culturally prescribed. In traditional Navajo Indian culture, the expression of grief lasts for four days following death; Orthodox Jews grieve for one year. In both cases the bereaved then returns to a normal life. Stroebe and Stroebe (1987) point to studies which demonstrate the positive part culturally determined rituals play in moderating the grief reaction and they suggest that the long-lasting grief and depression encountered in the bereaved in Britain is partly a result of the lack of death and bereavement rituals. One could also argue that British culture allows individuals to grieve indefinitely and does not impose an externally-based end to the process (see Seminar Question, p. 342).

To a certain extent cultural differences can be explained by the attachment model. For example, according to Stroebe and Stroebe (1987), Japanese women accept the death of their husbands with equanimity compared with Western women. This can be explained in terms of their strong belief in the afterlife, coupled with their view that their ancestors are always with them. Such assumptions lead to there being less to grieve about because they militate against feelings of complete loss.

---

mourning in advance may be helpful for the long-term adjustment of the bereaved, for the terminally ill patient it may cause problems. As loved ones come to accept the inevitability of death, they may begin to withdraw from the patient and begin to consider life after the patient's death. This is an understandable reaction but it may leave the dying patient feeling rejected and isolated. The reverse can also happen; the patient may begin to accept their own death and withdraw from their loved ones, who remain overwhelmed by grief. The patient's disengagement may only increase the grief of other family members. The phenomenon of anticipatory bereavement demonstrates the need to give care to the dying and the bereaved together. Loved ones and relatives will mourn in different ways. They will undoubtedly have an influence on each other, sometimes supporting each other but often finding it impossible to provide mutual support because of the consequent increases in their own feelings of loss.

Alarm and denial

Physiological and behavioural symptoms of alarm are produced in many animals by imminent threat or danger. The news of death can be the cause of an alarm reaction because the world suddenly becomes a threatening and unpredictable place. Parkes (1972) found the alarm reaction to be very common in the first few hours and up to

BOX 17.2   **TO TELL OR NOT TO TELL**

In the past, health professionals have tried to help patients cope with the pain of dying by not telling them that they were terminally ill (Cartwright *et al.*, 1973; Oken, 1961). Setting aside the question of whether a patient has a right to this information if they want it, Hinton (1972) has shown that most patients had a pretty good idea that they were dying despite not having been told directly. They gained the information indirectly, e.g. from overhearing conversations between staff or reading their own medical notes. Many of these patients felt that they had learned something that they were not supposed to know and were left quite alone with the news at a time when they most needed support. Glazer and Strauss (1965) call this phenomenon 'closed awareness'.

A reversal of opinion over this issue has taken place in the last thirty years. In the United States during the early 1960s 88 per cent of doctors did *not* tell their patients that they were dying. By 1979, 98 per cent of doctors said that they *did*. (Novack *et al.*, 1979; Oken, 1961). A similar finding was reported in the United Kingdom by Searle (1991), who replicated a large study by Cartwright *et al.* (1973). But Searle did find that there remained a third of patients who appeared not to have been told the seriousness of their condition. (It is possible that some of these patients had been told their poor prognosis but had denied the knowledge.)

The trend towards openness between patients and health professionals about death has prompted some writers (e.g. Armstrong, 1987) to suggest that patients are now being forced to confront their own death. The obvious solution is to tell those patients who want to know and not to tell those who don't. The problem lies in distinguishing these patients from each other, especially as, given the gravity of the news, most people will be in two minds about whether they want to hear it. It is possible to obtain clues from the way patients ask questions. For example, a seriously ill patient who says 'Am I going to die?' appears to be asking a straightforward question and should be given a straightforward answer. A patient who says; 'I'm not going to die, am I?' is concerned and aware of the possibility of death but is looking for reassurance. To give that reassurance would be to mislead the patient but to give the patient a straightforward answer would be to ignore the fact that the patient does not appear to want this information. The patient needs to be asked something like 'Are you very worried about dying?' in order to discover how strongly they want to have a conversation about their predicament. With questions like this, the patients who really do want reassurance will begin to find something else to talk about or something that you are able to give them reassurance about, e.g. there is no need for them to suffer pain.

Kubler-Ross (1969) advocates truthfulness, but points out that all patients, even those who had accepted their fate, hold on to some hope that they will survive. She suggests that it would be insensitive of health professionals to attempt to destroy such hope by demanding that patients accept their own death without reservation.

ten days following a bereavement. Most of the widows in his study were initially restless, panicky and in a state of high arousal. Two-thirds were jumpy and irritable. Many of the somatic changes these widows reported in the first days, such as headaches, muscle tensions, knots in the stomach, dryness of the throat, are a result of normal physiological reactions to threat. Appetite loss and insomnia were also experienced by most of the widows.

The task at this early stage is to begin to accept the reality of the loss. Anything that makes this loss unreal such as suddenness or unexpected, bizarre or unusual circumstances is likely to make accepting reality more difficult and to result in a more prolonged or complicated grief reaction (Parkes and Weiss, 1983). Thus, a loss that goes against the normal lifecycle (e.g. death of a child or a loss by violence or unusual circumstances) is especially traumatic. Nurses in Accident and Emergency Departments are likely to have to deal with a high proportion of such deaths.

Bereaved people who feel able to see the body of the deceased are likely to find the experience upsetting, but helpful in the long run because it makes the reality of death more apparent. Health professionals should bear this in mind, but ultimately be guided by the bereaved person's own wishes.

Kubler-Ross (1969) found that almost all the patients she interviewed initially denied that they had a life-threatening illness. Denial means deceiving yourself about something that another part of your mind knows to be true. Kubler-Ross found that only 3 out of 200 patients remained in a constant state of denial, with the remainder drifting in and out of the state. Denial was more common in patients who had been told their diagnosis or prognosis in an abrupt or insensitive way (or not told at all; see Box 17.2) or were surrounded by family and/or staff who were also denying the seriousness of their condition.

Searching

Parkes (1972) found that initial grief is often characterized by pangs of yearning for the dead person rather than a prolonged depression. These pangs began within a few hours and reached a peak between 5 and 14 days. The bereaved feel an intense wish to be with their loved one and an irresistible urge to search for them. Bowlby and Parkes describe this urge to search as instinctual; it is also evident in animals (Lorenz, 1963). Bereaved humans usually recognize that, rationally, a search is useless and so they find their overwhelming need to search as inexplicable, crazy and distressing. Many bereaved people describe very clear and upsetting pseudo-hallucinations of the bereaved person, which are explained by Parkes as experiences likely to help in the location of a lost object. Thus, other needs such as sleep and food, are ignored. Parkes and Weiss (1983) found that those bereaved people who experienced a high degree of pining were more likely to experience a prolonged or complicated grief reaction. Many of these people linked their pining with having been unduly dependent on their dead partner.

According to Kubler-Ross (1969) a common reaction of patients to the news of their life-threatening illness was to look for another opinion or look for reassurance that the information that they were hearing was not true. This is an understandable reaction given the devastating implications of the news. These patients have been catapulted into an unpredictable world and are desperately trying to change it back into the world they know and understand. They may, therefore, be very threatened by and dismissive of information or facts that the nursing staff find self-evident.

Anger and guilt

Anger was expressed by most of the bereaved people studied by Parkes. Anger was most common during the first month and may be seen as a reaction to the threat of a loss that has not fully been accepted. The periods of anger were interspersed with periods of apathy and depression and, as the first year progressed, these periods of apathy became more common.

Freud (1917) suggested that the adaptation of the bereaved to death is partly determined by the degree of ambivalent feelings the bereaved hold for the dead person. In a difficult relationship the bereaved will sometimes have unconsciously wished for the death of the person. If that wish becomes a reality, the bereaved believe, unconsciously, that they have brought about the death. They will then protect themself from the arising guilt by blaming others for the death. Parkes and Weiss (1983) provided support for Freud's suggestions. They found high levels of expressed anger and self-reproach were associated with a poorer adaptation. Parkes and Weiss noted that widows or widowers who had experienced an unhappy or conflictual marriage initially appeared to cope better with their bereavement, but as time went on they seemed unable to progress. They also suggest that these findings may have a more straightforward explanation. Perhaps those bereaved who have experienced a difficult marriage have more to grieve, they mourn 'not only for the marriage that was but also for the marriage that could have been' (Parkes and Weiss, 1983: 122).

Parkes (1972) found a tendency for widows to blame others for the death. Health professionals are particularly susceptible to being blamed as they are often present at the time of death and perceived as in a position of power over life and death. Likewise, Kubler-Ross (1969) found that as dying patients began to consider their predicament they became angry with and envious of the healthy people around them. If the patient is being well cared for, then it is important not to take these feelings of anger and envy personally. However, it is also worth considering whether the patient has a well-grounded reason for being angry. For example, patients who complain angrily that they are not receiving the attention they need may be right. Staff could indeed be avoiding these patients because they find being with a dying person uncomfortable.

Bargaining

Kubler-Ross noted that some patients used bargaining as a way of controlling the pain involved in accepting their own death. She found that patients would try to strike a deal with God, fate, the hospital, etc. They would agree to live an honest life if God reprieved them; or they would agree to die if they were given the time or energy to accomplish some final task. Kubler-Ross equated this period of bargaining with a child who initially reacts with anger when banned from doing something by her parents. Then, after some consideration, she thinks, 'Well, I haven't got what I want from being disagreeable. Let's try asking nicely.'

Kubler-Ross warns about taking these bargains literally. If staff can accede to patients' wishes, then there is no reason why they should not. However, do not expect the patients to keep their side of the bargain. Whether or not they accept the fact that they are dying is not really under their control.

Depression, apathy, acceptance and gaining a new identity

Bereavement involves a loss of identity. Our identities are determined by the relationships we have with people and objects. When a husband loses a wife he also loses a large part of the way he (and others) sees himself. He is now a widower, a person he knows nothing about. Parkes found that many bereaved described the loss of their spouse as a loss of part of themselves. It seems that during the first few weeks of bereavement, the bereaved learn that their way of dealing with the world no longer applies. There follows a period of apathy and aimlessness. Some react as if they had never lost their loved one and they avoid situations that will prove otherwise. The rest are caught in a vicious circle. Their apathy makes it difficult to learn a new identity, but they need one in order to interact with the world again.

Kubler-Ross (1969) and Hinton (1972) both found depression to be a common emotional reaction in the dying patient. Hinton cites evidence which shows that 18 per cent of suicides were principally a result of physical illness and 4 per cent of suicides were suffering from an illness that probably would have killed them within six months. Hinton (1972) reported that increased levels of anxiety and depression in younger patients and that patients' anxiety and depression levels increased with the duration of their illness. He also found an interesting relationship between anxiety and religious belief. Those who were actively religious or firm non-believers appeared to suffer less anxiety than those who professed belief in God but who did not practise.

Kubler-Ross divides the types of depression experienced into two forms. The first is reactive depression, which occurs in response to losses that have already occurred. For example, loss of job due to illness or loss of part of the body by amputation. In many respects such losses are likely to result in the sort of bereavement reactions outlined by Parkes and Weiss (1983). The second is preparatory depression. Dying patients review their life and mourn, in advance, the loss of different aspects of it. Elderly people who have lived a full life have relatively little to mourn. They have gained much and have lost few opportunities and so they may suffer little preparatory depression. On the other hand, people who review their life and perceive a life of mistakes and missed opportunities may paradoxically have more to mourn as they begin to realize that these opportunities are now lost forever.

Kubler-Ross identified some patients who feel neither anger nor depression. They seem content to spend long periods in silence and appear somewhat detached from those around them. Kubler-Ross called this stage acceptance. The families of patients in this stage often feel rejected and therefore it may be important to explain that this disengagement is a sign that the patient has been surrounded by loving and supportive relatives, friends and staff. Kubler-Ross is at pains to distinguish acceptance from resignation. In many ways a resigned patient will appear similar to one who has reached acceptance. Both will be quiet and still, demanding little. But the stillness of those who have accepted comes from calmness, while for those who have become resigned it comes from despair. Those in despair cannot accept death, nor can they deny its existence any longer. It is important for the nurse to distinguish between a person who is resigned to death and one who has accepted it.

Summary

Bereaved and dying people are faced with an old world that has been destroyed and a new one that is alien and unpredictable. Understandably, they usually react initially with disbelief and then by withdrawing emotionally and behaviourally. Periodically they emerge, sometimes in anger, to tackle the world again. But their expectations of life need to change so much that they are left with very few resources to enable them to deal with this new world and so usually they withdraw again, sad and disoriented. A pattern emerges of frightened withdrawal, followed by tentative exploration. Given time, the dying may be able to re-emerge in order to experience their life with its end in sight and the bereaved too can begin to learn an identity for themselves without the person they love.

The origins of stress in caring for dying and bereaved people

The previous section has outlined the reactions that nurses might expect from bereaved and dying people. This section considers the difficulties nurses can experience in this context. These difficulties have been divided into those arising from working in a stressful environment and those arising from the personal attributes of individual nurses (see also Chapter 16). However, as will be clear, these two areas interact.

The stressful environment

The central difficulty in caring for the dying and bereaved appears to be the strong sense that it imparts in carers of being quite unable to help. The following two quotations illustrate this:

> The loss of a loved person is one of the most intensely painful experiences any human being can suffer, and not only is it painful to experience, but also painful to witness, if only because we are so impotent to help. (Bowlby, 1980)

> Pain is inevitable in such a case and cannot be avoided. It stems from the awareness of both parties that neither can give the other what he wants. The helper cannot bring back the person who's dead, and the bereaved person cannot gratify the helper by seeming helped. (Parkes, 1972)

Despite this, in a large-scale study of death and coping in health professionals, Vachon (1987) found that six of the ten most frequently cited stressors encountered by staff appeared to have nothing directly connected with issues of death, but involved the structure or running of the organization. These stressors included problems of role ambiguity, role conflict, communication problems and inadequate staffing. These are problems that might be encountered in any setting. However, a closer consideration of the case studies given by Vachon demonstrates how it is death that has made these problems particularly stressful. For example, a staff nurse describes a problem of *communication*:

> An 18-year-old girl went for fairly minor surgery. . . . She appeared to be a 'street liver' . . . she was emaciated and unkempt. I called the intern and said, 'This girl doesn't seem quite right. She seems to be hallucinating and there seems to be something really strange about her. I think she's too sick to be here.' The intern said '. . . she's coming off drugs.' I said, '. . . she told me she never touched the stuff.' The intern said, 'She's full of shit.'
>
> Early next morning I called the intern again and said, 'This girl is really too sick to be here. She needs to be transferred to ICU.' He said it wasn't convenient to transfer her then. . . . When I came in that night I asked how she was. My colleagues told me she had died. . . . I wonder if we had communicated better . . . would she be dead?

The vulnerable nurse

Worden (1991) suggests three reasons why working with dying and bereaved people may be personally painful for the nurse. First, contact with a bereaved or dying person may remind nurses of their own previous bereavements. If these bereavements have reached a resolution, then that nurse's ability to understand and help others may be greatly improved. However, if grief remains unresolved, caring for a grieving or dying patient may be very difficult (see Hare and Pratt, 1989). This is particularly true if the experience of the patient is close to the experience of the nurse. If the nurse suffers from unresolved grief, the experiences of the bereaved or dying patient will serve only to remind the nurse of his/her own pain, not that of the patient. As a result, the nurse can be lost in his/her own grief and be quite unable to empathize with the patient.

Second, the experiences of a bereaved or dying patient may correspond to a nurse's own feared losses. For example, a nurse who finds the thought of losing her young son unbearable may be unable to provide good care to a family whose young son has leukaemia.

Third, contact with dying and bereaved people is likely to present nurses with the reality and inevitability of their own death. Some nurses will find this reality very frightening and attempt to avoid it, either literally or emotionally.

The implications of these difficulties have been misunderstood by some researchers (see Brockopp, King and Hamilton, 1991). For example, in two studies (Reisetter and Thomas, 1986; Thompson, 1985) it was hypothesized that nurses who expressed a negative attitude about death and who described themselves as anxious about matters relating to death were expected to retreat from dying patients. However, the opposite was found. In Thompson (1985) nurses who worked in hospice settings expressed more death anxiety than those who worked in curative settings. Despite this they felt more comfortable about working with dying patients. In Reisetter and Thomas (1986) nurses with higher levels of expressed anxiety and discomfort about death were found to be better able to communicate about death with their dying patients.

Why did this pattern of findings emerge? The studies divided nurses into those who expressed death anxiety and those who did not in both the studies. It was concluded that those who expressed no death anxiety did not suffer from any anxiety. Alternatively, it might be suggested that for some nurses their anxiety about death was so great that they could not admit it even to themselves, let alone anyone else. Such a nurse would not express any anxiety about death and yet avoid working with dying people or would find such work very uncomfortable. This was exactly what the studies found.

A number of writers have suggested that, for some caregivers, the need to feel helpful and the subsequent choice of profession is in part prompted by unhappy and unresolved past experiences of caring or being cared for. Malan (1979) calls this the 'helping profession syndrome'; Bowlby (1980) calls it 'compulsive care giving'. Both authors suggest that some carers are giving what they themselves unconsciously feel that they have missed or need. This sort of behaviour is defensive, but it fulfils an important function for these carers. The feeling that they have not been properly cared for or loved is painful. However, they can avoid these painful feelings by convincing themselves (and others) that they are strong, invulnerable providers of care. This self-deception may be successful, but it depends on these carers' receiving continual reassurance that they are indeed being helpful. But when dealing with death and dying, the overriding feeling is one of helplessness not helpfulness. Consequently, this defence mechanism is likely to break down, with the result that the caregivers begin to re-experience the very feelings they have been trying to avoid – feelings of being unloved and uncared for. The caregivers may then look at the care their patients are receiving from them and become envious because the patients are getting what these caregivers want. It is difficult to give patients care when you are made envious by the very thing you are giving. However, these feeling of envy can be avoided if the caregivers is able to distort reality again and perceive patients' genuine needs as unreasonable demands. These complex processes illustrate the types of difficulties nurses can face and also the difficulty of identifying and resolving the conflicts.

DISCUSSION POINT
What were your reasons for entering nursing? Are any of these reasons likely to make it particularly difficult for you to cope with painful experiences, such as the death of patients?

Summary

This section has presented a picture in which caring for the dying and bereaved is a difficult and demanding task which is likely to result in most responsible nurses feeling hopeless and useless at some time. Nurses react to this pressure in different ways. For some, their views on their own experiences of loss, of illness or of being cared for will make it very difficult to look after a particular dying or bereaved person and in some cases dying and bereaved people in general. The next section examines ways of coping with this difficult task.

Coping with the stress of caring for dying and bereaved people

The stress of caring needs to be addressed at two levels: the institutional and the personal. For reasons that will be outlined below, the institutional level should be the primary source of input and is considered first.

The institutional level

If nurses are expected to care for dying and bereaved people, then it must be accepted by their employers that nurses will be involved in upsetting, stressful work, which is potentially dangerous to mental health. It is the responsibility of the employers to provide safeguards to ensure that nurses are not damaged by their work. Holden's (1991) view is that many hospitals are not living up to these responsibilities: 'The structure of many hospital environments is such that they promote anxiety, depression, dependency, envy, emotional regression, guilt and grief on a global scale.'

A universally suggested solution to this problem is the setting up of support systems (Hines, 1989; Worden, 1991). It would be fair to say that all nurses who are working in an area in which death occurs regularly should have access, during working time, to a support system. The exact nature of the system will vary depending on the nature of the work and institution. For example, Wright (1990) outlines a support system that might be used in units where sudden deaths are a regular occurrence. Wright suggests that the nature of work in these units means that staff are susceptible to post-traumatic stress disorder, a collection of physical and psychological symptoms that have been found to be experienced by victims of violence, serious accidents or natural disaster (emergency service personnel who attend to the victims can also suffer similar symptoms). Wright's support system includes interventions that are useful in preventing or diminishing some of the negative effects of traumatic incidents.

Vachon (1987) describes the most commonly cited, institutionally-based coping mechanisms:

1. Belonging to a team which had clear goals both for the team and for each individual team member.
2. Being in a team which was able to support its members at times of stress.
3. Having good staff selection and staffing policies.
4. Having clear administration and decision-making policies, particularly over dealing with the dying, deceased and bereaved.

DISCUSSION POINT
What elements would you like to see in a support system?

Formal support groups are frequently cited as important components of a support system. Hines (1989) and Holden (1991) stress that the focus of these groups should not be on giving nurses personal support, but should be task-oriented. By this they mean the group should aim to improve working practices rather than intrude upon individual nurses personal lives and difficulties. Vachon (1987) found that support groups were infrequently mentioned by the interviewees in her survey and those who did mention them usually said that they were not useful.

Holden suggests that improvements in the education of undergraduate nurses might help an understanding of the process by which a seemingly honest desire to help others can turn into feelings of anger, envy, guilt and despair. However, Brockopp, King and Hamilton (1991) found inconclusive evidence for educational input improving attitudes to death and reducing death anxiety.

The personal level

As outlined above, nurses enter the profession for a variety of reasons and so past experiences may make caring for some patients difficult or impossible. Consequently, it is important for nurses to be able to recognize their own limitations, to consider how they cope with inevitable painful feelings and whether the method of coping negatively affects their own life or the care provided to patients.

Vachon (1987) lists the nine most frequently cited personal coping mechanisms:

1. Having a sense of competence or pleasure from work.
2. Having a sense of control over aspects of one's own practice.
3. Managing one's lifestyle.
4. Having a personal philosophy of illness and death.
5. Leaving the work situation if it became too stressful.
6. Avoiding or distancing oneself from patients or their families.
7. Continuing a programme of education.
8. Having a support system outside of work.
9. Using humour.

She is not presenting these as either good or bad, merely as common. Some (e.g. 5 and 6) are unhelpful to the patient. The effects of the remainder will depend entirely upon how they are used. For example, humour (9) can be used to convey truth and improve understanding or to humiliate and demean.

> DISCUSSION POINT
> What coping mechanisms do you use to help you with painful experiences? Are any of these likely to be damaging to you or your patients?

Summary

In this section, I have suggested that the responsibility for helping nurses cope with the stress of caring for the dying and bereaved lies primarily with their employers. Formal support systems should be in place which are relevant to the area and which are task-oriented. However, research indicates that existing systems are usually of doubtful efficacy. In addition to the responsibilities of the institution, individual nurses need to take responsibility for their behaviour and consider their limitations and how they cope when they are asked to work at or beyond their limit.

Summary

I began by noting that the reality of death and dying occupies a central position in nursing. I then considered the reactions of people who were dying or bereaved. Attachment theory was used to demonstrate that there was an understandable pattern of feelings and behaviour in response to the experience of dying or being bereaved. However, individuals find different routes through this pattern.

In the second half of the chapter I examined the stress of dealing with dying and bereaved people. The sources of stress were considered and two important areas identified. The first was the powerful sense of impotence that can be induced in staff who are working in this area. The second concerns the motivation for choosing to work in this area. It was suggested that some nurses may be attracted to the work, in part because they have unfulfilled needs concerning, for example, unmourned losses. They unconsciously see a possibility of having their needs met, but instead find themselves attempting to meet the needs of others and becoming envious and frustrated.

Finally, ways of coping with these difficulties were reviewed. At an institutional level, it was suggested that this area of work poses a potential danger to mental health and so safety mechanisms are necessary in the form of accessible support systems. At a personal level nurses should consider how they cope with the inevitable painful feelings associated with such work and whether their coping mechanisms are adaptive in the long term or likely to result in problems for themselves or those they care for.

Seminar questions

1. Does culture and ethnic origin influence bereavement reactions? Are there examples of culturally determined differences within the United Kingdom? Can rituals aid recovery?
2. What are the potential dangers of using models of dying and bereavement like the ones described to understand the behaviour of individual patients?

Further reading

Kubler-Ross, E. (1973) *On Death and Dying.* London: Tavistock.
Parkes, C.M. (1972) *Bereavement: Studies of grief in adult life.* Harmondsworth: Penguin Books.
Parkes, C.M. and Weiss, R.S. (1983) *Recovery from Bereavement.* New York: Basic Books.
Worden, J.W. (1991) *Grief Counselling and Grief Therapy*, 3rd edition. New York: Springer. These four books are useful for those interested in looking more fully into the area of which this chapter has been a summary.
Penson, J. (1990) *Bereavement: A guide for nurses.* London: Harper & Row. This book gives a very clear account of some of the more practical aspects of nursing dying and bereaved people, as well as good, understandable descriptions of the emotional and psychological problems encountered, with some solutions.

References

Armstrong, D. (1987) 'Silence and truth in death and dying', *Social Science and Medicine* **24**, 651–8.

Bowlby, J. (1969) *Attachment and Loss*, Vol. I. New York: Basic Books.

Bowlby, J. (1980) *Attachment and Loss*, Vol. III. New York: Basic Books.

Brockopp, D.Y., King, D.B. and Hamilton, J.E. (1991) 'The dying patient: A comparative study of nurse caregiver characteristics', *Death Studies* **15**, 245–58.

Caplan, G. (1964) *Principles of Preventive Psychiatry*. New York: Basic Books.

Cartwright, A., Hockey, L. and Anderson, J.L. (1973) *Life before Death*. London: Routledge & Kegan Paul.

Corr, C.A. (1993) 'Coping with dying: Lessons we should not learn from the work of Elizabeth Kubler-Ross', *Death Studies* **17**, 69–83.

Engel, G.L. (1962) *Psychological Development in Health and Disease*. Philadelphia: W.B. Saunders.

Erikson, E.H. (1951) *Childhood and Society*. New York: W.W. Norton.

Erikson, E.H. (1982) *The Life Cycle Completed*. New York: W.W. Norton.

Freud, S (1917) 'Mourning and melancholia', in *Metapsychology: The theory of psychoanalysis*. Harmondsworth: Penguin Freud Library.

Glazer, B.G. and Strauss, A.L. (1965) *Awareness of Dying*. Chicago: Aldine.

Hare, J. and Pratt, C. (1989) 'Nurses' fear of death and comfort level with dying patients', *Death Studies* **13**, 349–60.

Hines, N. (1989) 'Care for the carers', in L. Sherr (ed.) *Death, Dying and Bereavement*. Oxford: Basil Blackwell.

Hinton, J. (1972) *Dying*. Harmondsworth: Penguin Books.

Holden, R.J. (1991) 'An analysis of caring: Attributions, contributions and resolutions', *Journal of Advanced Nursing* **16**, 893–8.

Kubler-Ross, E. (1973) *On Death and Dying*. London: Tavistock.

Lindemann, E. (1944) 'The symptomatology and management of acute grief', *American Journal of Psychiatry* **101**, 141.

Littlewood, J. (1992) *Aspect of Grief: Bereavement in adult life*. London: Routledge.

Lorenz, K. (1963) *On Aggression*. London: McEwan.

Malan, D.H. (1979) *Individual Psychotherapy and the Science of Psychodynamics*. London: Butterworths.

Menzies-Lyth, I. (1988) *Containing Anxiety in Institutions*. London: Free Association Books.

Novack, D.H., Plumer, R., Smith, R.L., Ochitill, H., Morrow, G.R. and Bennett, J.M. (1979) 'Changes in physicians' attitudes towards telling the cancer patient', *Journal of the American Medical Association* **241**, 897–900.

Oken, D. (1961) 'What to tell cancer patients: A study of medical attitudes', *Journal of the American Medical Association* **175**, 1120–8.

Parkes, C.M. (1972) *Bereavement: Studies of grief in adult life*. Harmondsworth: Penguin Books.

Parkes, C.M. and Stevenson-Hinde, J. (eds) (1990) *The Place of Attachment in Human Behaviour*. Basic Books: New York.

Parkes, C.M. and Weiss, R.S. (1983) *Recovery from Bereavement*. New York: Basic Books.

Penson, J. (1990) *Bereavement: A guide for nurses*. London: Harper & Row.

Pincus, L. (1976) *Death and the Family*. London: Faber.

Reisetter, K.H. and Thomas, B. (1986) 'Nursing care of the dying: Its relationship to selected nurse characteristics', *International Journal of Nursing Studies* **32**(1), 39–59.

Searle, C. (1991) 'Communication and awareness about death: A study of a random sample of dying people', *Social Science and Medicine* **32**(8), 943–52.

Smith, C.R. (1976) 'Bereavement: The contribution of phenomenological and existential analyses to a greater understanding of the problem', *British Journal of Social Work* **5**(1), 75–92.

Stroebe, W. and Stroebe, M. (1987) *The Psychological and Physical Consequences of Partner Loss.* Cambridge: Cambridge University Press.

Thompson, E. (1985) 'Palliative and curative nurses' atitudes toward dying and death in hospital settings', *Omega* **16**, 233–43.

Vachon, M.L.S. (1987) *Occupational Stress in the Care of the Critically Ill, the Dying and the Bereaved.* Washington: Hemisphere.

Worden, J.W. (1991) *Grief Counselling and Grief Therapy*, 3rd edition. New York: Springer.

Wright, B. (1990) *Sudden Death: Intervention skills for the caring professions.* Edinburgh: Churchhill Livingstone.

Working with children

The material in Part IV is of special relevance to those such as midwives and health visitors who deal with parents and children, and to those who work in the community. However, the material has a more general relevance, as an appreciation of child development provides a foundation for the understanding of psychological processes in adults.

Chapter 18 considers the formation of relationships between parents and children. Historically, this has always been an important topic for those concerned with development. In the last fifty years the issue of separation from parents and the consequence of this for later personality has attracted much interest and this work has had implications for the way that health professionals care for children. Chapter 18 examines these issues by taking a critical look at research on bonding, separation and attachment.

Our models of children have changed over the years. Sometimes children have been seen as little, though unsophisticated adults. Current psychological views about children assume that the way children think about the world is different from adults, but that it has its own logic and assumptions. This viewpoint is reflected in Chapter 19, which discusses communicating with children and the related issue of children's understanding of illness and death.

In recent years we have seen massive changes in the treatment and attitudes to children with disabilities. Nevertheless, there is still scope for more progress to be made. Chapter 20 examines topics related to children with learning disabilities, including the issue of intelligence and the identification of learning disabilties; the way that learning disabilities can have an impact across the life span and an examination of specific disabilities.

Chapter 21 also considers the issue of disability in relation to children, in this case motor and sensory disability. The chapter outlines research findings about motor disability, visual impairment and hearing impairment. This chapter makes it clear that children can compensate for many types of physical disability if given the appropriate support and a suitable environment. Health professionals can play a crucial role in enabling such development.

CHAPTER 18

Bonding, attachment and separation

DAVID J. MESSER

Chapter outline

Introduction

The relationship between children and their parents (usually the mother) has been and continues to be an issue of interest to developmental psychologists. The attachment of child to mother was regarded by Freud as fundamental to the later development of other relationships and the issue of separation from parents came to prominence as a result of concerns during and after World War II. Today, issues of attachment and separation continue to be a topic of concern to parents and health professionals. In this chapter I shall first examine bonding, which is usually considered to be the relationship of mothers to their babies. Then the pattern of attachment of infants to their mothers will be outlined. This is followed by a discussion of theories about the formation of attachment relationships. Finally, the effects of children being separated from their parents are considered.

Bonding

Until the 1970s the usual hospital practice in the West was to separate newborn infants from their mothers after birth and to reunite them for their first feed. This was supposed to give the mother time to recover from labour. Today, hospital practice is very different; unless there are medical reasons for the separation, mother and baby are usually left together (with father) until the mother is taken to the maternity ward.

These changes can partly be attributed to the research work of Klaus, Kennell and their colleagues (1976). In one study they were able to randomly allocate mothers to either a treatment group, which had extra contact with their infant after birth, or to a control group, which followed the normal hospital procedure of separation until the first feed. When the two groups were seen at later ages various positive features were noted about the way the mothers in the treatment group reacted towards their children. These included: holding the baby closer; looking into the infant's eyes more often; more kissing; a more relaxed style of cuddling; being more likely to continue breast feeding, and at 2 years the mother asking more questions.

DISCUSSION POINT
Was the treatment group disadvantaged? Was the control group disadvantaged?

The findings of Klaus and Kennell (1976) created great interest, especially as the publication coincided with a movement to demedicalize birth and give women more say in the process. Klaus and Kennell pointed out that in other species such as goats and sheep the early exposure of the baby animal to the mother is necessary for her to bond to the infant. If this exposure does not take place, the mother is likely to reject her offspring. By implication it was being suggested that a similar process may occur in humans.

In the years following this work, hospital procedures were changed to allow for contact immediately after birth. In addition, the findings began to be interpreted as indicating that those mothers who did not experience early contact, perhaps for medical or other reasons, would be disadvantaged in developing a relationship with their baby and that a failure to 'bond' would have detrimental consequences for a child's development. It was even suggested that lack of this early bond might be a contributory factor in child abuse.

Subsequent work has questioned the role of early experience in bonding. One point that has often been made is that the social context of birth varies across human cultures and has varied across historical time. For example, in the Efé of Zaire, infant babies are often given to another mother to breastfeed for the first few days after birth. In addition, generations of mothers have successfully taken care of their children despite separation at birth. Further, some mothers, particularly those who experience a painful childbirth, may feel distant from their baby until some weeks after the birth, but they go on to develop strong bonds with their babies. More importantly, a number of studies failed to replicate Klaus and Kennell's findings (e.g. Carlsson *et al.*, 1979; Svejda, Campos and Emde, 1980), and where replications have been successful they tend to have been with mothers who are poorly educated and of a low social class; it may well be that these mothers feel less confident in hospitals and gain more benefit and confidence from the early contact (Vietze and O'Connor, 1980). Further, parents who have adopted a child and who have not experienced early contact nevertheless report strong relationships with their child.

In a recent review of this material, Schaffer (1990) criticizes the idea of bonding as 'super-glue'. He argues that the experimental studies do not provide support for the idea that early contact enhances mother–infant bonds, and that the idea of bonding fails to make allowance for the complexity of human relationships as well as the possibility of changing relationships during development. The story about bonding illustrates the dangers of changing policy on the basis of limited evidence from unreplicated studies, but in this case the ending seems to be a happy one.

The development of attachment of infant to mother

This section first considers the way newborn babies relate to people and in particular to their mother. Then the course of attachment is outlined.

A preference for adults?

Recent research has revealed that infants prefer the *sound*, *sight* and *movement* of adults to other comparable stimuli (see Messer, 1994). When we speak to young children we tend to use a higher pitch (similar to a higher musical sound), a more sing-song voice and shorter utterances. Newborns prefer to listen to this adult-to-child speech than to normal adult-to-adult conversation. Young infants find human faces attractive and this seems to be because human faces contain many general visual properties which make stimuli attractive for infants (high contrast between dark and light areas, vertical symmetry, movement and curved rather than straight lines). In addition, some investigators claim that infants may have a genetic predisposition to find human faces attractive. Infants are also interested in the movements of adults. Bertenthal and Proffitt (1986) attached light points to a person's limbs and recorded their movements in a darkened room. A computer was used to generate an equivalent set of movements which would not be possible for a human to make. Three-month-old infants preferred to watch the human movements rather than the computer-generated ones.

Thus, research investigations have discovered that the sounds, sight and movement of human adults are special to very young infants. As a result, they are attentive to the things people do and say, and this may be of assistance to the development of relationships with people. However, as we shall see in the next section, infants are also especially attracted to their mother from a very early age.

Interest in the mother

In the last decade there has been a series of investigations which have revealed that newborn infants show a preference for the *sound*, *sight* and *smell* of their mother. Day-old infants will suck harder and more frequently on a teat to hear their mother's voice rather than a stranger's voice (DeCasper and Fifer, 1980). This seems to be a result of *pre-natal learning*. Newborns show preferences for various sounds heard before their birth. These include nursery rhymes, speech transformed so that it sounds similar to what would be heard inside the womb and even the theme tune to the popular TV soap *Neighbours* (presumably a consequence of maternal interest in this programme during pregnancy; Hepper, 1992).

Even more remarkably, Bushnell, Sai and Mullin (1989) found that newborn infants, less than 24 hours old, looked longer at their mother than at another woman. This occurred even when all they could see were the adults' faces and when they were unable to smell their mother. The mechanism of this process is not yet established, but it may be an example of very quick learning based on the pre-natal preference of the baby for the mother's voice, and this preference is then generalized to a face soon after birth.

Infants are also attracted to the odour of their mother. MacFarlane (1975) placed, either side of babies' heads, a breast pad from their mother and one from another mother. By 10 days after birth infants showed a preference by turning towards the breast pad from their mother. The precise mechanism of this process is not yet clear, but it seems that familiarity with odours may result in preferences. Infants who were in a crib scented with either ginger or mint, later showed a preference for the scent they had experienced.

These findings indicate that infants within the first two weeks of life already show a preference for their mother. At present the indications are that this preference may be a result of familiarity – in this case, familiarity does not lead to contempt. However, it is important to emphasize that these preferences do *not* constitute attachment. Infants prefer the stimuli produced by their mother, but they are not necessarily distressed if she leaves them. Nor, as we shall see later, does it appear that these preferences are necessary for the development of close relationships with other adults.

The development of attachment

Infants are usually considered to be *attached* to someone when they show the following characteristics: distress at separation; an orientation to the person which involves responses such as gazing, following and vocalizing; and seeking the person in moments of stress.

At about 6–8 months infants start to show distress at the departure of familiar people and to seek their contact. However, the full range of attachment behaviours is not usually seen until about 8 or 9 months of age. (Most studies report quite a range of ages at which the characteristic develops.) In addition, at this age children often show fear and wariness of strangers. One of the first detailed studies of attachment revealed that although the mother was usually the main attachment figure, this was not always the case. Attachments were also formed to fathers, grandparents and others adults (Schaffer and Emerson, 1964). Obviously, in older children attachment to parents continues, but the behaviours which mark this attachment change. Furthermore, as verbal understanding increases so children are better able to cope with separations if they are told about and prepared for the events.

The attachment process

Theories of attachment

Why are children attached to their parents? Often we accept this process as being such a natural part of development that we do not think about the reasons why attachment develops. In the past an influential theory about attachment was derived from learning theory (see Box 7.2, p. 137). It was supposed that because mothers provided relief from hunger, thirst and cold, they became associated with rewarding circumstances and were valued in their own right. A similar idea is contained in Freud's description of the growth of attachment. Here the focus is on the way feeding provides oral gratification, which in turn provides a basis for the development of attachment. However, the basis of these theories was shown to be inadequate in the late 1950s and 1960s. Two studies which were very influential in changing views about attachment are given in Box 18.1.

The demise of learning theory explanations was accompanied by a growth of interest in Bowlby's theory of attachment. Bowlby (1958, 1969, 1973) believed that attachment is the result of evolutionary selection pressures. Young animals that stay close to their mother are more likely to avoid dangers such as becoming lost, being injured or attacked and, as a result, they are more likely to survive.

A powerful example of attachment in non-human species is *imprinting*, which occurs in ducks and geese. Shortly after hatching chicks will follow the first moving object that they see, whether this is their mother or, another animal, such as a human or even a dog. The chicks will seek this object when frightened and, when adult, sometimes display sexual behaviour towards it.

Findings from studies of animal behaviour were a powerful influence on Bowlby's thinking. However, although he believed that there was a strong biological basis to human attachment formation, he did not believe that the process was automatic as in some other species. Rather, he reasoned that the biological need for security has resulted in infants possessing a number of attachment behaviours, such as crying, following, proximity-seeking, smiling, clinging and sucking. He also believed that these are powerful stimuli in terms of their ability to gain an

BOX 18.1   **CARE AND ATTACHMENT**

The first and perhaps most famous study to show that attachment is not based on the supply of food was conducted by Harlow and Zimmerman (1959) on infant monkeys. The infant monkeys were placed in a cage with two wire mesh cylinders. On one cylinder the baby monkey could obtain milk from a teat, while the other cylinder was covered with cloth. If food was the cause of attachment then one would expect the monkeys to form an attachment to the bare cylinder which supplied the milk. In fact, the monkeys spent most of their time on the cloth-covered cylinder and would jump on this cylinder when frightened. Thus study (which would now be considered unethical) indicated that simply supplying food is not sufficient for the formation of attachment.

A second important study was conducted by Schaffer and Emerson (1964). They saw a group of 60 children every month during their first 12 months of life. Observations were conducted in the children's homes. Not only did the study reveal that children formed multiple attachments with mother, father, grandparents and other adults, but the study also revealed that attachments were formed when these other adults took little or no care of the infants' basic needs. Instead, attachments seemed to be formed to individuals who were prepared to play, be responsive and interact socially with the child.

Another interesting study was conducted by Fox (1977) in the kibbutzim of Israel. In the kibbutz, during the day, children are in a group with a 'metapelet', a trained carer. The children have contact with their parents in the late afternoon and in the evening. Thus, the metapelet provided training and care in a group setting, and the parents provided individual affection and attention. The attachment of the children to both the metapelet and the mother was assessed. The findings revealed that the children were attached to both individuals, but that in reunions after a separation the children showed a stronger affection for the mother. Thus, attachment developed to both individuals even though they provide different types of care.

adult response. Important to his theory was the idea that the mother provides a secure base for exploration and that as the infants' feelings of security increase so they are more prepared to move away from the mother. (Think about the difference in young children's activities when at home and when they visit a strange environment.)

A controversial aspect of Bowlby's work was his belief that mothers should be the most important carer and that this care should be provided on a continuous basis. An obvious implication is that mothers should not go out to work. There have been many attacks on this claim. One criticism has been that a wider perspective reveals that mothers are the exclusive carers in only a very small percentage of human societies (Weisner and Gallimore, 1977); similarly, van IJzendoorn and Tavecchio (1987) argue that a stable network of adults can provide adequate care and that this care may even have advantages over a system where the mother has to meet all her child's needs. In addition, there is evidence that children develop better with a mother who is happy in her work than with a mother who is frustrated by staying at home (Schaffer, 1990). Furthermore, studies such Suwalsky and Klein's (1980) have revealed that 1-year-olds' behaviour was not related to the number of separations or the different forms of care.

Assessing the quality of attachment

One problem with studying attachment was the need to devise a way to measure it. For instance, when children are prepared to wander away from their mother, does this indicate weak attachment or that the children have a secure relationship with their mother? Does the amount of crying on separation indicate a weak or strong attachment? Preliminary attempts to measure attachment in this way and treat it as a *quantity*, like the temperature of a person, were largely unsuccessful.

An important advance in measurement came from an investigation by Ainsworth and Wittig (1969), which indicated that there were different forms of attachment to a parent. Rather than measure the amount of attachment, Ainsworth observed the organization of attachment behaviour. The observations were made in a laboratory room (see Box 18.2) and have been used to classify children into one of three groups: *secure* (also known as type B), and two types of insecure attachment, *avoidant* (type A) and *ambivalent* (type C). In American samples the proportion of children in these three groups is approximately 70 per cent, 20 per cent and 20 per cent respectively. More recently, a further form, labelled *disorganized*, has been identified (type D).

Many studies have used the strange situation to investigate attachment. Originally, Ainsworth and Bell (1969) supposed that secure attachments were the result of mothers being responsive to children's needs. Their study claimed to show relations between responsiveness and the three types of attachment. However, there were flaws with this investigation. For example, the raters of maternal responsiveness knew about the eventual type of attachment developed by the child. As a result, their scoring of behaviour may have been biased (the raters should have been *blind* to (i.e. unaware of) the attachment classification).

More recently, Isabella, Belsky and von Eye (1989), in a better controlled study, have claimed to find a similar relationship between responsiveness and attachment, as predicted by Ainsworth. In particular, mothers and infants who tended to interact socially with each other at the same time at 1 month and later ages were more likely at 12 months to have a secure relationship. Those that had a more one-sided pattern of interaction tended to have insecure relationships. More surprisingly, Fonagy and his colleagues have found that mothers' pre-natal reports of their own relationship with their mother (concerning parental responsiveness, feelings, etc.) predict the security of attachment their child will have to them (Fonagy, Steele and Steele, 1991). It is important to realize that this finding

BOX 18.2 **THE STRANGE SITUATION**

The strange situation takes place in a laboratory with a set arrangement of attractive toys and furniture. The infants have to be independently mobile and the assessment is typically made with infants between 12 and 18 months of age. All the sessions, except the first one, are supposed to take 3 minutes.

In the strange situation the following sequence of events takes place:

1. The mother and child are introduced to the room.
2. The mother and child are left alone and the child can investigate the toys.
3. A stranger enters and stays.
4. The mother leaves the child alone with the stranger and the stranger interacts with the child.
5. The mother returns to greet and comfort the child.
6. The mother leaves the child with the stranger.
7. The stranger tries to engage the child.
8. The mother returns.

There is a detailed coding scheme to assign children to one of the three categories of attachment. In broad terms, *securely attached* infants tend to explore the unfamiliar room; they are subdued when the mother leaves and greet her positively when she returns. In contrast, *avoidant* infants do not orient to the mother while investigating the toys and room; they do not seem concerned by her absence and they show little interest in her when she returns. The *ambivalent* infants often show intense distress particularly when the mother is absent, but they reject the mother by pushing her away, often this occurs when the mother returns.

A further group of children has subsequently been identified, and this classification group is referred to as disorganized (Type D; Main and Cassidy, 1988). These children show inconsistent behaviour, confusion and indecision. They also tend to freeze or show stereotyped behaviours such as rocking. The methodology used in the strange situation has also been developed to assess attachment in the pre-school and school years (Cassidy and Martin, 1989; Main and Cassidy, 1988).

In general, studies have found that for a particular child the strange situation classification (SSC) is usually the same at different ages (i.e. reliable; see Box 7.4). When differences occur these are often associated with changes in the type of care children experience (Melhuish, 1993). Two studies have even found similar types of attachment at 1 year and 6 years (Main and Cassidy, 1988), and a study conducted in Germany found 78 per cent of the children were classified in the same way at these two ages (Wartner *et al.*, 1994).

concerns a mother's *perception* of her relationship with her mother and that this may or may not correspond to the reality of the relationship. Further research by this group has also revealed that mothers who are reflective about themselves and show interpersonal sensitivity are more likely to have securely attached children, whereas those who are non-reflective are likely to have insecurely attached children (Fonagy *et al.*, 1994).

Thus, it would seem that attachment patterns can, at least in part, be predicted from maternal characteristics and behaviour. Such predictability provides evidence for the validity (see Box 7.4, p. 140) of the strange situation classification (SSC); behaviour is related to attachment in a way that was predicted from Ainsworth's attachment theory. Another set of studies provides a different type of evidence about validity. These have found that the SSC is related to children's reactions when they are separated in more natural circumstances such as when a child is left with a babysitter (e.g. Smith and Noble, 1987).

Other sets of investigations have reported that the security of attachment predicts children's later abilities. Secure infants appear more cooperative with their mother at 2 years (Matas, Arend and Sroufe, 1978). In addition, infants rated as secure in their second year have been found to be rated by their nursery school teachers to be more popular, have more initiative, have higher self-esteem, be less aggressive and are social leaders. Secure children were also rated as more popular by other children (Sroufe, 1983). The children in Sroufe's study were seen again at 11 years. The secure infants were rated as higher in social competence, self-confidence and self-esteem (Elicker, Englunds and Sroufe, 1992). Thus, these and similar studies support the claim that the SSC is measuring a psychologically important characteristic.

How does attachment develop in families which have to cope with a child who has a chronic disease with its associated strains and extra demands? Studies have revealed, somewhat surprisingly, that there are as many infants with secure attachment in this group as in a control group of healthy infants. For example, Fischer-Faye *et al.* (1988) report this pattern of findings when considering infants with cystic fibrosis. Indeed, the secure infants with cystic fibrosis were chubbier than the secure infants in the control group (weight gain is a problem in children with cystic fibrosis). Secure infants with a congenital heart condition also seemed *healthier* in a study by Goldberg *et al.* (1990). In Fischer-Faye *et al.*'s study it was also found that infants diagnosed earlier tended to have insecure attachments. This may be because the emotion associated with the news of the diagnosis interferes with social interaction and attachment development. Such an interpretation is, however, only speculative.

A study conducted by Goldberg *et al.* (1990) of three groups of children (with cystic fibrosis, congenital heart conditions and no health problems) found no difference in attachment patterns across the three groups. At 2 years the children were observed undertaking problem-solving tasks with their mother. For the healthy infants, those who had a secure attachment tended to be more cooperative (as found in the study by Matas, Arend and Sroufe, 1978). However, there was no relationship between the earlier SSC and functioning in the problem-solving tasks for the other two groups. This may be because the stability of relationships is more uncertain in the children with disease so that early SSC does not necessarily predict later functioning.

Evaluation of the strange situation classification (SSC)

At first sight, all these findings about the strange situation suggest we should accept its usefulness without further question. However, it is important to note that there have been criticisms of some of the claims. It has been argued that behaviour in the strange situation is the result of children's inborn characteristics (temperament). For example, Kagan has suggested that avoidant infants are difficult to upset, ambivalent infants are easy to stress and that secure infants are somewhere between these two (see Campos *et al.*, 1983). Evidence to support the idea of infant temperament as the cause of the differences in behaviour in the strange situation come from a number of studies. It has been found that newborns who are less able to orient to people and objects are more likely to have insecure attachments at later ages (Waters, 1978). Similarly, low Apgar scores (an assessment of physiological status at birth) are associated with later insecure relationships. In addition, there are findings to suggest that providing support for parents with more difficult infants can result in secure patterns of attachment (Crockenberg, 1981). Thus, there is still controversy about whether or not infant temperament contributes to later attachment.

Another criticism of the SSC has been that, according to the culture being studied, there is variation in the proportion of children assigned to the three categories. Grossman *et al.* (1985), working in Germany, found a higher proportion of avoidant children (i.e. showing independence) and it was suggested that this may be a result of the greater value placed on this characteristic by parents in this culture. More worrying for the SSC are findings from Japan, where infants very rarely leave their mother and the strange situation is therefore an unusual and particularly stressful event. Many infants simply cannot cope with the strange situation and therefore their behaviour is very different from that seen in other studies (Miyake, Chen and Campos, 1985). Similarly, it has been questioned whether the SSC can be meaningfully applied to children who have extensive non-parental care (Belsky, 1988). Together, these findings indicate that we should not assume that secure attachments, as diagnosed by the SSC, are optimal for all cultures and it also seems to be the case that sometimes children react in ways not covered by the SSC.

More recent ideas about attachment

In the last decade many investigations of attachment have been concerned with the claim that the security of attachment is one part of a child's *working model* of herself and of her parents, involving conscious and unconscious thoughts (Bowlby, 1973; Main, Kaplan and Cassidy, 1985). According to this formulation, the SSC provides an assessment of the child's expectations about the way a parent will react during stressful events and the child's own feelings of security about being separated. It is also supposed that the working model that develops with the primary caregiver is likely to be extended to other adults.

Bretherton, Ridgeway and Cassidy (1990) suggest that secure children have developed a positive working model of themselves based on their feelings of security derived from a carer who is sensitive, emotionally available and supportive. In contrast, avoidant children have a carer who is rejecting, which results in their having a working model of themselves as unacceptable and unworthy. Ambivalent children have carers who are inconsistent and consequently the children have a negative self-image and exaggerate their emotional responses in order to gain attention. This hypothesis provides one explanation of the fact that early patterns of attachment are related to later child characteristics. The claim about the working model is not without controversy as any predictability could simply be due to certain positive or negative family characteristics having a continuing impact on attachment and later competencies. In a similar way arguments have been made that continuing child characteristics (e.g. adaptability and sociability) might be responsible for relationships between attachment and later abilities.

Summary

Research into the SSC has produced an impressive array of findings which suggest early attachment is a result of both parental and child characteristics. Findings also indicate that the SSC is a good predictor of later child characteristics. There still remains some uncertainty about the direction of causality (from infant or parents), but we now have a wealth of evidence about the psychological importance of this dimension of behaviour.

The effects of separating children from their families

Most of us assume that, unless it is necessary, young children should not be separated from their mother when, for instance, one of them has to go into hospital. This is such a prevailing assumption that it is easy to forget that thirty years ago attitudes were very different. Parental hospital visits were restricted, children were often placed in unfamiliar day nurseries when their mother went into hospital and there was little concern about the effects of these separations. One reason for these policies might have been the frequent disruption and anguish caused by children's distress at the end of any contact with their mother. However, as we shall see later, much can be done to minimize distress and some upset may be preferable to the effects of a complete separation.

The investigations conducted on the effects of separations have provided a scientific basis for the changes in hospital practice and the wider change in societies' attitudes to these matters. Much of the research was conducted some time ago when these separations were common, but the findings still have relevance to issues of today. The short-term and the long-term effects of separation have usually been studied separately.

Short-term effects of separation

Research has revealed that the immediate effects of separation on a young child are influenced by the age of the child and the type of care that is provided. As we have already seen, infants below about 5 months of age appear able to identify their mother, but do not show a marked preference for her presence. Therefore it is unsurprising that separations before this age do not seem to have a marked effect. For example, Schaffer and Callender (1959) observed few signs of distress in infants below 7 months when they were admitted to hospital, but above this age there was crying, together with disturbances in sleeping and feeding. In cases of complete separation because of adoption, some effects may occur at an even earlier age. Yarrow and Goodwin (1973) collected information about the reactions of infants who were being adopted into a new home. Their conclusion was that few infants show a reaction before 3 months; that between 3 and 6 months there is an increasing proportion of infants who show a reaction (e.g. sleep and feeding disturbances, emotional reactions), and that between 7 and 16 months all infants showed some reaction. On the basis of these and other studies we can have confidence that at about 7 months of age, there is an increase in disturbed behaviour following separation (Tennes and Lampl, 1966).

What are young children's reactions to separation? Robertson and Bowlby (1952) observed that there are three progressive reactions: protest, despair and detachment. The 1–4-year-olds in the study were placed by the parents in residential nurseries (often because their mother was entering hospital) or were themselves admitted to hospital. The initial *protest* involved crying, grizzling and calling the name of the mother, with the children appearing distraught and panic-stricken. These behaviours lasted from several hours to about a week. Protest reactions typically gave way to *despair* where children were apathetic, disinterested in their surroundings, cried occasionally and had a continuing need for their mother. This in turn was followed by *detachment* as the child cried less and became more alert and interested. The detachment at first sight appeared to indicate recovery, but the recovery seems to have been at the cost of suppression of feelings for the mother; when the mother returned the child responded to her with a lack of interest and often was angry and rejecting. If a child reacts in this way it is important to reassure the parents that the relationship will recover, but patience, reassurance and support are required. Subsequent work has confirmed that children from about 6 months to just before school age exhibit these reactions, but the process is somewhat varied and a range of behaviours are shown by children. It is interesting that Bowlby believed that these grief reactions are similar to those of bereaved adults (see Chapter 4).

In the past, very little used to be done to help children adjust to their new surroundings. An important study by Robertson and Robertson (1971) showed that given appropriate preparation and care, children could adjust to separation from their mother. The Robertsons were successful in minimizing the distress of four children whom they cared for on separate occasions in their own home.

DISCUSSION POINT

List the techniques the Robertsons might have used to help children adjust to separation in their temporary home (answers given at the end of the chapter). List current hospital practices which help to minimize the effects of separation.

Today, issues of separation are usually dealt with sensitively. However, it is important to remember that separation from a mother, because she is giving birth to another child, can still be stressful and disruptive to siblings, even if they stay at home in their usual surroundings. For example, Trause *et al.* (1981) have found firstborns show an increase in temper tantrums, excessive activity and sleep problems. They also found that visiting the mother in hospital was beneficial; it resulted in the older child being more responsive to the mother and new sibling. On the mother and baby's return home, older firstborn children had difficulties when left for short periods by the mother. They followed her around the house and had difficulty when playing with other children (Nadelman and Begun, 1982). Another study by Stewart, Mobley and Van Tuyl (1987) found that mothers tended to decrease the number of interactions with the older child dramatically, while fathers continued to interact at about the same rate. The firstborns in this study showed problems in behaviour even 12 months after the birth. However, there is also a positive side to these changes, with children being reported as being more 'grown up' and engaging in more advanced activities such as fantasy play (Dunn, Kendrick and MacNamee, 1981). Thus, if parents are separated from a young child, or if there is a new baby in the family, they should be advised to make allowances and provide additional preparation, explanations, security and comfort.

Long-term effects of separation

Concern about the long-term effects of separation were provided with a focus by Bowlby's (1946) report that delinquency was associated with young children's separation from their mother and claims that prolonged separation might lead to later inability to form relationships. However, Bowlby's study of delinquent boys was flawed. He found that most had been separated from their mother during early childhood and supposed that this was the cause of the delinquency. What he failed to do was find out whether a similar rate of separations occurred in similar adolescents who were not delinquent.

A later study by Bowlby *et al.* (1956) effectively showed that separations do not necessarily lead to later problems such as delinquency. The study concerned children under 4 years of age who had been isolated in TB units. In the units the children were not seen more than once a week by their parents, the nursing regimes tended to be strict and the care was impersonal. Information was obtained about these children when they were between 7 and 14 years old. A control group of children who had not been in the clinics was also studied. There were differences between the two groups, but they were not large and involved characteristics such as the tubercular group showing more daydreaming, being less sociable and less attentive. No differences were found in terms of delinquency or problems in forming social relationships.

A slightly less optimistic picture has been provided by Douglas (1975), who compared a large group of children admitted to hospital during their first 5 years with a group who had not been admitted. The time spent in hospital was usually about 3 weeks. Data collected in adolescence indicated that the children who had *repeated* hospital admissions had a higher rate of delinquency, poorer reading and more job changes. Clarke and Clarke (1976) have questioned whether there was a causal connection between repeated hospital admissions and later problems, using an analysis of Douglas's own data. Another analysis by Rutter (1976) of a different set of data revealed that repeated hospital admissions was a marker for disadvantage and this, rather than the separations themselves could account for the higher developmental risk. Thus in itself separation from parents does not necessarily lead to later problems; rather, the available evidence points to family stress and disruption as the cause.

Summary

Research in early childhood has led to a rejection of the more extreme claims made about bonding. However, the bonding hypothesis has resulted in beneficial changes in hospital practice. Research has also identified a number of reasons for the different forms of attachment between children and adults. There is evidence that differences at birth are related to later SSC. There is also evidence that the mother's characteristics, such as her 'working model' of her relationship with her own mother are related to the child's later pattern of attachment. Therefore, it is not surprising that early social interaction (which are likely to be influenced by both maternal and child characteristics) are also related to later SSC. We also have sound evidence that the SSC in the second year predicts children's later child characteristics. There is uncertainty about the precise reasons for this continuity, but such findings suggest early relationships are important for later development.

The findings about the short-term effect of separations are reasonable clear. If young children are not given adequate support, then protest, despair and detachment ensue. The longer-term effects are less clear, but the findings indicate that children should receive the best support possible when they are separated for any appreciable length of time from people to whom they are attached.

Seminar questions

1. Think about the studies of bonding. When should practice be changed in the light of research findings? When can we be confident about research findings?

2. Do you believe that psychologists can use the strange situation to classify children into different attachment types? If not, why not? If you are convinced, give your reasons.
3. Could more be done to help children adapt to a stay in a hospital with which you are familiar? Describe what could be done.

Answers to discussion point (p. 359)

- Meeting the child before the separation.
- Introduction of the child to the Robertsons' home.
- Keeping as far as possible to the same routines.
- Taking bed, blankets, clothes, cuddly toys and photograph of the mother to the Robertsons' home.
- Talking to the child about the mother during the separation.
- Fathers visited as often as they could.

Further reading

Schaffer, H.R. (1990) *Making Decisions about Children*. Oxford: Blackwell. A comprehensive review of the issues of separation, coupled with a concern for the issues which face health professionals.
Messer, D. (1994) *The Development of Communication*. Chichester: John Wiley. A good coverage of issues of early communication.

References

Ainsworth, M.D.S. and Bell, S.M. (1969) 'Attachment, exploration, and separation: Illustrated by the behavior of one-year-olds in a strange situation', *Child Development*, 49–65.
Ainsworth, M. and Wittig, B.A. (1969) 'Attachment and exploratory behaviour of 1-year-olds in a strange situation', in B.M. Foss (ed.) *Determinants of Infant Behaviour*, Vol. 4. London: Methuen.
Belsky, J. and Isabella, R.A. (1988) 'Maternal infant and social-contextual determinants of attachment security', in J. Belsky and T. Nezworski (eds), *Clinical Implications of Attachment*. Hillsdale, NJ: Lawrence Erlbaum.
Bertenthal, B.I. and Proffitt, D.R. (1986) 'The extraction of structure from motion: Implementation of basic processing constraints'. Paper presented at the International Conference on Infant Studies, Los Angeles, 1986. (Abstract in *Infant Behaviour and Development* 9, 36.)
Blacher, J. (1984) 'Attachment and severely handicapped children', *Journal of Development and Behavioural Pediatrics* 5, 178–83.
Bowlby, J. (1946) *Forty-Four Juvenile Thieves: Their characters and home life*. London: Baillière, Tindall & Cox.

Bowlby, J., Ainsworth, M., Boston, M. and Rosenbluth, D. (1956) 'The effects of mother–child separation: A follow-up study', *British Journal of Medical Psychology* **29**, 211–47.

Bowlby, J. (1958) 'The nature of the child's tie to his mother', *International Journal of Psycho-Analysis* **39**.

Bowlby, J. (1969) *Attachment and Loss*. Vol. 1, *Attachment*. London: Hogarth Press.

Bowlby, J. (1973) *Attachment and Loss*, Vol. II: *Separation, anxiety and anger*. London: Hogarth Press.

Bretherton, I., Ridgeway, D. and Cassidy, J. (1990) 'Assessing internal working models in the attachment relationship: An attachment story completion task for 3-year-olds', in M.T. Greenburg, D. Cichetti and E.M. Cummings (eds.) *Attachment During the Preschool Years*. Chicago: University of Chicago Press.

Bushnell, I.W.R., Sai, F. and Mullin, J.T. (1989) 'Neonatal recognition of the mother's face', *British Journal of Developmental Psychology* **7**, 3–15.

Campos, J.J., Caplovitz Barrett, K., Lamb, M., Goldsmith, H.H. and Stenberg, C. (1983) 'Socioemotional development', in P. Mussen (ed.) *Handbook of Child Psychology*. New York: John Wiley.

Carlsson. S.G., Fagerberg, H., Horneman, G., Hwang, C.P., Larson, K., Rodholm, M. and Schaller, J. (1979) 'Effects of various amounts of contact between mother and child on the mother's nursing behaviour: A follow-up study'. *Behaviour and Development* **2**, 209–14.

Cassidy, J., Martin, R. and The MacArthur Working Group on Attachment (1989) 'Attachment organization in three and four-year-olds: Coding guidelines.' Unpublished manuscript, University of Virgina and Pennsylvania State University.

Clarke, A.M. and Clarke, A.D.B. (1976) 'Studies in natural settings', in A.M. Clarke and A.D.B. Clarke (eds.) *Early Experience: Myth and evidence*. London: Open Books.

Crockenberg, S.B. (1981) 'Infant irritability, mother responsiveness, and social support mother–infant attachment', *Child Development* **52**, 857–65.

DeCasper, A.J. and Fifer, W. P. (1980) 'Of human bonding: Newborns prefer their mothers' voices', *Science* **208**, 1174–6.

Douglas, J.W.B. (1975) 'Early hospital admissions and later disturbances of behaviour and learning', *Developmental Medicine and Child Neurology* **17**, 456–80.

Dunn, J., Kendrick, C. and MacNamee, R. (1981) 'The reaction of first-born children to the birth of a sibling', *Journal of Child Psychology and Psychiatry* **22**, 1–18.

Elicker, J., England, M. and Sroufe, A.L. (1992) 'Predicting poor competence and poor relationships in childhood from early parent–child relationships', in *Family–peer relationships: Models of linkage*, Parke, Ross D. and Ladd, Gary W. (eds.), pp. 77–106. Hillsdale, NJ: Lawrence Erlbaum.

Fischer-Fay, A., Goldberg, S., Simmons, R. and Levison, H. (1988) 'Chronic illness and infant–mother attachment: Cystic fibrosis', *Journal of Developmental and Behavioural Pediatrics* **9**, 266–70.

Fonagy, P., Steele, H. and Steele, M. (1991) 'Maternal representations of attachment during pregnancy predict the organisation of infant–mother attachment at one year of age', *Child Development* **62**, 891–905.

Fonagy, P., Steele, M., Steele, H., Higgitt, A. and Target, M. (1994) 'The Emanuel Miller Memorial Lecture 1992: The theory and practice of resilience', *Journal of Child Psychology and Psychiatry* **35**, 215–30.

Fox, N. (1977) 'Attachment of kibbutz infants to mother and metapelet', *Child Development* **48**, 1228–39.

Goldberg, S., Morris, P., Simmons, R.J., Fowler, R.S. and Levison, H. (1990) 'Chronic illness in infancy and parenting stress: A comparison of three disease groups', *Journal of Pediatric Psychology* **15**, 347–58.

Grossman, K., Grossman, K.E., Spangler, G., Suess, G. and Unzer, L. (1985) 'Growing points in attachment theory and research'. In I. Bretherton and E. Waters (eds.) *Monographs of the Society for Research in Child Development*, Serial No. 209, Vol. 50, 3–35 monograph.

Harlow, H.F. and Zimmerman, R.R. (1959) 'Affectional responses in the infant monkey', *Science* **130**, 421–32.

Hepper, P.G. (1991) 'An examination of fetal learning before and after birth', *Irish Journal of Psychology* **12**, 95–107.

Isabella, R.A., Belsky, J. and von Eye, A. (1989) 'Origins of infant–mother attachment: An examination of interactional synchrony during the infant's first year', *Development Psychology* **25**, 12–21.

Klaus, M.H. and Kennell, J.H. (1976) *Parent–Infant Bonding*. St Louis: C.V. Mosby.

MacFarlane, A. (1975) 'Olfaction in the development of social preferences in the human neonate', in Ciba Foundation Symposium (ed.), *Parent–Infant Interaction*. New York: Elsevier.

Main, M. and Cassidy, J. (1988) 'Categories of response to reunion with the parent at age six: Predicted from infant attachment classifications and stable over a one-month period', *Development Psychology* **24**, 415–26.

Main, M., Kaplan, N. and Cassidy, J. (1985) 'Security in infancy, childhood and adulthood: A move to a level of representation', in I. Bretherton and E. Waters (eds.) *Growing Points of Attachment Theory and Research*. Monographs of the Society for Research in Child Development **50** (1–2, Serial No. 209).

Matas, L. Arend, R.A. and Sroufe, L.A. (1978) 'Continuity of adaptation in the second year', *Child Development* **49**, 547–56.

Melhuish, E.C. (1993) 'Behaviour measures: A measure of love? An overview of the assessment of attachment', *ACPP Review and Newletter* **15**(6), 269–75.

Miyake, K., Chen, S.J. and Campos, J.J. (1985) 'Infant temperament, mother's mode of interaction, and attachment in Japan: An interim report', in I. Bretherton and E. Waters (eds.) *Growing Points of Attachment Theory and Research*. Monographs of the Society for Research in Child Development **50** (1–2, Serial No. 209).

Nadelman, L. and Begun, A. (1982) 'The effect of the newborn on the older sibling', in M. Lamb and B. Sutton-Smith (eds.) *Sibling relationships: The nature and significance across the lifespan*. Hillsdale, N.J.: Lawrence Erlbaum.

Robertson, J. and Bowlby, J. (1952) 'Responses of young children to separation from their mothers', *Courier Centre International L'Enfance* **2**, 131–42.

Robertson, J. and Robertson, J. (1971) 'Young child in brief separation', *Psychoanalytic Study of the Child* **26**, 264–315.

Rutter, M. (1976) 'Parent–child separation: Psychological effects on the child', in A.M. Clarke and A.D.B. Clarke (eds.) *Early Experience: Myth and evidence*. London: Open Books.

Schaffer, H.R. and Callender, W.M. (1959) 'Psychologic effect of hospitalisation in infancy', *Pediatrics* **24**, 528–39.

Schaffer, H.R., and Emerson, P.E. (1964) 'The development of social attachments in infancy', Monographs of the Society for Research in Child Development **29**, (No. 3, Serial No. 94).

Sluckin, W., Herbert, M. and Sluckin, A., *Maternal Bonding.* Oxford: Blackwell.

Smith, P. and Noble, R. (1987) 'Factors affecting the development of caregiver–infant relationships', in L.W.C. Tavecchio and M.H. van IJzendoorn (eds.) *Attachment in Social Networks.* Amsterdam: North Holland.

Sroufe, L.A. (1983) 'Individual papers of adaption from infancy to preschool', in M. Perlmutter (eds.) *Minnesota Symposium on Child Psychology.* Hillsdale, NJ: Lawrence Erlbaum.

Stewart, R.B., Mobley, L.A. and Van Tuyl, S.S. (1987) 'The firstborn's adjustment to the birth of a sibling: A longitudinal assessment', *Child Development* **58**, 341–55.

Suwalsky, J.T.D. and Klein, R. (1980) 'Effects of natural-occurring nontraumatic separations from mother', *Infant Mental Health Journal* **1**(3), 196–201.

Svejda, M.J., Campos, J.J. and Emde, R.N. (1980) 'Mother–infant "bonding": Failure to generalise', *Child Development* **51**, 775–9.

Tennes, K.H. and Lampl, E.E. (1966) 'Some aspects of mother–child relationship pertaining to infantile separation anxiety', *Journal of Nervous and Mental Diseases* **143**, 426–37.

Trause, M.A., Voos, D., Rudd, C., Marshall Klaus, M.D., Kennell, J. and Boslett, M. (1981) 'Separation for childbirth: The effect on the sibling', *Child Psychiatry and Human Development* **12**(1), 32–9.

van IJzendoorn, M.H. and Tavecchio, L.W. (1987) 'The development of attachment theory as a Lakatosian research programme', in L.W.C. Tavecchio and M.H. van IJzendoorn (eds.) *Attachment in Social Networks.* Amsterdam: North Holland.

Wartner, U.G., Grossman, K., Fremner-Bombik, E. and Gucss, G.L. (1994) 'Attachment patterns in south Germany', *Child Development* **65**, 1014–27.

Waters, E. (1978) 'The reliability and stability of individual differences in infant–mother attachment', *Child Development* **49**, 483–94.

Weisner, T.S. and Gallimore, R. (1977) 'My brother's keeper: Child and sibling caretaking', *Current Anthropology* **18**(2), 169–90.

Yarrow, L.J. and Goodwin, M.S. (1973) 'The immediate impact of separation: Reactions of infants to a change in mother figures', in L.J. Stone, H.T. Smith and L.B. Murphy (eds.) *The Complete Infant.* New York: Basic Books.

CHAPTER 19

Communication and caring

Children and health

DAVID J. MESSER

Chapter outline

Introduction

This chapter addresses three interrelated issues. The first concerns the development of communication in children and the implications of this knowledge for health professionals when they are trying to obtain information from children or attempting to gain their cooperation. The second section briefly considers a related issue: children's understanding of health, disease and death. The final section examines the wider issue of the care of children with chronic or life-threatening diseases.

Communication

The development of communication

What is communication? Most people accept that it involves the transmission of information. This simple statement conceals a number of difficult issues: should non-intentional actions, such as the cry of a newborn or the nervousness of a person in an interview, be considered as communication? Should we be concerned about whether information is accurately received (e.g. when a parent changes a nappy in response to crying, but the baby needs a feed)? There are no agreed answers to these questions, but it is important to be aware of these and similar issues when thinking about communication.

Chapter 18 outlined the way that very young infants attend to the features of people, in particular the sound, sight and smell of their mother. Such abilities aid the process of communication by ensuring infants are attuned and attentive to what is probably the most important figure in their environment. In addition, young infants use a number of powerful signals that affect people. Both crying and smiling let carers know when a baby is distressed or is enjoying something.

Crying is present from the first few moments after birth and it is a powerful signal which is especially aversive to humans (Frodi, 1985). Indeed, so powerful is the signal that unremitting crying can be a precipitating factor in child abuse (Frodi, 1985). Different types of cry (e.g. pain, hunger and tiredness) can be identified from an early age (Wasz-Hockert *et al.* 1968). Crying typically results in adult attention and in attempts to remove the cause of the crying. Before speech is established, crying is one of the main signals that inform parents and health professionals that something is wrong with a young child. Furthermore, it is important for health professionals to know that abnormal acoustic patterns of crying can be associated with neurological impairment.

Reliable smiling in response to people and things does not typically emerge until about 2–3 months after birth. Before this, smiles are produced, but they are not as reliable as later ones; indeed, these early smiles have often been attributed to the effects of 'wind'. Smiling, like crying, is a powerful signal for adults. Adults will work very hard, engaging in all sorts of unusual facial expressions and voices to elicit a smile from a baby.

During the first six months of life, babies and adults tend to engage in social interaction which concerns only the participants themselves. Typical interaction involves body games, such as peek-a-boo and talk about emotions and feelings (Messer, in press). This early form of interaction may help to provide a basis for the development of attachment (see Chapter 18). There is some uncertainty about what sort of contribution infants are making to these social processes. Some theorists have argued that from a very early age, infants are able to identify other people as being similar to themselves (Meltzoff and Gopnik, 1993), that young infants can tune into the emotions of others (Hobson, 1993) and that young infants are making attempts to influence the course of social interaction (Trevarthen, 1982). These theorists maintain that young infants have some early understanding of people as being different from objects and that they engage in a form of communication with people. However, such claims are still the subject of debate. Others theorists (Leslie, 1987; Perner, 1991) believe that understanding that people have minds does not occur until about 18 months, and a fuller and more sophisticated understanding does not occur until about 4 years (see p. 368 below).

BOX 19.1 **WARINESS AND COMMUNICATION**

Chapter 19 shows that as specific attachments develop so does wariness of unfamiliar people. Wariness and shyness can continue until the school years. How should health professionals deal with and minimize such reactions? Obviously circumstances vary in terms of the age of child, as well as the place and urgency of any consultation.

Perhaps the first issue to deal with is to make the child feel as secure as possible. This can be best achieved if the child is near to, touching or sitting on a parent; if children feel secure, they will be less worried about unfamiliar people. It may also be necessary to set the parent(s) at ease. Anxious and fearful parents can convey their anxiety to children by non-verbal means, Favourite toys also provide security and can be used to provide a focus of joint interest. If possible, first make conversation with the parent(s). Children who see their parents being friendly with an unfamiliar person are likely to respond positively to this person. Studies have revealed that towards the end of their first year, infants engage in 'social referencing' when they check the reactions of parents to unfamiliar things or surprising events (Walden and Ogan, 1988). It also is a good idea to minimize your height and to avoid towering over a small baby. If possible keep your distance until rapport has been established. When at a distance, let children look at you by only occasionally looking at them (this gives the child a chance to study you) and smile when you look at the child. Often a side face rather than a full-face position seems less threatening to young children.

If the child appears settled and Is reacting to you positively, then it is appropriate to begin to interact with the child. This may take the form of presenting toys and asking questions which the child should be able to answer. If this is successful, you can move on to the purpose of the contact. At all stages it is important to remember the different effects of open and of closed questions on children. A closed question involves a simple reply such as 'yes' or 'no'. These are useful at first and can be effective in obtaining precise information. However, they can be leading and put pressure on children to giving false answers (see below). An open question allows the child to add information (compare 'Docs it hurt here?' with 'Tell me about what hurts'). If a child is not at ease, she may be more prepared to answer closed than open questions. However, a barrage of closed questions will make the interaction one-sided and the child could very well become unresponsive.

Do bear in mind that these are hints and there are no hard-and-fast rules about the best way to introduce yourself. Any technique will partly be based on the style of interaction that you enjoy and with which you feel comfortable.

Whatever the status of early communicative acts, as adults we modify our actions with young infants, moving closer to them and exaggerating our movements and voice in ways that are likely to maintain infant interest (see Messer, 1994). Often, simple games such as looking at the child and then hiding your eyes is sufficient to engage their attention. After about 6 months, infant interest in the environment becomes noticeable and adults often follow infants' interest in objects and events

(Trevarthen, 1982). At about 9 months there are important developments in communication with the use of conventional gestures such as pointing, the use of babbling and a little later the beginnings of one-word speech (i.e. the production of words like 'dada'). At this age and sometimes earlier, infants start to show wariness of strangers and this can make communication with them and enlisting their cooperation more difficult. Box 19.1 gives ideas about the way to overcome such difficulties.

During the second year, children's ability to understand adults' speech gradually increases and they can put their single word speech to more and more different uses, such as commenting on or requesting something. At about 18 months there are advances in a range of abilities. Children's vocabularies appear to expand rapidly. They start to produce two-word utterances and begin to engage in pretend play. It seems likely that these advances are due to children being able to form abstract and arbitrary representations about their world, but the precise nature of this cognitive advance is still the subject of discussion (Messer and Hasan, 1994).

Following these communicative advances, children begin to produce 'telegraphic speech', which consists only of words essential for the message; words that are less important for meaning are still omitted (e.g. a, the, very, there, here). At about 2 years children start to include the grammatical endings of words and to use 'functional' words (e.g. him, her, it, them) and this begins their acquisition of the grammar of language which continues for many years. The increase in verbal abilities means that between 24 and 30 months, one can begin to be reasonably confident that children can understand simple verbal messages.

A later development which has attracted a lot of recent interest is the idea that at about 4 years children start to develop a 'theory of mind'. This has been tested by stories similar to the following:

> A child called Maxi puts his chocolates in a green cupboard and then goes out to play. His mother tidies up and takes his chocolates out of the green cupboard and puts them in a blue cupboard. Maxi comes in from playing. Where do you think Maxi will look for the chocolate?

Children below 4 years typically think Maxi will look in the blue cupboard, whereas those above 4 years think Maxi will look in the green cupboard. These and similar stories identify an ability to understand that people's thinking may not always reflect reality. Interestingly, children with autism are usually unsuccessful with these tasks and they have difficulty communicating and interacting socially. Some studies suggest that these 'theory of mind' abilities can occur earlier than 4 years and there is debate about how important such skills are for the development of communication. However, the important point is that 4-year-olds are starting to have an appreciation that people can have different intentions from themselves and this type of knowledge means that they can start to relate to people in different and more sophisticated ways. One implication of this work is that after this advance children are also able to deceive and lie.

The role of context and non-verbal communication

When interacting with children of any age, it is important to recognize that they often give greater weight to non-verbal communication than to speech and that they may be trying to provide the answers they think the adult wants to hear rather then trying to say what they think and feel (see also Chapter 8). Many of the claims Piaget made about the age that children are able to understand and carry out cognitively complex tasks have been criticized because his methodology failed to take these two factors into account. (see Box 19.3 for an outline of his stages.)

Piaget and Inhelder (1956), for example, claimed that children are not able to understand the perspective of another person until about 8 years; instead children seem simply to assume that people think and see in the same way as themselves. One experiment which appeared to confirm this claim was the 'three mountains problem'. In this task a child was seated at a table on which there were three model mountains; at another side of the table an adult was seated. The child was asked to identify from a set of pictures what the adult could see. Typically, children below 6 years identified the view that they could see and not the view that could be seen by the adult.

The same types of ability were tested using a task which was made more simple and meaningful to children. In this task children were asked to tell the experimenter whether a policeman could see a thief (see Donaldson, 1978). The children were given a model policeman and a model thief, and the thief could hide behind brick walls which were shaped as a cross when viewed from above. Even some 4-year-old children could give accurate answers in this task. Other experiments have found that children are more likely to change their answer if asked the same question again, presumably because they infer that the first answer was incorrect (Rose and Blank, 1974). These and other studies have given a dramatic illustrations of the power of non-verbal and contextual cues on children's responses to questions. The implication of such studies is that questions and the context should be presented in a child-centred way as far as possible and made to appear neutral in terms of the demand characteristics of the situation (the non-verbal and contextual cues which suggest a certain answer is 'correct').

Child abuse and communication

Another serious issue related to the accuracy of communicating with children (and parents) is assessing the possibility that some injury or behavioural problem is the result of abuse. It is as well to remember that in the United Kingdom there is no consensus about whether discipline should, or should not, involve physical punishment such as smacking.

DISCUSSION POINT
Is physical punishment appropriate with children? Should health professinals give advice to parents about discipline and the use of physical punishment? Could this interfere with other objectives that health professionals have by alienating parents?

BOX 19.2 **CHILD ABUSE**

The distinction between physical punishment and physical abuse is sometimes unclear. At the extremes most of us (but not all) can accept a difference between a light tap and a blow that results in physical injury. However, such the distinctions are not always easy to make when account is taken of the frequency and context of the events. Not only can physical abuse occur, but there can also be neglect, emotional abuse and sexual abuse. Neglect involves failure to take adequate care of a child, often by a lack of care about feeding and health issues. Emotional abuse usually involves the verbal persecution of children with the result that they feel unloved and uncared. Sexual abuse is usually defined as the participation in sexual activities in which children are unable to give their informed consent and which violate family taboos. Again, with all these forms of abuse there is not always a hard-and-fast definition. (See Stainton Rogers, Hevey and Ash, 1989.)

There is a considerable literature on the identification, consequences and treatment of child abuse (see Box 19.2 for an introduction to this topic). In this chapter it is only possible to touch on some of these issues. In relation to detection it is important for health professionals to be alert to inconsistent or unusual behaviour in children. For example, children who suffer physical abuse may want to protect the family from detection and so wear long clothes in summer. It should not be assumed that because children have been abused that they are unatttached to their parent(s). Children may also react to abuse in very different ways. Some children may seek affection from almost anyone, while others may be withdrawn, fearful and wary. What should be borne in mind is that there is no fail-safe method of identifying abuse; what is necessary is a careful building up of information and evidence.

Summary

During the first two years of life children make dramatic advances in their ability to communicate. The communication of children and their cooperation will often be influenced by their feelings of security and by the social techniques used by health professionals. Furthermore, during the pre-school and early school years children rely on non-verbal information to help them understand communication and will often try to give the answer they think the adult wants to hear. As a result, health professionals need to be careful not to prompt children and to provide an open context for communication.

Children's understanding of diseases, illness and death

An important issue when communicating with children is the accuracy of their understanding of disease, illness and death. Some research has suggested that pre-

BOX 19.3	**PIAGET'S STAGES OF DEVELOPMENT (SEE FLAVELL, 1963)**

Age in Years	Stage	Cognitive abilities
0–2	Sensorimotor	The baby's understanding of the world is through sensations and motor activities. The baby is unable to engage in abstract thought.
2–6	Pre-operational	Children are able to think about symbols and use language. Children often lack appreciation of other's perspectives as in the 'three mountains task'.
7–12	Concrete operations	Children are much better at thinking in a logical manner. They are able understand reversable operations, e.g. when water is poured from a tall to a short glass they now understand there was the same amount in both containers despite differences in shape.
12+	Formal operations	The child has the ability to use scientific reasoning to think about the world.

school children have only a vague idea about the causes of illness so that it is sometimes seen as a punishment for bad behaviour (Kister and Patterson, 1980; Langford, 1948) or as a result of magic (Bibace and Walsh, 1981).

Bibace and Walsh (1981) suggest that children's ideas of illness change with age and with the Piagetian stage of cognitive development (see Box 19.3). During the pre-school years children were found to have only a hazy view of why illnesses are transmitted. At about 7 years, children start to accept that illnesses can be caused by factors external to themselves, that is by a process of *contamination*, so that their body can be affected by germs. Bibace and Walsh claim that this is followed by the understanding that the effects of this process are *internal* to the body and that illnesses can be cured by medication and treatment. During adolescence knowledge of biology learned in school combines with cognitive abilities so that accurate and sophisticated understanding of illness and disease can be achieved.

An interesting study by Brewster (1982) examined the beliefs of chronically ill children. A three-stage model was identified which was linked to cognitive development in terms of Piaget's stages. Children between 5 and 7 years thought that illness was a consequence of some human action (e.g. eating something, not taking care); older children between 7 and 10 years believed that illness was due to some physical cause such as germs; while children over 9 years tended to recognize that there are a number of causes of illness (e.g. bodily susceptibility and pathogens). More worrying was the report that these stages were linked to the way young children viewed medical procedures. At 5 and 6 years all children saw medical procedures as punishments, then at 7 to 10 years they were viewed as beneficial but that medical staff knew about pain only if the child cried or screamed, and at a still older age children appreciated that medical procedures were for beneficial purposes and the health professionals understood the feelings of the child. As we shall see, there are reasons to believe that general cognitive development does not always determine the level of a child's understanding of illness. Interestingly, Brewster argued that care needs to be taken when explaining these issues to children as the resulting cognitive gain may result in the child feeling more vulnerable and less able to cope.

In a similar way one can trace a growing awareness of children's understanding of death. Kane (1979) reports that 3-year-olds have some awareness of the meaning of death. By 5 years many children understand that death involves separation and a year later many appreciate that there is a biological cause of death and that certain biological processes such as breathing stop. Eight-year-olds usually understand that all biological entities die and that pain ceases with death.

Issues of communication between health professionals, the family and the child about illness and death can be made even more stressful by differences in opinion about what the child should be told (see also Chapter 9). At present, the general policy is to respect the parents wishes; this can, however, be difficult if the child is asking searching questions. It is also the case that children may avoid talking about these issues because of the fear of upsetting adults. Claflin and Barbarin (1991) investigated the communication to children with cancer about their condition. They found that youngsters over 9 years were told more about their disease, but younger children had similar levels of adjustment to those who were told more and that some children who were not told about their condition made inferences about themselves. In addition, there are reports that some young children appear less distressed than their parents about the idea of their own death. It should also be remembered that children may differ in their understanding of the implications of death, depending on their parents' religious beliefs and their culture. Health professionals should be aware of such differences and adapt their responses to the needs of the families.

The limitations of a purely cognitive account of children's understanding of illness is becoming increasingly recognized. Although cognitive abilities may limit some types of knowledge, it is apparent that children can acquire and understand new information if it is presented carefully, repeatedly and, perhaps most importantly, if it is the type of issue that is disucussed by those around the child. *Socioecological* approaches stress the way these influences can play a part in shaping children's understanding of the world, so that the family, school, hospital and the wider social context that the child experiences can all be seen as playing a part in what children know and understand about illness (and other matters). Similarly, the *alternative conceptions movement* predicts that children's understanding of health matters does not go through a series of universal stages, but that understanding and knowedge largely depend on the type of information and culture to which the child is exposed.

As adult conceptions of health, illness and death have changed radically over the years, one would also expect these changes to be reflected in children's knowledge and thinking. It is not so surprising then that Kendrick *et al.* (1986) found that 2 and 3-year-olds with cancer acquired a surprising amount of knowedge from overhearing conversations and through talking to other children. Similarly, Eiser (1993) gives an impressive example of a 3-year-old girl's understanding of her leukemia:

> I got leukemia. It just happens. I full of bad blood. Blood is red cells which make new blood; white cells which fight infection, and platelets which stop bleeding. Sometimes the platelets don't come and then you keep bleeding.

DISCUSSION POINT
In your experience, how much understanding do you think that children of different ages have about their illness and death? How could you assess a child's level of understanding without causing distress?

Summary

An important message from this literature is that one cannot assume that just because a child is of a certain age he or she will have a given level of understanding about illness, disease and death. Children acquire their understanding not only from what adults explain and tell them, but also from what they overhear, the salience of processes related to these matters in their lives and also from other children. Therefore, it is always necessary to check the nature of a child's understanding of these matters, as well as bearing in mind and working within the cultural assumptions of the family.

Family care for children with an illness

Communication between members of a family also impinges on the broader topic of the care of a child with an illness and the reaction of the family to this illness. Often it is claimed that open communication helps provide a sense of control and wellbeing. Recent research with adults suggests that psychological wellbeing can have important consequences for health, as in the case of prolonging the life of cancer patients and reducing the risk of a heart attack (see Chapter 15). Little is known about the direct medical benefits of psychological wellbeing in children, but it would be unlikely for them to unaffected by such variables. Furthermore, we saw in Chapter 18 that distress and anxiety in children increases the risk of later behavioural problems. Thus, the adequate care of children is not only desirable because of their vulnerability, but may also help their health and minimize any long-term psychological consequences.

What are the consequences of children being diagnosed as having chronic or life-threatening diseases for themselves and their family? It is important to recognize that any answer to this question will consist of generalizations based on fairly limited research evidence. However, this information does provide a useful background for health professionals. The initial parental reactions to the news about a child's condition is likely to consist of shock, grief, anxiety, denial, anger, adaptation and finally seeking help and managing day-to-day issues (see Chapters 20 and 21). Furthermore, it is useful to note that this grief reaction is similar to bereavement (see Chapter 17). However, it should be remembered that not all these reactions necessarily occur, and if they do, they may not occur in this order (Blacher, 1984).

Care, stress and coping

The family situation where there is a child with a severe illness fits the circumstances described as 'normal person, abnormal situation' (Russo and Varni, 1982). Armstong (1992) has argued that a prominent feature of such situations is that children often have painful experiences as a result of medical interventions which are outside their control and without obvious immediate benefits. Furthermore, the lack of escape from painful and aversive stimuli is likely to produce anxiety and avoidance. When avoidance behaviour occurs, such as crying and complaining, he supposes that this may be maintained by the rewards of parental attention. Similarly, providing treats and presents for these children can also be seen as providing a reward for behaviour which involves a lack of coping. Armstrong argues that this should not be interpreted as parents and child colluding to prevent treatment, but rather as patterns of behaviour which are appropriate in other circumstances. These are difficult issues and we still have an indaequate understanding of the psychological processes occurring in these situations; thus dogmatic advice about what should or should not be done needs to be treated with great caution. A more appropriate perspective is to recognize and be open to the problems that the families face in relation to medical procedures and the abnormality of the situation for the family.

How parents cope with a child who has a chronic or life-threatening illness is covered in Chapter 4 and Chapter 14 provides an overview of the issues of stress and coping. One finding from this literature is that the ability to cope may depend more on perceived demands and supports than on objective circumstances. This makes it less surprising that a number of studies which have revealed that mothers' beliefs about the severity of their child's medical condition are more predictive of their behaviour (e.g. own stress ratings) and children's emotional adjustment than the severity of the condition as identified by medical diagnosis (Appolone-Ford, Gibson and Driefuss, 1983; DeMaso et al., 1991).

A distinction is often made between the type of coping that involves dealing with the *environment* (e.g. discovering more about treatment and in this way developing stronger feelings of control; or taking a greater interest in medical procedures) and the type of coping that involves dealing with *emotions* (e.g. avoiding thinking about pain or trying to relax before a medical intervention, Eiser, 1993). Various terms and theoretical orientations are used to describe these processes (e.g. cognitive-appraisal,

Lazarus and Folkman, 1984; monitoring–blunting, Miller, 1980; primary–secondary control, Murphy and Moriarty, 1976). With increasing age there appears to be an increase in the use of coping strategies that involve emotions and thoughts and this may be associated with progress to formal operational thought in adolescence (Band, 1990; Worchel, Copeland and Barker, 1987; see Box 19.3). In addition, older children may be better able to adopt the coping strategies of others and they may be better at recognizing that emotions can be controlled (Compas, Worsham and Ey, 1992). One study of the coping strategies to deal with pain has been conducted by Gil *et al.* (1992) on sickle cell disease. Parents who used adopted positive coping strategies appeared to have beneficial effects, since their children adopted similar strategies. Further, children who adopted negative thinking and utilized passive adherence as a way of coping with pain tended to be less active and more distressed.

Although emotion-focused coping appears more developmentally advanced, there are various indications that it is not necessarily the best strategy. Children with diabetes who adopted an environment-focused approach appeared to have a higher health status and be better adjusted to their disease than those who used emotion- and thought-based strategies (Band, 1990); although the complications of other stresses which occur during adolescence were a confound in this association. In addition, it could simply be that the children with the less severe conditions adopt this approach.

The wider family and environment

Another feature of the family care of children with illnesses is that mothers and fathers tend to adopt different roles. Mothers are often involved in the physical care of the child, e.g. they take them to medical appointments and are involved in administering medicines (Nagy and Ungerer, 1990). Fathers often have been reported to be distant and uninvolved in the care process. However, they can play a crucial role in providing psychological support to mothers and may be more involved in the care of the other children in the family (Klein and Simmons, 1979; Nagy and Ungerer, 1990). This, of course, follows the stereotyped roles in our society, but clearly some families will function in different ways. Not surprisingly, mothers who are caring for a child who is chronically ill are more likely to have poor mental health (anxiety and depression) and poor physical health compared to mothers with healthy children (Cadman *et al.*, 1991; Wallander *et al.*, 1989).

There have also been suggestions that there are higher rates of divorce in families with ill children. However, in reviewing a range of investigations, Eiser (1993) points to the difficulty of obtaining a clear answer to this proposal. Furthermore, families can react in very different ways. Anecdotal evidence suggests that sometimes the presence of an ill child can provide the additional strain on a family which leads to the separation of the parents. In other cases, parents will report that the illness brought them closer together and has helped their relationship (see also Chapter 4 for a discussion of this issue).

The presence of a severely or chronically ill brother or sister will have effects on the other healthy children in a family. Healthy children are likely to receive less attention. They may be exposed to the worries and stresses of their parent(s), as well as worrying about what will happen to their sibling. In addition, they may have concerns about their own health (whether or not they will 'catch' the condition). Often, these children are not seen by health professionals or their needs are low on the list of priorities.

The problems of healthy siblings are reasonably well documented in studies using *parental* reports. These include emotional behaviour, attention-seeking, declining academic performance, social withdrawal and behavioural problems such as poor sleeping (Carpenter and Sahler, 1991; Lobato, 1990). Other studies have found higher rates of psychosomatic problems such as sleep disturbance, feeding problems, headaches and stomach aches (Powazek *et al.*, 1980). It is unclear whether these effects are due to modelling the behaviours seen, whether they are used as instrumental ways of obtaining attention or whether they are the response to stress. However, some caution must be exercised in relation to these findings. An extensive study of the children themselves by Cadman, Boyle and Offord (1988) revealed lower rates of difficulties and also that the problems were mainly confined to emotions (depression, anxiety, etc.) and poor relationships with peers. Similarly, Lobato *et al.* (1988) found that measures from the siblings revealed no difference between them and peers, but that mothers rated their ill child as more depressed and aggressive. There are also suggestions that the experiences associated with having an ill sibling can result in the development of positive qualities such as social skills, empathy and consideration (Ferrari, 1984; Horwitz and Kazak, 1990). In addition, the degree of communication about the illness in the family is related to the adjustment of the patient and siblings (Townes and Wold, 1977; Veldhuizen and Last, 1991).

In many cases parents do not give healthy siblings information about the medical problem of the ill child. This may be because parents do not want to distress the other children or because they find it difficult to discuss a painful topic. Menke (1987) interviewed parents and healthy siblings of an ill child who had a chronic or life-threatening disease. Over half the children were worried about their ill sibling, with the usual concerns being about the child's feelings, the use of medication and prognosis. Nearly three-quarters of the healthy children experienced problems because of the attention given to the ill child. However, the majority said they did not resent this. When the parents' and children's perceptions were compared it became apparent that parents tended to underestimate the worries of the healthy siblings about the ill child and they also lacked awareness of the concerns of the healthy siblings about their own health and academic success (see also Walker, 1988).

The culture of the health care that the family receives may also provide an important influence on coping and functioning (Mercer, 1994). Nor should it be forgotten that the health professionals will have their own psychological needs in relation to dealing with these families (see Chapters 1, 14 and 16). In addition, the reactions of friends and fellow pupils can be important to children with life-threatening diseases; in particular, adolescents complain of being avoided or 'babied' (Claflin and Barbarin, 1991).

Summary

Feelings of wellbeing and control are likely to be important to facilitate physiological reactions to illness and disease, as well as being important in terms of later development. There are suggestions that coping methods that focus on environmental rather than emotional dimensions may be more effective, although there is still uncertainty about this issue. Not surprisingly, the rest of the family are usually affected by the presence of an ill child. Typically, most of the physical burden of care falls on mothers and this seems to result in more health and psychological problems for them. In addition, there are indications that the healthy children of the family may be more susceptible to psychosomatic problems and that the problems of these children are often unrecognized.

Summary

The development of communication is an important intellectual achievement; problems in communication can alert health professionals to general cognitive delays. Effective communication with children requires an appreciation of different levels of ability, the need to make children feel secure and the appreciation of the role of non-verbal sources of information. When communicating with children, one cannot simply assume that because they are a certain age they will have predictable ideas about disease, illness and death. A number of studies report that understanding of these issues increases with age. However, there are also indications that in some circumstances children will be much more knowledgeable than others. The chronic or terminal illness of a child obviously affects the whole family. There are suggestions that the normal reactions to these abnormal circumstances may be one cause of difficulties in reactions to treatment and poor adjustment to illness.

Seminar questions

1. What general principles should be considered when trying to gain the cooperation of children in medical settings?
2. What is the most important practical consideration when trying to gain the cooperation of children in a medical setting? Can a single one be identified?
3. 'All children are different': Is this a useful principle or a cry of despair? Identify how health professionals should take account of this when dealing with children in relation to their duties.

Further reading

Douglas, J. (1993) *Psychology and Nursing Children.* Basingstoke: Macmillan/
  BPS. A comprehensive and easy-to-read introduction to the issues health
  professionals face when dealing with children.
Eiser, C. (1993) *Growing up with a Chronic Disease.* London: Jessica Kingsley.
  A useful and thoughtful review of this topic.
Messer, D.J. (1994) *The development of communication.* Chichester: Wiley.
  A thorough coverage of issues about early non-verbal and verbal
  communication.

References

Appolone-Ford, C., Gibson, P. and Driefuss, F. E. (1983) *Pediatrics: Epileptology,
  classification and management of seizures in the child.* Littleton, Mass.: PSG Publishing.
Armstrong, F.D. (1992) 'Psychosocial intervention in pediatric cancer: A strategy for
  prevention of long-term problems', in T. Field *et al. Stress and Coping in Infancy and
  Childhood.* Hillsdale, NJ: Lawrence Erlbaum.
Band, E. (1990) 'Children's coping with diabetes: Understanding the role of cognitive
  development', *Journal of Pediatric Psychology* **15**(1), 27–41.
Bibace, R. and Walsh, M.E. (1981) 'Children's conceptions of illness', in R. Bibace and
  M.E. Walsh (eds.) *New Directions for Child Development: No.14. Children's Conceptions
  of Health, Illness and Bodily Functions.* San Francisco: Jossey-Bass.
Blacher, J. (1984) 'Attachment and severely handicapped children', *Journal of
  Developmental and Behavioural Pediatrics* **5**, 178–83.
Brewster, A.B. (1982) 'Chronically ill hospitalized children's concepts of their illness',
  Pediatrics **69**, 355–62.
Cadman, D., Rosenbaum, P., Boyle, M. and Offord, D. (1991) 'Children with chronic
  illness: Family and parent demographic characteristics and psychosocial adjustment',
  Pediatrics **87**, 884–9.
Cadman, D., Boyle, M. and Offord, D. R. (1988) 'The Ontario Child Health Study: Social
  adjustment and mental health of siblings of children with chronic health problems',
  Journal of Development and Behavioural Pediatrics **9**, 117–21.
Carpenter, P.J. and Sahler, O.J.Z. (1991) 'Sibling perception and adaptation to childhood
  cancer: Conceptual and methodological considerations', in J.H. Johnson and S.B.
  Johnson (eds.) *Advances in Child Health Psychology.* Gainesville, Fla.: University of
  Florida Press.
Claflin, C. and Barbarin, O. (1991) 'Does "telling" less protect more? Relationships among
  age, information disclosure, and what children with cancer see and feel', *Journal of
  Pediatric Psychology* **16**, 169–91.
Compas B.E., Malcarne, V.L. and Fondacaro K.M. (1988) 'Coping with stressful events in
  older children and young adolescents', *Journal of Consulting and Clinical Psychology*
  56(3), 405–11.
Compas, B.E., Worsham, N.L. and Eye, S. (1992) 'Conceptual and developmental issues in
  children's coping with stress', in A.M. La Greca, L.J. Siegel, J.L. Wallander and C.E.
  Walker (eds.) *Stress and coping in child health.* New York: Guilford Press.

DeMaso, D.R., Campis, L.K., Wypij, D., Bertram, S., Lipshitz, M. and Freed, M. (1991) 'The impact of maternal perceptions and medical severity on the adjustment of children with congenital heart disease', *Journal of Pediatric Psychology* **16**, 137–50.

Donaldson, M. (1978) *Children's Minds*. Glasgow: Fontana.

Eiser, C. (1993) *Growing up with a Chronic Disease*. London: Jessica Kingsley.

Ferrari, M. (1984) 'Chronic illness: psychosocial effects on siblings. Chronically ill boys', *Journal of Child Psychology and Psychiatry* **25**, 459–76.

Flavell, J. H. (1963) *The Developmental Psychology of Jean Piaget.* Princeton, NJ: Van Nostrand.

Frodi, A. (1985) 'Variations in parental and nonparental response to early infant communication', in M. Reite and T. Field (eds.) *The Psychobiology of Attachment and Separation.* New York: Academic Press.

Gil, K., Williams, D., Thompson, R. and Kinney, T. (1992) 'Sick cell disease in children and adolescents', *Journal of Pediatric Psychology* **16**, 643–64.

Hobson, R.P. (1993) 'Perceiving attitudes, conceiving minds', in C. Lewis and P. Mitchell (eds.) *Origins of an Understanding of Mind*. Hillsdale, NJ: Lawrence Erlbaum.

Horwitz, W.A. and Kazak, A.E. (1990) 'Family adaptation to childhood cancer: Sibling and family system variables', *Journal of Clinical Child Psychology* **19**, 221–8.

Kane, B. (1979) 'Children's conceptions of death', *Journal of Genetic Psychology* **134**(1), 141–53.

Kendrick, C., Culling, J., Oakhill, T. and Mott, M. (1986) 'Children's understanding of their illness and its treatment within a paediatric oncology unit', *Association for Child Psychology and Psychiatry* (Newsletter) **8**, 16–20.

Kister, M.C. and Patterson, C.J. (1980) 'Children's conceptions of the causes of illness: Understanding of contagion and use of immanent justice', *Child Development* **51**, 839–46.

Klein, S. and Simmons, R. (1979) 'Chronic disease and childhood development: Kidney disease and transplantation', in R. Simmons (ed.) *Research in Community and Mental Health*, Vol. 1. Greenwich, Conn.: JAI Press.

Langford, W. F. (1948) 'Physical illness and convalescence: Their meaning to the child', *Pediatrics* **33**, 242–50.

Lazarus, R.S. and Folkman, S. (1984) *Stress, Appraisal and Coping*. New York: Springer.

Leslie, A.M. (1987) 'Pretence and representation: The origins of "Theory of Mind".' *Psychological Review* **94**, 412–26.

Lobato, D., Faust, D. and Spirito A. (1988) 'Examining the effects of chronic diseases and disability on children's sibling relationships', *Journal of Pediatric Psychology* **13**(3), 389–407.

Meltzoff, A. and Gopnik, A. (1993) 'The role of imitation in understanding persons and developing a theory of mind', in S. Baron-Cohen, H. Tager-Flusberg and D. Cohen (eds.) *Understanding Other Minds: Perspective from autism*. Oxford: Oxford University Press.

Menke, E.M. (1987) 'The impact of a child's illness on school-aged siblings', *Children's Health Care* **15**, 132–40.

Mercer, A. (1994) 'Psychological approaches to children with life-threatening conditions and their families', *Association of Child Psychology and Psychiatry Review and Newsletter* **16**, 56–63.

Messer, D. and Hasan, P. (1994) 'Early communication and cognition in children with Down's syndrome', *Down's Syndrome Research and Practice.*

Messer, D.J. (in press) 'Referential communication: Making sense of the social and physical worlds', in G. Bremner, G. Butterworth and A. Slater, *Advances in Infancy Research*. Hillsdale, NJ: Lawrence Erlbaum.

Miller, S. (1980) 'When is a little information a dangerous thing? Coping with stressful life events by monitoring vs blunting', in S. Levine and H. Ursin (eds.) *Coping and Health.* New York: Plenum Press.

Murphy, L.B. and Moriarty, A.E. (1976) *Vulnerability, Coping and Growth.* New Haven, Conn.: Yale University Press.

Nagy, S. and Ungerer, J. (1990) 'The adaptation of mothers and fathers to children with cystic fibrosis: A comparison', *Children's Health Care* **19**, 147–54.

Perner, J. (1991) *Understanding the Representational Mind.* Cambridge, Mass.: MIT Press.

Piaget, J. and Inhelder, B. (1956) *The Child's Conception of Space.* London: Routledge & Kegan Paul.

Powazek, M., Schijring, J., Goff, J.G., Paulson, M.A., and Stegner, S. (1980) 'Psychosocial ramifications of childhood leukemia: One year post diagnosis', in H. L. Schulman and M. J. Kupst (eds.) *The Child with Cancer.* Springfield, Ill.: Charles C. Thomas.

Rose, S.A. and Blank, M. (1974) 'The potency of context in children's cognition: An illustration through conservation', *Child Development* **45**, 499–502.

Russo, D.C. and Varni, J.W. (1982) 'Behavioral pediatrics', in D.C. Russo and J.W. Varni (eds.) *Behavioral Pediatrics: Research and practice.* New York: Plenum Press.

Stainton Rogers, W., Hevey, D. and Ash, E. (1989) *Child Abuse and Neglect: Failing the challenge.* Milton Keynes: Open University Press.

Townes, B.D. and Wold, D.A. (1977) 'Childhood leukemia', in E. Pattison (ed.) *The experience of dying.* Englewood Cliffs, NJ: Prentice Hall.

Trevarthen, C. (1982) 'The primary motives for cooperative understanding', in G. Butterworth and P. Light (eds.) *Social Cognition.* Hemel Hempstead: Harvester Wheatsheaf.

Veldhuizen, A.M. and Last, B. *Children with Cancer.* Amsterdam: Swets and Zeitlanger.

Walden, T.A. and Ogan, T.A. (1988) 'The development of social referencing', *Child Development* **59**, 1230–40.

Walker, C.L. (1988) 'Stress and coping in siblings of childhood cancer', *Nursing Research* **37**(4), 208–12.

Wallander, J.L., Varni, J.W., Babani, L., DeHeen, C.B., Wilcox, K.T. and Banis, H.T. (1989) 'The social environment and the adaptation of mothers of physically handicapped children', *Journal of Pediatric Psychology* **14**, 371–88.

Wasz-Hockert, O., Lind, J., Vuorenkoski, V., Partanen, T. and Valanne, E. (1968) 'The infant cry: A spectrographic and auditory analysis', *Clinics in Developmental Medicine* **29**.

Worchel, F., Copeland, D. and Barker, D. (1987) 'Control-related coping strategies in pediatric oncology patients', *Journal of Pediatric Psychology* **12**, 25–38.

CHAPTER 20

Health professionals and people with learning disabilities

JULIE DOCKRELL AND PAT HASAN

Chapter outline

Introduction

People with learning disabilities undergo the same life transitions as other people. But these life transitions are often accentuated because of the individual's learning difficulty. In this chapter the cognitive difficulties experienced by people with learning difficulties are described. The implications for special needs and additional support are outlined. The chapter concludes by highlighting key topics which are central to service provision in the 1990s.

The focus of this chapter is children and adults who are often described as 'mentally handicapped'. The term mental handicap is applied to a group of individuals who show a wide range of intellectual functioning and social skills. Recently, there has been an attempt to dispense with terms that have pejorative overtones, such as 'mentally retarded', 'mental handicap' and so forth, and to use the term

---

BOX 20.1   CHARLES' AND KATRINA'S LIFE OPPORTUNITIES

Charles

Charles is 4 years old. He was brought to the attention of the consultant paediatrician at the age of 18 months. At this point he was diagnosed as being developmentally delayed. Regular assessments have continued. His most recent assessment suggests that his cognitive and social skills are equivalent to those of a 2-year-old and his language and communication skills are further delayed. His IQ score is 55. Charles is not toilet-trained and he has difficulties in feeding himself. He shows no interest in books and when given a crayon manages a wild scribble. It has been recommended that he attend a developmental nursery.

Katrina

Katrina is 37 and lives at home with her parents in a small village. Katrina has Down's syndrome. As a child Katrina was slow to develop a range of skills. She did not walk until she was 4. She started using words about the same time and even now her communication skills are limited. Katrina is very happy in her village. All the residents know her. She goes out by herself and shops locally, provided there is help with the payments. Twice a week Katrina joins her friends at the local adult training centre some 25 miles away. She is particularily fond of one young man at the centre. She has no special friends in the village and much of her leisure time is spent with her parents or watching TV.

'learning disabled'. This is now, generally speaking, the accepted term in service provision and will be used in this chapter.

When individuals are diagnosed as having a learning disability this does not mean they all experience the same type or degree of problem. Nor is a learning disability an illness or a disease. Learning disabilities, however, may be caused by illness or disease, such as rubella. When individuals have a learning disability they have some difficulty in acquiring and using information. Learning disabilities are often distinguished by the level of their severity – mild, moderate or severe. This classification of the learning disability relates to a particular range of scores on an intelligence test. In addition, problems may be experienced with the demands of daily living.

Learning disabilities are usually identified for the first time in childhood as Charles' case illustrates (see Box 20.1). This slow potential for learning continues into adulthood and can have quite marked effects on life opportunities, as Katrina's case shows (see Box 20.1). Charles and Katrina have very different needs. Their needs are determined both by their intellectual limitations and their chronological age. In 1971, the United Nations adopted a declaration of rights, which stated:

> the mentally retarded person has the same basic rights as other citizens of the same country and the same age . . . each mentally retarded person has a right to such education, training, habilitation and guidance as will enable him (her) to develop his (her) ability and maximum potential.

The principles of normalization guide professionals in this task (O'Brien and Tyne, 1981; Wolfensberger, 1972). *Normalization* refers to the use of culturally valued activities and resources for enabling people to cope and behave in culturally valued and appropriate ways. The principle of normalization entails that we offer people with learning disabilities the same types of services and facilities that we ourselves would like and value; services that will encourage individuals to behave and respond in a socially appropriate fashion and services that reflect a typical community life. To do this effectively, it is important to understand the nature of the problems experienced by the individual with learning disabilities and how an individual's needs will change over the lifecycle.

In the following sections we shall consider:

- The nature of a learning disability.
- The contexts in which nurses may encounter people with learning disabilities throughout the lifespan.
- Some of the specific problems experienced by people with learning disabilities.

DISCUSSION POINT
List the range of contacts between health professionals and individuals with learning disabilities. What is the nature of the relationship in these contacts?

What are general learning disabilities?

Definition and IQ

The American Association on Mental Deficiency (AAMD) has provided a very influential definition of 'mental retardation' as 'significantly sub-average general intellectual functioning existing concurrently with deficits in adaptive behaviour, and manifested during the developmental period'. Sub-average general intellectual functioning is defined by a score on an intelligence test (see Box 20.2 for details of the notion of IQ). Individuals with an IQ score below 70 are classified as learning disabled. This does not mean that individuals with scores below 70 behave in a qualitatively different way from individuals above 70. Rather, it is a choice arrived at for statistical reasons. Until recently this was the common cut-off point in Britain to warrant education in special schools.

The two most popular classification schemes, the AAMD and DSM-IIIR, classify by IQ scores. However, there are limitations in placing too much emphasis on an IQ score. Intelligence test scores provide a measure of current intellectual functioning. These scores do not tell us which cognitive processes are affecting an individual's performance, nor do they address what adaptive problems may be experienced. In Britain, the actual allocation of a child with mild learning disabilities to special educational facilities depends as much on regional provision as it does on a child's performance on intelligence tests (Tomlinson, 1982). Moreover, IQ scores can change over time, although the extent of this change may not be as great as originally

---

BOX 20.2   IQ SCORES AND RELATED MEASURES

IQ is the standard abbreviation for intelligence quotient. It is a score derived from an individual's perfomance on a set of tests designed to measure intelligence.

What is measured?

The definition of intelligence continues to be a problem. There are many definitions of this construct and these differences are reflected in the ways tests are constructed. Each intelligence test contains different subtests which, summed together, give a score that is transformed into an intelligence quotient. It is possible to get the same overall score on an intelligence test either by being very good at some items and very poor at others or by scoring in the same range on all the items. For example, if there were 10 tests and a score of 5 out of 10 on all of the subtests, the average score would be 5. An average score of 5 would also be achieved if the subject scored 9 on five tests and 1 on five tests. Carefully designed tests of intelligence take these issues into account in the way the final score is derived.

How the score is derived

The IQ is a standard score with a mean of 100 and a standard deviation of 16. The normal distribution curve can be used to interpret scores thoughout the scale. An IQ score of 116 is one standard deviation above the mean and an IQ score of 70 is two standard deviations below the mean. This cut-off point, 2 standard deviations below the mean, marks the point for learning disabled in many classification systems and is a statistical rather than functional criterion.

Mental ages (MA)

Mental ages provide the age equivalent for a subjects score. Before IQs were in usage this was the common measure in assessing an individual's performance on intelligence tests. An 8-year-old performing with an MA of 4 is thought to be performing at the same level generally as a child who is 4 years of age. The caveat 'generally' is important. Since these scores are made up by the child's result on a series of tests there is no reason to assume that the pattern of results will be the same across the age levels. Many factors will need to be taken into account in interpreting MA scores.

---

assumed (Moffitt *et al.*, 1993). For practitioners, the critical aspect is whether the score says anything important about behaviour and the individual's needs.

The observation that many academically disadvantaged individuals functioned adequately in society after their school years led clinicians in the 1960s to redefine 'retardation' to include social and practical as well as academic disabilities. Thus, learning disabilities are viewed as both a significant impairment in the ability to learn *and* to adapt to the demands of society (President's Committee on Mental Retardation, 1973).

There is considerable debate about what makes up adaptive behaviour (see Coulter and Morrow, 1978) and whether it is a valid concept. In effect, adaptive behaviour is rarely used as a criterion by researchers for identification of groups or in the diagnostic process by clinicians. This is partly a result of the uncertainty surrounding the reliability and validity (see Chapter 7) of tests of adaptive behaviour. However, it can play a central role in considering the likelihood of successful placements for people with learning disabilities or integration into mainstream schools for children with learning disabilities. For example, it is more important to know whether an individual can maintain her or himself in the community and abide by socially acceptable standards of behaviour than it is to know her or his IQ score. IQ does not provide the descriptive information necessary for decisions about appropriate support in the community.

Prevalence, aetiology and classification

Determining the number of people with a learning disability is very difficult (Mittler, 1979). Prevalence studies need to consider the population at large, not simply children and adults in special centres or hospitals. For example, some people never come to the attention of the services until their carer dies and statutory services become involved.

Several studies have used standardized assessment devices and considered the child population at large (e.g. Drillien *et al.*, 1966; Rutter, Tizard and Whitmore, 1970). The general population estimate of children with IQs below 70 is between 2 per cent and 2.5 per cent. It has been estimated that half show a severe language deficiency, disorders in speaking (articulation) or a combination of the two (Enderby and Davies, 1989; Rutter, Tizard and Whitmore, 1970).

While there is a consensus about which individuals are experiencing severe learning disabilities, the situation with respect to milder problems is not always clear cut (Gillham, 1986; Mittler, 1979). The National Child Development Study (Kellmer-Pringle *et al.*, 1966) found that at the age of 7 years, 0.4 per cent of the children in the survey were attending special schools; 5 per cent were receiving help in the ordinary classroom because of educational or 'mental' backwardness; while there were a further 8 per cent who, their teachers considered, would benefit from some help. The Warnock Report (Warnock, 1978) suggests that children who have 'limited ability' and children who are 'retarded' by other conditions would amount to approximately 10 per cent of the school population. This figure excluded those with severe learning problems. Thus, the range of children who might be included in such a category is broad and harder to define than a criterion based on IQ would suggest.

A distinction is frequently drawn between those individuals whose difficulties are of organic origin and those whose difficulties are of unknown aetiology. Over the last thirty years advances in biomedical research have greatly increased our ability to identify some causes of general learning disabilities. Grossman (1983) notes that there are now 200 identified causes of 'mental retardation'. For those individuals experiencing *severe* learning disabilities (IQ of approximately less than 50) aetiological causes can be identified in 85–90 per cent of the cases (Fryers, 1984). Organic insults are generally of three kinds: those occurring before birth such as genetic abnormalities or problems *in utero*; those occurring at the time of birth, such as anoxia; those occurring postnatally, such as childhood encephalitis.

By contrast, for those individuals experiencing *mild* or *moderate* learning disabilities aetiological implications are less clear. For many individuals who are diagnosed as 'mentally retarded' there are no obvious organic aetiologies. IQ levels of this group tend to fall in the moderate to mild range (50–70). Zigler and Hodapp (1986) estimated that only 45 per cent were of unknown aetiology. This figure is continually changing due to advances in identification procedures and the increased numbers of infants being kept alive despite serious CNS (central nervous system) damage.

People who show no evidence of organic brain dysfunction are referred to by the AAMD as suffering from 'retardation' due to psychosocial disadvantage. The older and more widely used description is cultural-familial disadvantage. This description reflects the combination of environmental and genetic factors which might account for individuals who had no definite organic pathology (Zigler, 1969). Thus, the mild level of learning difficulty (IQ in the range 50–70) is viewed primarily as academic dysfunction or a deficiency in learning ability with aetiology unknown, while severe learning difficulty (IQ below 50) is often viewed as a physiologically caused handicap.

Deciding whether an individual is experiencing a learning disability is not always straightforward. The more severe problems are easy to identify and this generally occurs in the first year of life. However, the diagnosis of milder problem is much more complex and depends on the community where the individual lives and the demands that exist in that specific context. Generally diagnosis happens in the preschool years or at school. However, some individuals remain undetected until adulthood, possibly until they come into contact under the purview of the criminal justice system (see Dockrell *et al.*, 1993). For example, John was arrested by the police for trying to set fire to a building. He was 17 years of age and had spent much of his last years at school absconding. In primary school he had experienced great difficulty learning to read and his reading age was 7 years 6 months; he could barely write. He was unemployed and living at home with an elderly mother, who looked after his daily needs. Psychological assessment indicated that John had a mild learning difficulty and was in need of support to lead his life in the community.

Nurses and learning disabilities over the lifespan

Nurses may become involved with individuals with learning disabilities and their families and carers in many different situations and about many different issues:

- pre-natal screening and early injury,
- family reactions to learning disability,

- school children,
- issues of sexuality,
- care in the community,
- challenging behaviour,
- ageing with a learning disability.

Pre-natal screening and early injury

An area of particular relevance to nurses, where the issue of potential learning disabilities is raised, is that of pre-natal screening. In this context the focus is on detection and possible prevention of some better-known examples of learning disabilities caused by organic problems. For example, Down's syndrome is the result of a genetic abnormality caused by abnormal division of the 21st chromosome pair. It causes learning disabilities which range from mild to severe.

Nurses and particularly midwives are likely to be involved in pre-natal screening procedures such as amniocentesis, which is carried out by a doctor at approximately 15–16 weeks' gestation. Chorionic villus sampling, carried out even earlier to detect Down's syndrome and other abnormalities in the developing foetus, involves the nurse practitioner too. An additional role for the nurse may be to counsel parents both before and after these sensitive clinical procedures. Pre-natal screening also can detect certain maternal diseases which, if transmitted to the foetus *in utero*, could result in learning disabilities. Specific examples include rubella, alcoholism (which may cause foetal alcohol syndrome) and, more rarely nowadays, syphilis. Even severe malnutrition in the mother during pregnancy may affect the infant's learning potential.

Preventive screening procedures are also used with neonates. An important example relates to the detection of phenylketonuria (PKU), a metabolic disorder which makes the infant unable to digest many varieties of food, including milk products. If this is not detected and the infant placed on a special diet, severe learning disabilities are likely to develop. An important preventive measure is the Guthrie test, which involves taking a sample of blood from a pinprick in the infant's heel. This test is carried out by the midwife approximately five days after birth.

It is important to realize that learning disabilities may result from causes associated with the labour and delivery process itself. Trauma associated with the birth of the infant may cause damage to certain areas of the brain. Anoxia or prolonged deprivation of the oxygen supply is particularly dangerous. The degree of severity will obviously depend to a certain extent on the nature of the trauma.

Family reactions to learning disability

Again, nurses and midwives may find themselves involved at the time when parents are first told that their child has a learning disability. This may happen shortly after birth or perhaps sometime later, when the diagnosis is more certain. Richard and Reed (1991) state: 'the way in which parents are told of their children's condition affects the way they adjust to the situation, the way they treat the child and their attitudes to future service provision.' One line of research has focused on parents' psychological responses to information of such an emotive and sensitive nature. MacKeith (1973) suggests that a complex set of 'feelings' are invoked, which may include almost instinctive 'biological' reactions such as the desire to protect the helpless infant, or conversely, a revulsion at the 'abnormal' aspect of the birth. In addition, in terms of reproduction and childbearing, the parents may feel that they have failed and are inadequate as a result of their apparent inability to produce a perfect child. This may mean that they view the situation as the 'loss' of the perfect baby which they had hoped for; consequently psychological processes normally associated with loss and bereavement become relevant in this context (see Chapter 4). Most research uses models which describe various stages of adaptation by which parents come to terms with the child's disability, e.g. denial, anger, depression, acceptance. There seems to be a consensus in the literature that a stage-like model such as this is the most efficient way of conceptualizing parental responses and most researchers provide some variation on this basic theme with models which vary from three to five stages (Drotar *et al.*, 1975; Mattson, 1972; Richmond, 1973). The fact that there may be a 'denial' stage when the news is first broken explains in part why parents often need to be told the same information on several occasions before it really 'sinks in'. While they are busy 'denying' that the situation is really happening to them and their child, they are unable to process and internalize the information efficiently. However, it is possible that parental reactions may not always develop through such rigidly defined stages and particularly not within clearly defineable time constraints. Gath (1978), for example, found that 90 per cent of parents of children with Down's syndrome were still grieving over the birth of their child six years later.

Maxwell (1993) describes some of the problems related to adjusting to life with a child with a learning disability. From the perspective of both a parent of a child with Down's syndrome and a nurse, she highlights the sense of loss and also the needs of the parents. She notes that it is not surprising that parents refuse services if they feel badly treated by professionals.

Any one of the psychological responses mentioned above is likely to result in particular behavioural outcomes which will affect the parents' relationship with their child, e.g. acceptance, overprotection, overpressure or rejection, of which the first two are the most common (Bowley, 1967; Sheridan, 1965). In any event, the consequences of feelings such as guilt, self-blame and anxiety are almost certain to disturb the normal pattern of mother–infant interaction in particular (Bentovim, 1972).

Some research has addressed the issue of which factors might mediate the nature and intensity of the parental reaction and the subsequent degree of adaptation. Goddard and Rubissow (1977) suggest that parental shock is greater and recovery slower when the affected child is their firstborn. Steinhauer, Mushin and Rae-Grant

(1974) suggest that a variety of factors, including prognosis, affect parental adaptation. This finding presents additional problems because in many cases of learning disability a precise and accurate prediction of the child's potential cognitive and adaptive functioning cannot be made at birth. For example, children with Down's syndrome appear to be a fairly homogeneous group in terms of organic aetiology, but there are considerable individual differences between them in the level of functioning which they achieve. Therefore, although parents seek reassurance or at least demand the 'truth', a realistic assessment of prognosis often cannot be made at the same time as the initial information concerning the child's learning disability is conveyed to them.

School children

The recognition that special educational provision needs to be made for children with learning disabilities is of comparative recent origin (Pritchard, 1963). Before the middle of the nineteenth century, so called 'mentally defective' children requiring custodial care were placed in workhouses or infirmaries. The first special educational provision was introduced at the end of the nineteenth century, but the emphasis was on occupational activities rather than formal education. This idea was carried forward into the late twentieth century under the rubric of Adult Training Centres (ATCs).

The Royal Commission (1889) drew attention to the needs of 'mentally handicapped children' and distinguished between 'feeble-minded', 'imbeciles' and 'idiots'. The Royal Commission decided that these terms referred to 'mental handicaps' of different severity but the distinction was one of degree, not of kind. There was considerable dispute among the committee about whether the distinction should be drawn on medical or educational grounds (Pritchard, 1963). The decision was that a doctor should select children for special education. To this day, a doctor's report is still required to complete a Statement of Special Educational Needs.

A Statement of Special Educational Needs (in Scotland, The Record of Needs) is a formal document which specifies the educational provision required to meet a child's needs (see Stow and Selfe, 1989). The concept of educational need has superseded earlier categorization schemes based on IQ or type of school attended, i.e. remedial, special or mainstream. Integration with non-disabled peers is seen as an important element of special provision, but provision covers the full range from children who are supported in ordinary classrooms, various part-time arrangements between special and ordinary schools or full-time segregated facilities where a child's needs cannot be met in mainstream school.

Although the general aim has been to avoid categorization, the terms *mild*, *moderate* and *severe* are used to refer to the child's teaching and curricular requirements. Children with severe learning difficulties are defined as those who require a developmental curriculum, covering a range of educational experience but more selectively and sharply focused on the development of personal autonomy and social skills. Children with moderate learning difficulties are defined as those who need a modified curriculum similar to that provided in ordinary schools but with modified objectives. Children with mild learning difficulties should cope with the normal curriculum and most are likely to manage with normal support in the ordinary classroom.

Issues of sexuality

The move from childhood to adulthood places a range of new demands on young people with learning disabilities. Having left full-time education, many young people with learning disabilities depend for their daily activities on segregated facilities such as day centres and for their social lives on their parents (Aull, Davies and Jenkins, 1993). In general, these young people's lives are much more uniform than would be expected from their non-disabled peers.

Adolescence brings changes in physical maturity. The vast majority of young people will develop secondary sex characteristics and will need help in understanding these changes. More individuals with learning disabilities are living in the community, marrying and raising children (Dowdney and Skuse, 1993). Education, counselling and support are needed to help develop personally satisfying and socially acceptable relationships. Relevant issues concerning the sexuality of adolescents are of central concern.

One of the major problems facing young people with learning disabilities is having to come to terms with their growing awareness of their sexuality. As a result of their cognitive skills people with learning disabilities are often regarded as perpetual children, and therefore any expression of sexuality is seen as inappropriate. It often appears that family and professional carers collude to protect these young adults from the normal expression of sexual feelings and behaviour (Fairbrother, 1983). However, as Craft and Craft (1985) note: 'Sexual ignorance is not bliss: it opens people to damaging and exploitative situations.'

A particular area of concern for nurses is in relation to contraceptive needs. Occasionally individuals have been subjected to sterilization at the request of their carers, apparently without the informed consent of the individual concerned.

DISCUSSION POINTS

In what ways does the issue of 'informed consent' raise issues about the nature of the learning disability itself? Who decides whether an individual is incapable of giving informed consent? What criteria should be used in making that decision? Who has the right to make a decision on behalf of an individual who cannot give informed consent?

At present the usual requirement is for the surgeon to be satisfied that the patient understands what is involved in the procedure and what is known about the consequences of the intervention. This should occur for all medical interventions experienced by people with learning disabilities. The only exception to this ruling is when the patient is a minor. There may, of course, be situations when sterilization is the preferred course of action (after MacLean, 1979), but this should only be considered in the light of the individual's needs and appropriate counselling. Some of the issues you should consider if asked to counsel a person with learning disabilities about birth control are the following:

1. Do they understand the procedures for using birth control and the various advantages and disadvantages of the chosen method?
2. Do they want children?
3. The age of the woman.
4. The cause of the learning disability, particularly whether there is an associated genetic component.
5. Will the individual be able to meet a child's emotional and physical needs?
6. What do they feel are the advantages and disadvantages of parenthood?
7. How financially independent are the parents of the child likely to be?

Care in the community

Since the early 1970s there have been major changes in services for people with learning disabilities. In many countries the large institutions that have traditionally provided living accommodation for people with learning disabilities have been replaced by the provision of residential accommodation within the community, with access to the facilities and resources offered in local areas. Korman and Glennester (1990) studied the closure of one large institution in the south of England. Their results are, on the whole, positive. All clients moved to accommodation that was of a much higher standard, following traditional domestic arrangements which provide a degree of privacy. Residents gained in other ways. A greater respect was shown to them by the care staff. Moreover, staff were more aware of the residents' rights to be involved in decisions about their lives. However, a great deal more was required for residents to reach their potential.

The White Paper on Community Care (1989) establishes the right of people with learning disabilities to normal patterns of life within the community. Service users are to be treated as individuals. Both the exercise of choice and the importance of supporting users to achieve the maximum possible degree of independence is emphasized.

The social system through which resources and personal support are made available to people with learning disabilities is diffuse and complex. At least three levels of provision are involved:

1. Formal, through statutory agencies like social work.
2. Informal, through churches, lunch centres, etc.
3. Benefits, financial aid through care allowances.

The relationships between these levels causes serious gaps in service provision. Comprehensive, community-based services are still in their infancy. They will need to be carefully supported if individuals are to lead as full a life as possible. There are two groups of residents where particular problems exist in providing adequate resources and support: those with challenging behaviour and those who are elderly.

Challenging behaviour

Challenging behaviour is the term that has come to replace the 'behaviour problem' category. There were sound ideological reasons for this change in terms. Effectively, the problem is shifted from the individual to the service providers. A widely accepted definition is to be found in the King's Fund Report, *Facing the Challenge* (1987):

> severely challenging behaviour refers to behaviour of such intensity, frequency or duration that the physical safety of the person or others is likely to be placed in serious jeopardy, or behaviour which is likely to seriously limit or delay access to and frequent use of ordinary community facilities.

Estimates of the prevalence rates of difficult and disruptive behaviours vary considerably. Some authors suggest that in the United Kingdom 10–15 people with learning disability per 100,000 of the population present a serious challenge to services (Kiernan, 1987; Lewis *et al.* in Emerson *et al.*, 1987) while others estimate rates of 31 per 100,000 (Kushlick, Blunden and Cox, 1973). Harris and Russell (1989) found evidence of 45.5 per 100,000 displaying aggressive behaviour in their district health authority survey. Problems of definition and a reliance on the records of service agencies have made accurate estimates difficult to establish. There is some evidence that the term 'challenging behaviour' covers two quite different categories of behaviour: 'problem' and 'dangerous' behaviours. Problem behaviours tend to be experienced frequently but pose few serious difficulties (e.g. verbal abuse, pestering others). Dangerous behaviours are qualitatively different, serious, infrequent, and fit into the first clause of the definition (e.g. arson, physical violence). These behaviours pose serious difficulties but are relatively infrequent. Many such dangerous behaviours come within the purview of the criminal justice system and, as such, reflect a societal and consensual definition of the unacceptable. Problem behaviours, those that may limit the 'use of community facilities' are generally manageable within the local services. Dangerous behaviours, sometimes, are outside the range of experience and skills of a local facility. It is for these behaviours that specialist inputs may be necessary (see Gaskell, Dockrell and Rehman, in press).

Ageing with a learning disability

Better provision means that more individuals are surviving into old age. This raises concerns for families, especially for parents where a child might survive them, and

Table 20.1   *Behavioral Characteristics of Learning Disabled People Throughout the Life Span*

Type	Characteristics from birth to adulthood		
	Birth through Five	*Six through Twenty*	*Twenty-one and Over*
Mild (IQ 53–69)	Often not noticed as delayed by casual observer but is slower to walk, feed him- or herself, and talk than most children.	Can acquire practical skills and master reading and arithmetic to a third- to sixth-grade level with special education. Can be guided toward social conformity.	Can usually achieve adequate social, vocational and self-maintenance skills, may need occasional guidance and support when under unusual social or economic stress.
Moderate (36–52)	Noticeable delays in motor development, especially in speech; responds to training in various self-help activities.	Can learn simple communication, elementary health and safety habits, and simple manual skills; does not progress in functional reading in arithmetic.	Can perform simple tasks under sheltered conditions; participate in simple recreation; can travel alone in familiar places; usually incapable of self-maintenance.
Severe (20–35)	Marked delay in motor development; little or no communication skill; may respond to training in elementary self-help, such as self-feeding.	Usually walks, barring specific disability; has some understanding of speech and some response; can profit from systematic habit training.	Can conform to daily routines and repetitive activities; needs continuing direction and supervision in protective environment.
Profound (below 20)	Gross disability; minimal capacity for functioning in sensorimotor areas; needs nursing care.	Obvious delays in all areas of development; shows basic emotional responses; may respond to skilful training in use of legs, hands, and jaws; needs close supervision.	May walk, need nursing care, have primitive speech, usually benefits from regular physical activity; incapable of self-maintenance.

also for social and medical services. As yet, we have very little knowledge about the needs of older people who have a learning disability. Their needs will have to be addressed both in the community and in sheltered and residential accommodation (see also Chapters 22–25).

In fact, the fastest growing group of people with a learning disability is the elderly. They have been described as having a double jeopardy: age and learning disability. Anderson (1988) noted that the trend towards an increasingly aged population of individuals with learning disabilities is expected to continue well into the future and will have a marked impact on the models of residential care and support services provided.

There are very few studies of this population, perhaps surprisingly, because there are special problems for people ageing with a learning disability. Older people with learning disabilities have higher mortality rates than their age-matched contemporaries. Suggestive data indicate that there is an increased likelihood of decreased motor functioning, mobility and daily living skills in this population, as well as hearing loss (Cooke, 1988) and fractures (Jancar, 1989).

Much of the data reflects the patterns of ageing and the needs of a population that spent the majority if not all of their lives in an institutional setting. More information is required to address the needs of individuals who live in the community using mainstream services. Nursing services and nursing homes for older people will need to widen their range of skills and expertise to cope with these needs. In addition, preparing the individual for some of the changes of the later years will demand special skills.

It should be clear from this review that a nurse's career will lead to contact with people with learning disabilities. This may occur at any stage of the lifespan, from birth to old age. The consequences of the disability and the individual's needs will change according to their age (see Table 20.1). For nurses to work effectively they need to understand both the criteria for diagnosing a learning disability and the social and cognitive consequences of such a diagnosis.

Specific disabilities experienced

One of the defining characteristics of people with learning difficulties is intellectual impairment. Yet there is still much uncertainty about the nature of the specific skill deficits that accompany leaning dificulties. In the past, many practitioners have found theoretical models to be inappropriate as they were not easily translated into practice and often emphasized unmodifiable aspects of cognition. Contemporary models are more relevant to practitioners because they emphasize aspects of information-processing that can be modified through instruction.

Cognitive skills

Intelligence tests can serve as a useful screening device, but they do not tell us about the nature of the cognitive problems. Nor can they offer direct predictions of what sorts of other difficulty may exist (e.g. in language). The relationship between cognition and language is unclear. For an individual to use symbols to communicate that individual must possess a certain level of cognitive functioning (Owens, 1989), but there is only a moderate relation between language and intelligence (Bellugi *et al.*, 1988; Clark and Clark, 1974).

Researchers have attempted to clarify the types of difficulty experienced by examining the ways in which individuals process information (Weiss, Weisz and Bromfield, 1986). Persistent problems have been identified in several different cognitive areas, including speed of information processing, memory and strategic behaviour (for a review see Dockrell and McShane, 1993). There are marked difficulties in identifying and maintaining attention to the relevant stimulus dimensions (Owens, 1989). These problems have direct implications for assessing learning disabilities and language skills in particular (Kahmi and Masterton, 1989) and for designing intervention programmes. At the most basic level it must be established that the individual with learning disabilities is actually focusing on the relevant task dimensions.

In addition, there has been extensive work on memory (Campione, Brown and Ferrara, 1982), which shows that individuals with learning disabilities fail to employ strategies that help in learning new material (see Chapter 8). Individuals can be taught to employ strategies and are most likely to generalize a new strategy if they understand the reasons for its use. Such problems of generalization can have important implications for interventions. For example, if an individual is taught the meaning of a word in one situation, it may need to be relearnt and reinforced each time it occurs in a different context. This could be very important for successful adaptation.

While memory performance can be improved by training, some difficulties may remain and there is some indication that the speed at which information is retrieved from memory is a limiting factor in general cognitive performance (Kail, 1990). Most findings concern individuals experiencing mild learning disabilities; the evidence suggests that extrapolating from the findings to individuals with severe learning disabilities may be inappropriate (Broman et al., 1987). None the less these problems highlight the complexities of cognition and the need to be clear about which skills are being tapped in any specific situation.

To date, more similarities than differences have appeared when children with general learning disabilities have been compared with normal children on cognitive tasks. General reviews of the relevant research conclude that children categorized as 'cultural-familial' have similar cognitive structures to their normally developing peers whereas organically retarded children do not (Weiss, Weisz and Bromfield, 1986; Weisz, Yeates and Zigler, 1982). Such conclusions are still contentious. Children with mild, moderate and severe learning disabilities are a heterogeneous group.

Given the range of difficulties that may be experienced, it is important to be sensitive to the different ways these problems may manifest themselves. Specifically they may:

- have difficulty remembering new information,
- find it difficult to generalize what has been learned to new situations,
- have great difficulty in understanding complex or abstract ideas,
- may finish jobs more slowly or not complete tasks.

Communication skills

That people with learning disabilities, in general, have distinct problems with language has been recognized for some time. Studies of the development of language and language-related skills in association with learning disabilities has highlighted the need for careful examination of both the individual and the various components of the linguistic system. In general, the more severe the level of cognitive impairment the more likely it is that the individual will experience problems in the expression and comprehension of language. There is evidence that language development does not proceed in a uniform fashion. So, for example, some individuals may have specific problems with the grammar of the language and others with language as a communicative tool; that is, the pragmatic factors. There are also indications that parents may use functionally different language with a child with disabilities and are less likely to follow the child's initiative. This latter point highlights the need to consider environmental mediators and the communicative potential in the environment when working with individuals who have learning disabilities. Enough is now known to suggest that language does not develop merely by providing a stimulating, enriched environment.

It is very important that assessment procedures focus on individuals, with the awareness that unexpected patterns of development may occur. For example, language development can still occur after puberty in some individuals (Rondal, 1987). Recent studies show a high incidence of speech problems in children with learning disabilities. In particular, the severity of the learning difficulty and the high level of hearing problems increase the incidence of speech problems. It is essential when talking to individuals with learning disabilities that one's language is understandable but not patronizing.

Down's syndrome children have been studied in great detail and experience specific difficulties with language. Their linguistic impairments appear to be most evident in the grammatical as opposed to the single word (lexical) or pragmatic aspects of language (Beeghly and Cicchetti, 1987). Their problems become particularly acute as language becomes more complex. Great difficulties are often experienced in constructing questions and understanding sentences which contain a number of elements.

Some individuals will not acquire language or develop functional speech. In such cases the aim of developing communication skills to a level adequate to meet communicative needs will be dominant. It is inaccurate to assume that the individual with severe learning disabilities has nothing to communicate. There are a range of systems that can be used in such circumstances. A sign language like Makaton (derived from British Sign Language) can be particularly helpful, but various techniques which rely on the use of concrete aids can also support communication (e.g. Bliss symbolics).

Social skills

As more and more individuals with learning disabilities strive to live independent lives in the community, an added emphasis has been placed on social skills.

Inappropriate responses or lack of social responsiveness can lead to social isolation. To some extent this has been tackled by the development of specialized social skills training packages. The role of monitoring such training programmes and liaising with the relevant institutions will sometimes fall to the community nurse. When considering an individual's social skills it is important to analyze the skill components. Skills required for personal competence will not necessarily be the skills required for community competence. An example will serve to illustrate this point:

> Paul is 21 years old and has a mild learning disability. He was having difficulties with his personal relationships with young women and with this need in mind, a psychologist taught Paul the skills needed for asking someone out. These included being friendly, paying compliments and discussing interests. These sessions culminated in Paul learning the appropriate words to use to suggest an evening meeting. Following the sessions with the psychologist Paul was very satisfied and felt he had learnt a lot. Shortly after this Paul caused some upset at church. Apparently he saw a young lady he was attracted to there and approached her. Everything he learnt was put into practice in a few minutes, even though he had never met her before. Paul was very upset by the young woman's response. He had, after all, done everything he was taught.

The issue of communication is also important in relation to legal processes. Individuals living in the community may come into contact with the police, either as a suspect or as a victim of crime. One question which needs to be considered is how reliable their reports of a particular incident will be. Preliminary evidence suggests that recall is poorer among groups of individuals with learning disabilities (Clare and Gudjonsson, 1993). Moreover, people with learning disabilities are more susceptible to leading questions and more acquiescent in their responses. People with learning disabilities are more vulnerable than average ability peers. It becomes particularly important when questioning an individual in such situations that the use of all facilities to support an accurate reporting of an incident be made.

Summary

In this chapter, the transition points in the lives of individuals with a learning disability have been outlined. Nurses will encounter these individuals in many different contexts. Individuals with learning difficulties vary in their intellectual skills and communicative skills. Above all they are individuals with individual needs. If the cognitive and communication limitations are adequately understood, it will be possible to provide appropriate services, both specialized and generic. Nurses may play a central role in coordinating some of these services.

Seminar questions

1. What features characterize a learning disability?
2. How would you counsel an individual with learning disabilities about birth control?
3. How would you involve individuals with learning disabilities in identifying their service needs and evaluating service provision?

Further reading

Jahoda, A. and Cattermole, M. (in press) 'Leaving home: A real choice for people with learning disabilities', in G. Wilson (ed.) *Community Care: Asking the user.* London: Chapman & Hall. This chapter explores the fears and beliefs of a group of individuals who are leaving hospital to live in the community for the first time. The authors provide a clear picture of the issues that cause concern for the participants and their fears for the future.

Mittler, P. (1979) *People not Patients: Problems and policies in mental handicap.* London: Methuen. The emphasis of this book is on how we can help people with learning disabilities. It covers the lifespan, from childhood to adulthood, examining at each stage critical factors in the life of the handicapped person.

Towell, D. (1988) *An Ordinary life in Practice: Developing comprehensive community-based services for people with learning disabilities.* London: King's Fund Publishing Office. This book brings together the experiences of a range of practitioners involved with people who have learning disabilities. There is a general commitment to three fundamental principles – 1. People with learning disabilities have the same human value as anyone else and the same human rights; 2. Living like others within the community is both a right and a need; 3. Services must recognize the individuality of people with learning disabilities. Within this framework the various chapters cover issues ranging from designing high quality services to the mechanisms needed for achieving large-scale change.

Zigler, E. and Hodapp, R.M. (1986) *Understanding Mental Retardation.* New York: Cambridge University Press. This book provides a clear, up-to-date discussion of the field of 'mental retardation'. There is a historical analysis as well as a discussion of mechanisms responsible for the learning difficulties. Readers are provided with a context to understand the changes in philosophy and provision that have occurred in recent years.

References

Anderson, D. (1988) 'Elderly mentally retarded persons: Policy issues and trends'. Paper presented at VIIIth Congress of IASSMD, Dublin.

Aull, C., Davies, C. and Jenkins, R. (1993) 'Young people with learning difficulties: The transition to adulthood', *Social Care Research Findings* **35**.

Beeghly, M. and Cicchetti, D. (1987) 'An organisational approach to symbolic development in children with Down syndrome', in D. Cicchetti and M. Beeghly (eds.) *Symbolic Development in Atypical Children: New directions for child development.* San Francisco: Jossey-Bass.

Bellugi, U., van Hoek, K. Lillo-Martin, D. and O'Grady, L. (1988) 'Disassociation between language and cognitive functions in Williams syndrome', in D. Bishop and K. Mogford (eds.) *Language Development in Exceptional Circumstances.* Edinburgh: Churchill Livingstone.

Bentovim, A. (1972) 'Handicapped pre-school children and their families: Effects on child's early emotional development', *British Medical Journal* **3**, 634–7.

Bowley, A. (1967) 'A follow-up study of 64 children with cerebral palsy', *Development Medicine and Child Neurology* **9**, 172–82.

Broman, S., Nichols, P., Shaughnessy, P. and Kennedy, W. (1987) *Retardation in Young Children.* Hillsdale, NJ: Lawrence Erlbaum.

Campione, J. C., Brown, A. L. and Ferrara, R. A. (1982) 'Mental retardation and intelligence', in R.J. Sternberg (ed.) *Handbook of Human Intelligence.* Cambridge: Cambridge University Press.

Clare, I.C.H. and Gudjonsson, G.H. (1993) 'Interrogative suggestibility, confabulation and acquiescence in people with mild learning disabilities (mental handicap): Implications for reliability during police interrogations', *British Journal of Clinical Psychology* **32**, 295–301.

Clark, A.M., and Clarke, A.D.B. (1974) *Mental Deficiency: The changing outlook*, 3rd edition. London: Methuen.

Cooke, L. (1988) 'Hearing loss in the mentally handicapped: A study of its prevalence and association with ageing', *British Journal of Mental Subnormality* **34**, 112–6.

Coulter, W.A. and Morrow, H.W. (eds) (1978) *Adaptive Behavior: Concepts and measurement.* New York: Grune & Stratton.

Craft, A. and Craft, M. (1985) 'Sexuality and personal relationships', in M. Craft, J. Bicknell and S. Hollins (eds.) *Mental Handicap: A multidisciplinary approach.* London: Baillière Tindall.

Department of Health (1989) *Caring for People: Community Care in the Next Decade and Beyond.* London: HMSO.

Dockrell, J.E., Gaskell, G., Rehman, H. and Normand, C.E.M. (1993) 'Service provision for people with mild learning disabilities and challenging behaviour', in C. Kiernan (ed.) *Research to Practice? Implications of research on the challenging behaviour of people with a learning disability.* Avon: BILD.

Dockrell, J. E. and McShane, J. (1993) *Children's Learning Difficulties: A cognitive approach.* Oxford: Basil Blackwell.

Dowdney, L. and Skuse, D. (1993) 'Parenting provided by adults with mental retardation', *Journal of Child Psychology and Psychiatry* **34**, 25–47.

Drillien, C.M., Jameson, S. and Wilkinson, E.M. (1966) 'Studies in mental handicap, Part 1: Prevalence and distribution by clinical type and severity of defect', *Archives of Disease in Childhood* **41**, 528–38.

Drotar, D., Baskiewicz, Irvin, N., Kennell, J. and Klaus, M. (1975) 'The adaptation of parents to the birth of an infant with a congenital malformation: A hypothetical model', *Pediatrics* **56**(5), 710–17.

Emerson, E., Barrett, S., Bell, C., Cummings, R., Toogood, A. and Mansell, J. (1987) *Developing Services for People with Severe Learning Difficulties and Challenging*

Behaviours. University of Kent at Canterbury, Institute of Social and Applied Psychology.

Enderby, P. and Davies, P. (1989) 'Communication disorders: Planning a service to meet the needs', *British Journal of Disorders of Communication* **24**, 301–32.

Fairbrother, P. (1983) 'The parent's viewpoint', in A. Craft and M. Craft (eds.) *Sex Education and Counselling for Mentally Handicapped People.* Tunbridge Wells: Costello Press.

Fryers, T. (1984) *The Epidemiology of Severe Intellectual Impairment: The dynamics and prevalence.* London: Academic Press.

Gaskell, G., Dockrell, J.E. and Rehman, H. (in press) 'Community care for people with challenging behaviours and mild learning disability: An evaluation of an assessment and treatment unit', *British Journal of Clinical Psychology.*

Gath, A. (1978) *Down's Syndrome and the Family: The early years.* London: Academic Press.

Gillham, B. (1986) *Handicapping Conditions in Children.* London: Croom Helm.

Goddard, J. and Rubissow, J. (1977) 'Meeting the needs of handicapped children and their families', *Child: Care, Health and Development* **3**, 261–73.

Grossman, H. (ed.) (1983) *Classification in Mental Retardation,* 3rd edition. Washington, DC: American Association of Mental Retardation.

Harris, P. and Russell, O. (1989) *The prevalence of aggressive behaviour among people with learning difficulties (mental handicap): Interim Report.* University of Bristol: Norah Fry Research Centre.

Jancar, J. (1989) 'Fractures in older people with mental handicap', *Australia and New Zealand Journal of Developmental Disabilities* **15**, 321–7.

Kahmi, A. and Masterson, J. (1989) 'Language and cognition in mentally handicapped people: Last rites for the difference–delay controversy', in M. Beveridge, G. Conti-Ramsden and I. Leudar (eds.) *Language and Communication in Mentally Handicapped People.* London: Chapman & Hall.

Kail, R. (1990) *The Development of Memory in Children*, 3rd edition. New York: W.H. Freeman.

Kellmer-Pringle, M., Butler, N.R. and Davie, R. (1966) *11,000 Seven-Year-Olds.* London: National Children's Bureau.

Kiernan, C. (1987). *Dilemmas: Services for Mentally Handicapped People with Challenging Behaviours.* Paper presented at BIMH conference, Llantrisant, Wales.

King's Fund Centre (1980) *An ordinary life: Comprehensive locally-based residential services for mentally handicapped people*, (Project Paper 24). London, King Edward's Hospital Fund for London.

Korman, N. and Glennester, H. (1990) *Hospital Closure.* Milton Keynes: Open University Press.

Kuschlick, A., Blunden, R. and Cox, G. (1973) 'A method of rating behaviour characteristics for use in large-scale surveys of mental handicap.' *Psychological Medicine* **3**, 466–78.

MacKeith, R. (1973) 'The feelings and behaviour of parents of handicapped children', *Developmental Medicine and Child Neurology* **15**, 524–7.

MacLean, R. (1979) 'Sexual problems and family planning needs of the mentally handicapped in residential care', *British Journal of Family Planning* **4**(4), 13–15.

Mattson, A. (1972) 'The chronically ill child: A challenge to family adoption', *Medical College of Virginia Quarterly* **8**, 171–5.

Maxwell, V. (1993) 'Look through the parents' eyes: Helping parents of children with a learning disability', *Professional Nurse*, 200–2.

Moffitt, T.E., Caspi, A., Harkness, A.R. and Silva, P.A. (1993) 'The natural history of change in intellectual performance: Who changes? How much? Is it meaningful?' *Journal of Child Psychology and Psychiatry* **34**, 455–506.

O'Brien, J. and Tyne, A. (1981) *The Principle of Normalisation: A foundation for effective services.* London: CMH.

Owens, R. (1989) 'Cognition and language in the mentally retarded population', in M. Beveridge, G. Conti-Ramsden and I. Leudar (eds.) *Language and communication in mentally handicapped people.* London: Chapman Hall.

Philp, M. and Duckworth, D. (1982) *Children with Disabilities and Their Families: A review of research.* Windsor: NFER-Nelson.

President's Committee on Mental Retardation (1973) *MR-72: Islands of Excellence.* Washington DC: Government Printing Office.

Pritchard, D.G. (1963) *Education of the Handicapped, 1760–1960.* London: Routledge & Kegan Paul.

Richards, C. and Reed, J. (1991) 'Your baby has Down's syndrome', *Nursing Times* **87**(46), 60–1.

Rondal, J. (1987) 'Language development and mental retardation', in W. Yule and M. Rutter (eds.) *Language Development and Disorders.* Oxford: MacKeith Press.

Royal Commission on the Blind and the Deaf and Others of the United Kingdom, vol. 2, Appendix 26 cited in Pritchard (1963) reference above.

Rutter, M., Tizard, J. and Whitmore, K. (eds.) (1970) *Education, Health and Behaviour.* London: Longman.

Sheridan, M.D. (1965) *The Handicapped Child and His Home.* London: National Children's Home.

Steinhauer, P.D., Mushin, D.N. and Rae-Grant, Q. (1974) 'Psychological aspects of chronic illness', *Pediatric Clinics of North America* **21**(4), 825–40.

Stow, L. and Selfe L. (1989) *Understanding Children with Special Needs.* London: Unwin Hyman.

Tomlinson, S. (1982) *A Sociology of Special Education.* London: Routledge & Kegan Paul.

Warnock, H.M. (1978) 'Special Education Needs: Report of the Committee of Enquiry into the Education of Handicapped Children and Young People. London: HMSO.

Weiss, B., Weisz, J. and Bromfield, R. (1986) 'Performance of retarded and nonretarded persons on information-processing tasks: Further tests of the similar structure hypothesis', *Psychological Bulletin* **100**, 157–75.

Weisz, J., Yeates, K.O. and Zigler, E. (1982) 'Piagetian evidence and the developmental–difference controversy', in E. Zigler and D. Balla (eds.) *Mental Retardation: The developmental–difference controversy.* Hillsdale, NJ: Lawrence Erlbaum.

Wolfensberger, W. (1972) *Normalization: The principles of normalization in human services.* Toronto: National Institute of Mental Retardation.

Zigler, E. (1969) 'Developmental versus difference theories of mental retardation and the problem of motivation', *American Journal of Mental Deficiency* **73**, 536–56.

Zigler, E. and Hodapp, R.M. (1986) *Understanding Mental Retardation.* New York: Cambridge University Press.

CHAPTER 21

Physical and sensory disabilities in childhood

VICKY LEWIS

Chapter outline

Introduction
Disability in childhood
Physical disability
Visual impairment
Hearing impairment
Implications for health professionals
Summary

Introduction

Health professionals come into contact with children who have many different disabilities: some will be severely affected psychologically, while others will be developing normally. Contact varies depending on the nature of the work. It may be in hospital with a family and their newborn baby or when hospital treatment is necessary. It may be as a health visitor working with children and families at home. It may be in a surgery or school. Whatever the health professionals' involvement, this chapter gives some idea of how a disability may affect development and indicates some of the implications for families and professionals.

First, I shall raise some issues relevant to all children with disabilities. I shall then consider some consequences for psychological development of physical disability, visual impairment (VI) and hearing impairment (HI). Finally, I shall examine some of the implications for professionals who work with children with disabilities and their families.

Disability in childhood

Childhood is a period characterized by rapid psychological development. Although babies are surprisingly competent (see Chapter 19; also Bremner, 1994), a great deal of change occurs over the first seven or eight years of life (see Chapter 19). A disability will affect this development. Box 21.1 lists some general issues which are relevant to the impact of a disability on psychological development.

BOX 21.1 **GENERAL ISSUES**

Onset time

An acquired disability will have less effect on psychological development than an equivalent disability present from birth or shortly after. For example, HI acquired after speech has developed will affect communication less than either congenital HI or HI acquired before the onset of spoken language.

Cause

The cause of a disability is often unknown and parents may worry that something they did or did not do was responsible. Knowing the cause can provide a focus for parents' anger and distress. If a disability is inherited, development may proceed more smoothly than if the impairment is acquired, as the parents may have personal experience of the disability and will have come to terms with it. Also, a child of a parent with a known inherited disability is more likely to be given tests (e.g. for HI), so that earlier diagnosis and support may therefore occur.

Nature of the disability

This varies enormously and may differ greatly in children with ostensibly the same disability: three children may have VI but one may be unable to see anything, another may have light perception and the third may have a narrow field of central vision. In addition, many children have more than one disability: 33 per cent of children with either VI or HI and most children with moderate to severe motor problems have some additional disability.

Effect on development

This is very varied and a disability in one area may affect many aspects of psychological development. However, all children grow up in different environments and have different experiences. Having a disability does not remove the individuality of a particular child: children with the same disability will have more in common with members of their own families than another child with the same disability.

Society's view

Society values normality and often expresses negative attitudes towards people with disabilities. As a result, when parents discover their child has a disability they may mourn the normal child they have lost and initially may reject their child. Society also holds limited expectations of people with disabilities and often makes unjustified assumptions. Thus, people with limited spoken language are often assumed to be intellectually disabled. Such assumptions may restrict opportunities for development.

Children with a particular type of disability such as VI tend to be grouped together and as a result the individuality of each child and family and the context in which the child is growing up may be overlooked. For professionals working with such children, it is crucial to be conscious of individual differences. Nevertheless an awareness of how a disability may or may not affect psychological development is of obvious use and in the next three sections I have provided an overview of the psychological impact of three types of disability.

Physical disability

Many children have some form of motor impairment, although the actual incidence is uncertain. In some cases there may be a specific neurological diagnosis, such as spina bifida (SB) or cerebral palsy (CP). In others there may be no identifiable neurological problem; for example, children described as clumsy. The incidence of SB is about 20 per 10,000 (less than 1 per cent) of the school population, although SB occulta, which normally has no consequences for psychological development, may affect as many as 1,000 per 10,000 (10 per cent). The incidence of CP is about 25–35 per 10,000 (less than 1 per cent), while clumsiness may affect 700–1,000 per 10,000 (7–10 per cent) of the school population. In addition, a small number of children are born with other types of physical disability and others will become physically disabled as a result of accidents.

Psychologists have been interested in children with motor impairments because their development should illuminate the role of action in thinking and cognition. However, the study of children with physical disabilities is fraught with problems. Even those children who are very severely disabled physically can usually act on the environment in some way and, if development is impaired, this may be a consequence of an additional disability rather than the physical impairment.

In terms of impaired motor skills, children identified as clumsy probably form the largest group. These children, mainly boys, have motor impairments but no known intellectual, sensory or neurological impairments, although it has been suggested that they may have minimal brain damage and perhaps lie on the CP continuum. Their motor impairments involve difficulty with skilled purposive movements resulting in problems with fine motor tasks (e.g. writing and drawing), gross motor tasks (e.g. running and jumping), throwing and catching and with general balance and posture (e.g. Hulme and Lord, 1986; Smyth, 1992). By late childhood their motor skills may show a delay of four to five years. These problems are likely to persist into adolescence, by which time they may show below average verbal IQs, low academic achievement and increased social and emotional problems (e.g. Losse *et al.*, 1991).

Since the mid-1980s a number of studies have examined possible explanations for these difficulties, in particular the relationship between clumsiness and visual perception and movement perception (kinaesthesis). Although the relationship is not clear (e.g. Hulme and Lord, 1986) there is some evidence that training kinaesthetic ability can improve motor ability (e.g. Laszlo and Sainsbury, 1993).

In contrast, children with SB or CP are likely to have problems additional to their motor impairments. In CP, the motor problems result from brain damage and therefore there is an increased likelihood of sensory and intellectual impairments. In about 85 per cent of people with myelomeningocele SB, hydrocephalus occurs which, if not treated surgically quickly and effectively, can result in brain damage. Box 21.2 lists some of the main types of CP and SB, their causes and consequences for motor ability.

BOX 21.2   CEREBRAL PALSY AND SPINA BIFIDA

Cerebral palsy

In about 90 per cent of cases the brain is damaged at birth, usually because of insufficient oxygen reaching the brain (although it has been suggested that the brain may be damaged before birth and the damage causes the asphyxia at birth, rather than vice versa). Other causes include rhesus incompatibility, maternal rubella and, postnatally, meningitis, encephalitis and various traumas. There are three types of CP, all characterized by uncontrolled movements, which may co-occur:

1. Spastic (50 per cent of cases). Characterized by abnormal posture and rigidity of one or more limbs.
2. Athetoid. Characterized by writhing, involuntary uncoordinated movements. Often the muscles involved in speaking are affected.
3. Ataxic (relatively rare). Balance, coordination and ability to integrate spatial information affected.

Spina bifida

SB results from incomplete closure of the spinal column somewhere along its length during the first two months of pregnancy. The cause is uncertain but may involve a genetic predisposition plus some environmental factor, possibly maternal diet, before and during early pregnancy. In SB occulta the vertebrae do not fuse completely but the spinal cord and surrounding tissue are undamaged and development is usually normal. In SB cystica the cord is involved. There are two types of SB cystica:

1. Meningocele (15 per cent of cases). The spinal cord is undamaged but the meninges and cerebrospinal fluid protrude into a sac-like cyst on the back. This has little or no effect on motor ability.
2. Myelomeningocele (85 per cent cases). Part of the cord and associated nervous tissue protrudes into the cyst with serious consequences for motor ability. Since muscles innervated by nerves originating below the lesion are usually paralyzed, the higher up the spine the damage, the more extensive the paralysis.

BOX 21.3 **JOHN (SELFE AND STOW, 1981)**

John was born after a protracted labour. He was found to be blue at birth and had to be resuscitated; it was feared that he had cerebral palsy. He was very ill for many weeks after birth and was diagnosed as suffering from hemiplegia affecting the left side of his body and diplegia affecting both his legs . . . John was able to walk with the aid of a wheeled frame by the age of two-and-a-half years . . . He had difficulty controlling his tongue and throat musculature but, as he was attempting to communicate, speech therapy was arranged.

At the age of four John . . . was now speaking in short sentences and was able to communicate with his mother although strangers had some difficulty in understanding him. By the age of six . . . [h]e had acquired a small sight vocabulary as a basis to reading. . . . He was also able to write with his right hand. . . . John is now sixteen. He has obtained three 'O' level passes and is hoping to attend a Manpower Services Residential Training School for vocational training in clerical employment.

The presence of additional disabilities makes it difficult to examine the consequences of physical disabilities for psychological development. However, since some very severely physically disabled people are intellectually able, it is clear that a physical disability does not necessarily lead to intellectual impairments. Box 21.3 gives extracts of Selfe and Stow's (1981) account of a boy with quite severe physical problems who achieved several 'O' level passes.

Most children with SB and CP are delayed in reaching major motor milestones and some children may never be able to carry out certain actions. For example, Hewett (1970) reports that less than half of a group of children with CP could walk by 5 years. They may have problems with fine motor movements, especially if athetoid. Interestingly, poor fine motor control has also been reported for children with SB whose arms are not affected. This is possibly because they use their arms to help maintain balance while sitting, etc. and so have fewer opportunities to develop fine motor control.

Children with physical disabilities may have perceptual difficulties. Many children with spastic CP and children with SB and hydrocephalus appear to have problems understanding spatial relationships (e.g. Abercrombie, 1964; Anderson and Spain, 1977). They may orient letters and copy designs incorrectly, misplace parts of the body when drawing a person, misjudge distances and have difficulties dressing (e.g. putting the wrong arm in a sleeve). Given that these sorts of difficulty are seldom found in children with athetoid or ataxic CP, it seems possible that the stiff and jerky movements characteristic of spastic CP may limit a child's understanding of space.

If action is important for understanding, children with physical problems should be impaired cognitively. However, the literature indicates that even a profound physical impairment need not impair cognitive development (e.g. Lewis, 1987). Nevertheless the majority of children with CP and SB do have below average IQs. This may result from brain damage or limited experiences because of the physical limitations. Thus any intellectual impairment is unlikely to result directly from an inability to act on the environment.

DISCUSSION POINT

Discuss the types of social and intellectual experiences that may be denied to a child with CP or SB.

Many children with CP have poor speech which, if understood at all, may be understood by only a few people. Such children, even if of average intelligence, may be presumed to be of below average ability. This was well illustrated by the television documentary of Joey Deacon who had athetoid CP. No one except his mother, who died when he was young, and Ernie, a friend he made many years later when institutionalized, understood him. Ernie and others helped Joey write a book about his life (Deacon, 1974). The process was laborious: Joey spoke a sentence; Ernie repeated it; someone else wrote it down; a nurse corrected the spelling; Joey spelled out each letter and punctuation; Ernie repeated each letter and punctuation and another person typed what Ernie said.

The opposite may occur in children with SB. Their verbal skills may seem quite good and in advance of other areas of development. Nevertheless, when listened to carefully, it often appears that, although speaking fluently, what they say is inappropriate to the context (e.g. Anderson and Spain, 1977).

These communication problems are likely to make interaction with the child difficult. This, plus society's generally negative attitude towards people with physical disabilities, particularly those whose speech is unintelligible and who move in uncontrolled ways, may make acceptance of the disability by both the family and the child difficult.

Visual impairment

About 4 per 10,000 of the school population have VI. Some will have had impaired vision from birth, others will have acquired their impairment. However the majority will be able to see something. There are many different causes of VI, although in possibly 50 per cent of congenital VI the cause is unknown. Box 21.4 lists some of the main types of VI, their causes and effect on vision.

Vision may be impaired in many ways and, with the exception of conditions such as anopthalmia, no two children are likely to have exactly the same impairment. Also in many cases (e.g. macular degeneration, retrolental fibroplasia), the impairment may go undetected for some time and, even if suspected, the nature of the impairment may be unknown for many months.

Although VI can restrict experiences and opportunities throughout life it is in childhood that many of the major difficulties occur. The child has to learn about the environment through the intact senses. As with all disabilities, any residual ability can make a marked difference. However, in the following discussion, I shall concentrate on the development of children with little or no sight from birth.

BOX 21.4   VISUAL IMPAIRMENTS

Congenital cataract

The lens of the eye is cloudy. It can be inherited or caused by the mother having rubella in early pregnancy. An extremely opaque lens may be removed and glasses provided. However the resulting vision is likely to be poor.

Congenital glaucoma

This is usually inherited and results from a buildup of vitreous humour within the eye which destroys retinal cells from the periphery inwards.

Albinism

This inherited condition results in a partial or total absence of pigmentation. The child is very light-sensitive since the iris cannot screen out bright light, but may be able to read print.

Congenital atrophy of the optic nerve

This is seldom inherited and the effect on vision depends on the number and location of the damaged fibres.

Macular degeneration

The cells in the central portion of the retina are destroyed by disease or fail to develop, resulting in peripheral vision.

Anopthalmia

Complete absence of one or both eyes, probably caused by some environmental factor affecting early foetal development.

Retinoblastoma

A malignant tumour on the retina, which can be inherited. Not necessarily congenital. The eye is removed to prevent the tumour from spreading.

Retrolental fibroplasia

An excess of oxygen in the newborn period causes the retinal blood cells to grow abnormally. This occurred frequently 50 years ago in premature babies who were administered high levels of oxygen to minimize brain damage. Since not all the retina is affected equally the child may have restricted vision.

BOX 21.5   **TONI (FRAIBERG, 1977)**

She was five months old . . . When her mother went over to her and called her name, Toni's face broke into a gorgeous smile, and she made agreeable responsive noises. I called her name and waited. There was no smile. . . . [A]t eight months . . . [s]oon after she heard our voices, strange voices, she became sober, almost frozen in her posture. Later, when I held Toni . . . she began to cry, squirmed in my arms, and strained away from my body. . . . At ten months Toni demonstrated for the first time her ability to reach and attain an object on sound cue alone. . . . Between eight and ten months . . . we would see Toni stretched out on the floor, prone on the rug, and for long periods of time lie quite still, smiling softly to herself. . . . [A]t ten months . . . [s]he was still unable to creep . . . [A]t thirteen months . . . she began walking with support – and now also creeping . . . she had a small and useful vocabulary, she was using her hands for fine discriminations, and she was now expert in reaching and attaining objects on sound cue . . . [B]eginning in the second year . . . [w]hen Toni became anxious . . . she would fall into a stuporous sleep. . . . In all other respects she was a healthy, active little girl, able to ride a trike, play ball, join in children's games. Her speech was good . . .

An account of the early development of a child by Selma Fraiberg from her excellent book *Insights from the Blind* (1977) is given in Box 21.5. If you know a young child with severe VI compare your observations. Fraiberg's observations are fairly representative of children with profound VI but no other problems (Warren, 1984). They can be bright, responsive children, although they may show odd behaviours (e.g. Toni fell asleep when anxious). Nevertheless, they develop attachments with familiar people, recognizing their voices and how they hold them, etc. By 5 months, Toni could discriminate between her mother and strangers. However, she may not have shown other features of attachment – holding up arms to be picked up, distress when a familiar person leaves. In the absence of vision these behaviours depend on children understanding that they are surrounded by objects and people. This understanding is difficult without sight.

Sight continuously provides information about the environment. Touch indicates nothing about out-of-reach objects and sounds are seldom continuous. However, it is through these senses that children with VI have to understand their world. This more difficult route can explain the delayed reaching and mobility characteristic of many children with VI (e.g. Bigelow, 1986). Sighted children see something and reach or crawl towards it. Children with VI do not have this incentive and, until they realize that objects and people are permanent and continue to exist, they will not seek them out.

It is often suggested that the intact senses of people with sensory impairments are more acute. However, there is no clear evidence for this (e.g. Warren, 1984). In reality, children with VI are often poor at discriminating sounds and tactile patterns, although this improves with age (Gomulicki, 1961). It may be that with experience they get better at using their intact senses, which may give the impression that their intact senses are more acute.

Interestingly, reliance on intact senses may explain the limited play of children with VI (Fraiberg and Adelson, 1975). Sighted children perceive dolls or toys as miniature versions of people or objects. For children with VI, the doll does not feel, smell or sound like a person; children with VI may have felt the door, window and seat of a car and heard the engine, but have no overall impression which corresponds to a toy car. For children with VI, toys may not represent real objects and this may explain their reduced play.

Unlike children without a disability (see Chapter 19), young children with VI may appear to show little interest in their environment with lowered, silent, blank faces (e.g. Fraiberg, 1977). However this posture, which might indicate boredom in sighted children, may indicate the opposite in children with VI: they may be concentrating on listening, trying to make sense of the sounds they can hear. Children with VI may also indicate interest in other ways. Fraiberg noted that during their first year children with VI made small hand movements towards objects they had dropped or towards sounds.

Being unable to see also influences language development and interaction with others. We rely heavily on vision to initiate and regulate interactions. We signal interest in something by pointing or looking. Children with severe VI cannot respond to the visual interest of others and cannot convey interest in things to others in this way. Similarly, when sighted children begin to talk their first words are usually associated with what can be seen: naming and requesting objects, commenting on events, etc. These opportunities are limited in children with VI and, because of this, some may be delayed in starting to talk, although any delays are usually made up quickly once language begins. However, their language may differ from that of sighted children in various ways. For example, certain words may have different meanings, although the meanings may be appropriate to the children's experience (e.g. Tobin, 1992). For example, Urwin (1981) reports a child with VI describing a coal shed as 'dark'. But for her, dark meant 'Sort of still. And cold. Like when it's raining.' Landau and Gleitman (1985) observed a child with VI manually exploring an object when asked to 'look' at an object, but just touching the object when asked to 'touch but not look'.

Other differences include asking many questions or repeating what others have said. Interestingly, both of these may be a way of establishing and maintaining contact with others (e.g. Urwin, 1981). They may be using language to check who is present and what is happening. Another frequently reported difference is a delay in the correct use of personal pronouns: when asked 'Would you like a biscuit?' children with VI may reply 'You would like a biscuit' (e.g. Fraiberg, 1977). Their difficulty probably reflects the fact that they have not experienced other people's nonverbal signals which often accompany pronouns and indicate the person referred to.

It is clear that children with severe VI and no other disability can become able and competent individuals. Nevertheless, because they experience their environment without the benefit of sight, much of their development follows different routes from that of sighted children (e.g. Ittyerah and Samarapungavan, 1989). The challenge for parents and for professionals working with such children is to tap into these routes to maximize development.

Hearing impairment

There are two main types of chronic HI in childhood: conductive, due to an abnormality of the middle ear, and sensorineural, resulting from damage to the sensory hair cells of the inner ear or to the auditory nerve. The incidence is about 9 per 10,000. Some of these children will have had impaired hearing from birth; others will have acquired their impairment, either before or after they have learned to talk. Most will be able to hear something, although they may be unable to make sense of spoken language using sound alone. In addition, as many as two-thirds of all children may experience at least one episode of otitis media (inflammation of the middle ear) before the age of 3 years resulting in transient HI. However, this seldom has any long-term effect on psychological development (e.g. Schilder *et al.*, 1993).

There are many different causes of HI, although in many cases (possibly 40 per cent) the cause is unknown. Box 21.6 lists the main types of HI, known causes and consequences for hearing.

Sounds are described in terms of amplitude and pitch and HI is assessed by presenting sounds of different pitch/frequencies (measured in Hertz, Hz) at different amplitudes (measured in decibels, dB) and noting responses. As with VI,

---

BOX 21.6   HEARING IMPAIRMENT

Sensorineural loss

The most common type. In about 50 per cent of cases caused by inheritance of a recessive gene from both parents. Also caused by the mother having rubella in early pregnancy, by incompatibility in the rhesus factors in maternal and foetal blood and by the baby experiencing an oxygen deficiency at birth. After birth sensorineural damage can result from severe viral infection, notably meningitis. In all cases the HI is severe and permanent.

Conductive loss

Caused by an air bone gap in the middle ear, usually because of recurrent bouts of otitis media during childhood. Unless the infections are frequent and untreated, the loss is seldom total and usually reversible. Nevertheless, during and immediately after an infection children may experience marked variations in hearing.

Auditory pathway damage

This is relatively infrequent. However, it can be caused by exposure to a teratogen during early pregnancy, such as the thalidomide tragedy of the late 1950s.

assessment is difficult with very young children and, unless HI is anticipated (as in 10 per cent of cases where one or both parents have HI), it may go undetected for many months. Nevertheless parents may suspect something. Fletcher (1987) comments: 'there is something not quite right, but the feeling is vague, unspecific, confirmed by nothing visible, though we watch him very closely.' Her son, Ben, had profound bilateral HI which was finally diagnosed at 10 months. However developments such as the auditory response cradle may enable an earlier diagnosis. This is based on the observation that a baby may either still or move more when a sound is heard. The baby lies in a specially designed cot and sounds of various frequencies and intensities are presented. Any changes in the baby's movements are detected through movements of the cot. In this way, the range of sounds which can be heard can be examined.

Perfect hearing is defined as a 0 dB loss across the normal frequency range of 20–20,000 Hz. Losses of up to 25 dB have negligible effect, but beyond this increasing problems will arise especially when the frequency range for speech (250–4,000 Hz) is affected. If the loss exceeds 55 dB little will be heard and spoken language will be understood primarily via lip-reading. However, the loss may differ across the frequency range and, since consonants give more information about spoken language than vowels and have frequencies above 1,000 Hz (vowels have lower frequencies and also have a 15 dB advantage so are easier to hear) a high frequency loss impairs speech perception more than a low frequency loss. Hearing aids can assist, particularly if the loss is under 50 dB or occurs after spoken language has been acquired. Unfortunately, hearing aids are of little use to children with losses above 70 dB which are either congenital or acquired pre-lingually.

Box 21.7 describes a child who acquired severe HI after beginning to talk. If you know a young child with severe HI compare your observations. Joe's acquired HI affected subsequent language development. Not surprisingly, acquiring spoken language can be very difficult for children with severe prelingual HI. In the rest of this section, I shall concentrate on such children.

Children with severe HI and no other disability attain early motor milestones at about the same time as children who can hear, although they may not be as good at tasks requiring certain types of coordination (e.g. Wiegersma and van der Velde, 1983). Also, like children with VI, there is no clear evidence that their intact senses are more acute.

The cognitive abilities of children with HI have received much attention from psychologists because it was thought that they could answer the enduring question of whether understanding precedes language, or vice versa. However, this assumes that children with HI do not develop language. While some children with HI do not develop speech, many do, and others will acquire sign language. Sign languages, such as British Sign Language (BSL), are now accepted as real languages, each with its own grammatical features distinct from other spoken or signed languages (e.g. Kyle and Woll, 1985). This is in contrast to some sign systems which follow the grammar of a spoken language (e.g. Signed Exact English, Makaton). Despite this, the effect of HI on cognition is still an important issue.

BOX 21.7   **JOE (SELFE AND STOW, 1981)**

Joe had meningitis at twenty-one months. Before his illness his language was developing well and he was a bright, alert child. He had a large vocabulary of single-word utterances. After his illness he relapsed into a passive baby-like state for many months. By . . . two-and-a-half he was beginning to take an alert interest in the world around him again but the language . . . had disappeared altogether. Motor co-ordination . . . had returned completely, and he was agile and curious.

By the age of three Joe was attempting to vocalise, but his words were very poorly articulated . . . he had a 70 decibel bilateral hearing loss . . . a sensorineural deafness associated with his early illness.

He was fitted with hearing aids and his language ability improved dramatically although his articulation remained poor. From the age of four Joe was given intensive help from a peripatetic teacher of the deaf. . . . [O]n . . . psychological tests [he] was found to be above average on visual/spatial skills, just below average in verbal comprehension, but well below average on any task that required verbal expression. . . . His spoken language slowly improved and he learned to lip-read and to use his residual hearing to the best possible advantage. He learned to read . . . Socially he has become withdrawn and shy . . .

Children with HI develop a similar understanding of people and objects as hearing children although they will not know certain things (e.g. the noises particular objects or animals make). Their play is similar (e.g. Gregory, 1976), although older children with HI may engage in less joint play, primarily because of communication difficulties. On intelligence subtests of visual and spatial ability, provided they have no additional problems, they perform within the normal range (e.g. Conrad and Weiskrantz, 1981). However, they perform below average on subtests of verbal ability.

The early language environments of children with profound HI markedly affect language acquisition. If one or both parents have HI, interaction from early on seems to proceed more smoothly (Gregory and Barlow, 1989). If the parents sign, the children begin to use signs earlier than hearing children start to talk, although in other respects acquisition of the two languages is fairly similar (e.g. Schlesinger and Meadow, 1972).

However, most children with congenital HI have hearing parents and language acquisition will be painfully slow. Gregory and Mogford (1981) describe two children with fewer than 10 words by the age of 4, compared with an expected vocabulary for hearing children of 2,000. Hearing children add new words every day whereas each new word is a struggle for children with HI. Also, adults talk less to children with HI, providing information and answers rather than asking questions and seeking opinions. Parents may have difficulties explaining things, such as plans for the future, or why children cannot do something (Gregory, 1976). Interestingly, Wood *et al.* (1986) found that when teachers focused more on the communicative intent of children with HI and less on correcting their speech, the children spoke more.

Reading can also present problems. Conrad (1979) found that only 2.5 per cent of school leavers with profound HI had reading ages comparable with their chronological age, compared with 50 per cent for hearing school leavers. Conrad also reported that over half of the school leavers with HI had reading ages below 8 years. Wood *et al.* (1986) suggest that this depressing finding may be because teachers focus on reading accuracy rather than comprehension.

Given the problems with communication, it is not surprising that many children with HI have social and behavioural problems (Denmark *et al.*, 1979). However it seems likely that these problems will be mitigated in children who have access to a sign language.

Unlike children with VI who have to discover alternative routes, there is a readily available route for children with profound HI. However, unless one or both parents already sign, this language is not usually easily available. The Fletchers (Fletcher, 1987) did not sign themselves and eventually obtained the help of a native signer when their son was 4. As Fletcher writes:

> So many parents emerge tearstained from their deaf child's diagnosis, feeling a tragedy has occurred. So many profoundly deaf children reach the age of five with little or no language. This need not and should not happen. The tragedy is not that some people are born deaf, but that they are denied a means of communication appropriate to their needs.

Implications for health professionals

The material I have discussed in this chapter has many implications for professionals who come into contact with children with disabilities and their families.

DISCUSSION POINT

Review what you have learned about children with (1) a physical disability, (2) VI, and (3) HI. What are the implications for health professionals working with a child with each of these disabilities? For example, what needs might arise for such a child who is admitted to hospital for surgery or a painful investigation? How might a health professional try to provide for these needs?

One of the important implications is that we all acknowledge that we are part of society and as such have our own views of and attitudes towards disability. If you are to be able to help and support children with disabilities and their parents, you need to explore your own attitudes and how you react or might react towards people with disabilities.

How parents react to the news that their baby or child has a disability varies. Those who have feared something very serious was wrong may feel relieved by the diagnosis (e.g. Gregory, 1991). For others, such as parents with HI which their child also has acquired genetically, the diagnosis may present little problem. However, those families where the diagnosis is not expected often go through phases which have been characterized as shock, denial, sadness and anger, adaptation and re-organization (Drotar *et al.*, 1975). The length and nature of these phases may vary. Nevertheless, sadness almost inevitably accompanies the news and this may inter-fere with the parents' comprehension of what they are told. How this period is handled by health care workers may influence parents' reactions to the news and to their child (e.g. Cunningham, Morgan and McGucken, 1984). They should be told as soon as possible by a relevant professional and given plenty of time. The baby or child should be present, preferably held by the parents or professional. Although information should be given on this first occasion it is crucial that other oppor-tunities are arranged within a day or two for the parents to ask questions and have the information repeated. The information which is given needs to be realistic but balanced. Everyone involved needs to be very careful what they say to families at this very difficult time.

Although some disabilities are diagnosed at the time of birth or very shortly afterwards, others do not become apparent until later. Nevertheless, during this time the parents may suspect that something is wrong. They may share their worries with professionals or may keep them to themselves. It is important that profes-sionals encourage parents to share any worries. Most of these worries will turn out to be unfounded and reflect the normal variability of development; some may indicate a disability. All should be taken seriously (see Chapter 20).

One of the difficulties for health workers is that they are likely to see a wide range of disabilities, some having a minor effect on development, others having a profound effect. Nevertheless, for a family, any disability, however minor, may cause distress and require some readjustment. It is important that the disability is seen from the family's point of view, rather than from the health worker's wider perspective on disability. Only empathy with the family will gain their trust. Similarly, some disabilities are much more frequent than others. This should not be allowed to influence the health worker's reaction. The diagnosis of clumsiness in a child may be just as distressing to a family as the diagnosis of some less frequent physical disability. For each family the problems are very real and unique. However, families and their reactions vary and professionals need to be sensitive to these differences.

DISCUSSION POINT
If you have any family, friends or colleagues who have a physical or sensory disability and who are prepared to talk to you about this, ask them about their childhood experiences. Compare notes with your fellow students or colleagues. How might the knowledge you have gained from this activity influence how you would care for a child with a disability?

Support for families is crucial to help them come to terms with their child's disability. This is essential if they are to develop a positive attitude towards their child. If the disability is not accepted, it is difficult to help parents to help their child. Some may turn to professionals for support; others may have their own support mechanisms. As a health professional, your main role will be the health care of the child, rather than their psychological development. Nevertheless your advice may be sought about psychological development. Perhaps the main implication of the material covered in this chapter is that there are many routes to development. A conventional route may not be available because of a disability; nevertheless the child may still develop, albeit by a different route. Awareness of this is important for all professionals. Similarly, it is important to be aware that a psychological ability may be present but be expressed in a different way in a child with a disability. It is also important for professionals to facilitate ways of helping children to express themselves and not to assume that lack of expression of an ability means absence of that ability. Parents of a child with a disability need to be encouraged to think about how their child experiences the environment and how to relate to this experience. This is particularly relevant to children with a physical or sensory disability.

Summary

This chapter has examined the impact on psychological development when a child has a physical disability, severe visual impairment or profound hearing impairment. Although different children may be identified as having the same disability, it is important to consider each child as an individual with unique experiences and opportunities. Some of the implications for health professionals working with children with disabilities have been examined. In particular the professional's own attitude to disability, the reactions of the child's family to the disability and the possibility of development occurring via a number of different routes are identified as important factors.

Seminar questions

1. How does a physical or sensory disability in a child affect that child's relationships with other people?
2. In what ways does a physical or sensory disability affect the child's perception and understanding of objects?
3. Design an ideal hospital policy to meet the needs of children with disabilities who have to come into hospital. How could this be implemented?

Further reading

Bishop, D. and Mogford, K. (1988) *Language Development in Exceptional Circumstances*. Edinburgh: Churchill Livingstone. Examines the development of language in children with a range of disabilities, including the three types of disability discussed in this chapter.

Delight, E. and Goodall, J. (1990) 'Love and loss: Conversations with parents of babies with SB managed without surgery, 1971–1981', *Developmental Medicine and Child Neurology*, Supplement No. 61. Reports interviews with 44 families whose child with SB myelomeningocele died before 5 months. The interviews were retrospective, carried out between 5 and 15 years after the child had died. Useful for professionals working with families with children with different disabilities.

Fletcher, L. (1987) *Language for Ben: A deaf child's right to sign*. London: Souvenir Press. A hearing parent's account of the development of her profoundly deaf son who learnt to sign. While giving a very positive view of disability, this book also illustrates many of the problems and challenges facing parents with a child with a disability.

Fraiberg, S. (1977) *Insights from the Blind*. London: Souvenir Press. One of the best accounts of the development of children with VI.

Lewis, V. (1987) *Development and Handicap*. Oxford: Basil Blackwell. Describes and discusses in some detail the consequences of different disabilities for psychological development and examines the practical and theoretical implications.

References

Abercrombie, M.L.J. (1964) *Perceptual and Visuo-Motor Disorders in Cerebral Palsy*. Little Club Clinics in Developmental Medicine No. 11. London: Spastics Society and Heinemann.

Anderson, E.M. and Spain, B. (1977) *The Child with Spina Bifida*. London: Methuen.

Bigelow, A. E. (1986) 'The development of reaching in blind children', *British Journal of Developmental Psychology* 4, 355–66.

Bremner, J. G. (1994) *Infancy*, 2nd edition. Oxford: Basil Blackwell.

Conrad, R. (1979) *The Deaf School Child: Language and cognitive function*. London: Harper & Row.

Conrad, R. and Weiskrantz, B.C. (1981) 'On the cognitive ability of deaf children of deaf parents', *American Annals of the Deaf* 126, 995–1003.

Cunningham, C.C., Morgan, P.A. and McGucken, R.B. (1984) 'Down's syndrome: Is dissatisfaction with disclosure of diagnosis inevitable?' *Developmental Medicine and Child Neurology* 26, 33–9.

Deacon, J. J. (1974) *Tongue Tied: Fifty years of friendship in a subnormality hospital*. London: National Society for Mentally Handicapped Children.

Denmark, J.C., Rodda, M., Abel, R.A., Skelton, U., Eldridge, R.W., Warren, F. and Gordon, A. (1979) *A Word in Deaf Ears. A study of communication and behaviour in a sample of 75 deaf adolescents*. London: Royal National Institute for the Deaf.

Drotar, D., Baskiewicz, A., Irvin, N., Kennell, J. and Klaus, M. (1975) 'The adaptation of parents to the birth of an infant with a congenital malformation: A hypothetical model', *Pediatrics* 56, 710–7.

Fletcher, L. (1987) *Language for Ben: A deaf child's right to sign*. London: Souvenir Press.

Fraiberg, S. (1977) *Insights from the Blind*. London: Souvenir Press.

Fraiberg, S. and Adelson, E. (1975) 'Self-representation in language and play: Observations of blind children', in R. Lenneberg and E. Lenneberg (eds), *The Foundations of Language Development: Multi-disciplinary approach*, Vol. 2, New York: Academic Press.

Gomulicki, B.R. (1961) 'The development of perception and learning in blind children', The Psychological Laboratory, Cambridge University. Cited by J. Juurmaa (1973) *Transposition in mental spatial manipulation: A theoretical analysis.* Research Bulletin, American Foundation for the Blind **26**, 87–134.

Gregory, S. (1976) *The Deaf Child and his Family.* London: George Allen & Unwin.

Gregory, S (1991) 'Challenging motherhood: Mothers and their deaf children', in A. Phoenix, A. Woollett and E. Lloyd (eds.) *Motherhood: Meanings, practices and ideologies.* London: Sage.

Gregory, S. and Barlow, S. (1989) 'Interaction between deaf babies and deaf and hearing mothers', in B. Woll (ed.) *Language Development and Sign Language.* Monograph No. 1, International Sign Linguistics Association, Centre for Deaf Studies, University of Bristol.

Gregory, S. and Mogford, K. (1981) 'Early language development in deaf children', in B. Woll, J.G. Kyle and M. Deuchar (eds.) *Perspectives on BSL and Deafness.* London: Croom Helm.

Hewett, S. (1970) *The Family and the Handicapped Child: A study of cerebral palsied children in their homes.* London: Allen & Unwin.

Hulme, C. and Lord, R. (1986) 'Clumsy children: A review of recent research', *Child: Care, Health and Development* **12**, 257–69.

Ittyerah, M. and Samarapungavan, A. (1989) 'The performance of congenitally blind children in cognitive developmental tasks', *British Journal of Developmental Psychology* **7**, 129–39.

Kyle, J. G. and Woll, B. (1985) *Sign Language: The study of deaf people and their language.* London: Cambridge University Press.

Landau, B. and Gleitman, L. R. (1985) *Language and Experience: Evidence from the blind child.* Cambridge, Mass.: Harvard University Press.

Laszlo, J. I. and Sainsbury, K. M. (1993) 'Perceptual-motor development and prevention of clumsiness', *Psychological Research – Psychologische Forschung* **55**, 167–74.

Lewis, V. (1987) *Development and Handicap.* Oxford: Basil Blackwell.

Losse, A., Henderson, S.E., Elliman, D., Hall, D., Knight, E. and Jongmans, M. (1991) 'Clumsiness in children: Do they grow out of it? A 10-year follow-up study', *Developmental Medicine and Child Neurology* **33**, 55–68.

Schilder, A.G.M., van Manen, J.G., Zielhuis, G.A., Grievink, E.H., Peters, S.A.F. and van der Broek, P. (1993) 'Long-term effects of otitis media with effusion on language, reading and spelling', *Clinical Otolaryngology* **18**, 234–41.

Schlesinger, H. and Meadow, K. (1972) *Sound and Sign: Childhood deafness and mental health.* Berkeley, Calif.: University of California Press.

Selfe, L. and Stow, L. (1981) *Children with Handicaps.* Sevenoaks: Hodder & Stoughton.

Smyth, T. R. (1992) 'Impaired motor skill (clumsiness) in otherwise normal children: A review', *Child: Care, Health and Development* **18**, 283–300.

Tobin, M. (1992) 'The language of blind children: Communication, words, and meanings', *Language and Education: An international journal* **6**, 177–82.

Urwin, C. (1981) 'Early language development in blind children', *The British Psychological Society Division of Educational and Child Psychology Occasional Papers* **5**, 78–93.

Warren, D.H. (1984) *Blindness and Early Childhood Development*, 2nd edition, New York: American Foundation for the Blind.

Wiegersma, P.H. and van der Velde, A. (1983) 'Motor development of deaf children', *Journal of Child Psychology and Psychiatry* **24**, 103–11.

Wood, D., Wood, H., Griffiths, A. and Howarth, I. (1986) *Teaching and Talking with Deaf Children.* Chichester: John Wiley.

PART V

Working with elderly adults

In 1900, only 25 per cent of people in Western countries were expected to reach their 65th birthday. Today, about 70 per cent of people will live to this age and between 30 per cent and 40 per cent will live beyond the age of 80 years. With good health care and economic prosperity, these extra years of life will provide much enjoyment and fulfilment for many people (see Chapter 23). On the other hand, we need to acknowledge that senescence, 'the general biological impairment which increases the likelihood of death', is the companion of longevity. Inevitably, therefore, those in the later years of life are more likely to call on the resources of the health care services. It is vital, for this reason, that health professionals are knowledgeable about the ageing process and do not fall prey to the prevalent negative stereotypes that exist about elderly people.

Cognitive changes (Chapter 22) and wellbeing (Chapter 23) in older people are considered first. While some individuals do experience a degree of intellectual decline as they age, the overwhelming body of evidence supports a model of adaptation and change in intellectual and social functioning for most people as they grow older. Chapter 24 examines the nature of dementia and how psychology has contributed to the care of those who develop this condition. Practical advice is offered to those who work with patients or family members who are dementing.

The final chapter of the book (Chapter 25) adopts a systems approach to looking at the care of individuals who are elderly within our society, locating their care within a wider social context. Thus, this last chapter serves to remind us of the point made by the first chapter, that in trying to provide good individual care one cannot afford to lose sight of wider social and organizational considerations.

CHAPTER 22

Cognitive changes in normal ageing

CLAIRE MELDRUM

Chapter outline

Introduction

As the number of elderly people increases in society, nurses will inevitably spend more of their time, both in hospitals and in the community, catering to the needs of older patients and clients. For some nurses this will involve caring for those with dementia (see Chapter 24). However, in the majority of cases, nurses will be interacting with elderly patients who are mentally healthy.

In this chapter I shall consider to what extent nurses should make allowances for the impaired mental power or different cognitive style of their elderly patients or clients. How inevitable is the negative stereotype of the increasingly inflexible and mentally slow, forgetful older person? Is there a qualitative or quantitative change in the cognitive (intellectual) functioning of older people? Where changes can be detected, should these be construed as cognitive deterioration or rather as adaptations to changing life circumstances? How might research findings be used to ensure good nursing practice?

In order to address these questions, I shall consider:

- The different ways in which age can be defined.
- The research methods employed in studies of cognitive ageing.
- The types of cognition that have been studied and how much age-related stability and change have been found.

These considerations comprise the first three sections of the chapter. The last section deals with interventions and some implications for nursing practice. Throughout the chapter, however, you will be encouraged to relate the theoretical issues to practical nursing concerns.

Types of ageing

According to Birren and Renner (1977) there are three different ways in which the age of an individual can be meaningfully described:

1. *Biological age.* This has two aspects: the first relates to the relative condition of the individual's organ and body systems, e.g. heart and lung capacity. It is clear, when using this criterion, that biological age need not be synonymous with chronological age. Some 70-year-olds may be fitter in terms of body systems than 50-year-olds. The second aspect of biological age refers to an estimate of an individual's potential lifespan. Such an estimate (based on biological, social and psychological factors) enables comparisons between individuals of the same chronological age in terms of their life expectancies.
2. *Psychological age.* This refers to how well an individual can adapt to the demands made by a changing environment. In addition, this type of age includes the notion of subjective awareness about one's capabilities. Psychological age may be related to chronological and biological age, but it cannot be adequately encompassed by either or both. A person may be 80 years old and suffering from chronic arthritis, but nevertheless be as alert and well informed as someone much younger.
3. *Social age.* This refers to how satisfactorily an individual adheres to the social roles, habits and attitudes which a society expects of someone of that age. Social age may be related to chronological, biological and psychological age. However, this relationship is not entirely predictable. For instance, some elderly people enjoy music and sporting activities that are more commonly associated with a younger age bracket. We become aware of the existence of social age stereotyping when we hear expressions such as 'dirty old man' or

---

BOX 22.1   WHEN DOES COGNITIVE AGEING START?

'All the age trends . . . begin early and are usually progressive from the middle twenties onwards.' (Welford, 1966: 5)

'all available objective data on cognitive ageing suggests that cognitive decline is slight up to the age of 50.' (Rabbitt and Abson, 1990: 11)

'most intellectual abilities begin to decline in the 60s.' (Cunningham, 1987: 126)

'most abilities tend to peak in midlife, plateau until the late fifties or sixties, and then show decline, initially at a slow pace, but accelerating as the late seventies are reached.' (Schaie, 1989: 66)

'limitations of mental functioning occurs precipitously in individuals over the age of 65 or 70 and is closely related to health status.' (Birren, 1968: 19)

'the decline is continuous rather than abrupt and thus the loss of intellectual ability may be as important a consideration in a comparison of 50-year-olds with 30-year-olds, as it is in a comparison of 70-year-olds with 50-year-olds.' (Salthouse, 1982: 82)

'mutton dressed as lamb'. In these cases, the individuals described have violated the accepted social norms associated with older people.

The notion of *functional age* is also becoming popular and can be defined as 'an index of one's level of capacities or abilities relative to those of others of similar age. Such skills can range from job performance to the condition of various organ systems' (Hayslip, 1989: 12). Again, there is no exact correspondence between chronological and functional age. For instance, an elderly individual living alone may be more, or less, self-sufficient than a 20-year-old. In assessing health care needs a measure of this type of ageing may be the most pertinent.

Despite the acknowledged status of these different types of ageing, it is still *chronological* age that is most commonly used as a classifying variable (means of allocating people to 'age groups') in research on the effects of ageing.

Bromley (1988) has discussed the difficulties of trying to distinguish *normal* from *pathological* ageing. Normal patterns of ageing can be seen as distinct from pathological conditions, or alternatively ageing can be viewed as 'an accumulation of pathological processes which eventually kill off the individual' (p. 81). In reality, however, no one is entirely free from all pathology. Most researchers of cognitive change during normal ageing either, at worst, assume a lack of serious pathology in their participants or, at best, select them from 'healthy' populations on the basis of their medical records or self-reports. That some subjects might have undiagnosed depression or early stage dementia remains a problem particularly in research on the old-old (usually defined as those aged 75 years and over). As Rinn (1988) has reported, half the cerebral infarcts which are discovered at autopsy were undetected during the person's life. He recommends that those collecting normative data on test performance in elderly people should check on the status of participants about three years after the data have been collected. Thus the distinction between normal and pathological patterns of ageing is particularly difficult to make.

DISCUSSION POINTS

When do you think the ageing process begins? Compare your answers with the quotations in Box 22.1. What factors might influence when cognitive processes start to decline? What abilities would you wish to know about if you were caring for someone whose chronological age was not known?

Research methods

The three research methods employed in studies of ageing and cognition have been the cross-sectional, the longitudinal and the cross-sequential. In general, results from longitudinal studies have tended to minimize age differences in cognitive functioning. Cross-sectional results, however, paint a gloomier picture of decline in those abilities that require abstract reasoning. In an attempt to understand these sometimes contradictory findings, Schaie (1965) devised the cross-sequential method that takes account of the shortcomings of the two earlier approaches.

Cross-sectional and longitudinal

The majority of studies of ageing and cognition have, until fairly recently, used the *cross-sectional* method where individuals of different ages are compared at the same point in time. For example, one may compare a group of 20-year-olds with a group of 70-year-olds. Cross-sectional investigations have the advantage of allowing data to be collected rapidly. As a consequence this type of study is common.

However, such designs also have several disadvantages. The most important of these is that people of different ages have had different experiences so that, for example, today's 20-year-olds have had a very different education and diet compared to today's 70-year-olds. Schaie (1965) first used the term 'cohort effects' to describe these non-maturational variables. Cohort effects are defined as a unique input from the environment for a particular generation, including such things as type and length of formal education, nutrition habits and prevailing social customs. Such factors may have a confounding effect, in that they influence cognitive functioning, independent of any ageing effects that may arise. It has been suggested that many age differences noted in cross-sectional studies can be explained in terms of these generational (cohort) influences.

Since cross-sectional studies are so bedevilled by problems, it would seem sensible to abandon them and resort to longitudinal designs. *Longitudinal* studies are those in which the same individuals are tested repeatedly over a period of time. Schaie (1983) and Salthouse (1982) have detailed the advantages of this method. The most important of these is that individual ageing trends as well as inter-individual variability can be studied. However, several difficulties attach to the longitudinal approach. The long timescale involved acts as a disincentive to some researchers who wish to know the results of their work before they die! Additionally, these studies are expensive and may suffer from inconsistent use of measurement tools over long periods of data collection.

The biggest problem of all for longitudinal studies is *selective attrition*. This refers to the situation when the participants who remain in a longitudinal study are no longer representative of the individuals who were originally recruited. Those who drop out tend to be less intellectually able than those who remain. Despite this selective attrition, many longitudinal studies nevertheless do show decline in cognitive functioning in elderly people, although the onset appears to be later than that indicated by cross-sectional studies (Botwinick and Siegler, 1980).

Another potentially confounding factor is the amount of *practice* that participants undergo. Necessarily, there are repeated assessments and so older individuals will become more practised in the testing procedures. As with selective attrition, this practice effect may positively bias the performance of participants as they grow older (Salthouse, 1991).

In 1965, Schaie combined aspects of both cross-sectional and longitudinal methods in such a way as to take into account both practice effects and selective attrition. He aimed to establish whether or not age differences in cognitive processing could be explained entirely in terms of cohort effects.

The cross-sequential method

In his Seattle Longitudinal Study (SLS) of adult development which spanned 21 years, Schaie and his colleagues used a sequential method. The first longitudinal sample of 162 participants was tested in 1956 and thereafter at 7-year intervals. Participants came from one of seven birth cohorts. At each measurement point (i.e. 1956, 1963, 1970 and 1977) different samples were selected from each cohort for participation in the longitudinal study. This meant that practice effects could not happen and that selective attrition posed much less of a problem. Cross-sectional samples were also drawn at each testing point. The main results of this study will be returned to later.

DISCUSSION POINTS
List some cohort effects that might distinguish your generation from your parents'. Do you think these cohort effects have influenced intellectual functioning?

Cognitive processes and ageing

Cognitive processes

The term *cognitive processing* relates to the mental activities of perceiving, remembering and information processing that enable us to acquire information, to make plans and to solve problems. Therefore the study of cognitive ageing is concerned with how these abilities change or remain stable as we grow older.

Most studies of ageing and cognitive ability have been concerned with the decline and loss of function. Only more recently has interest turned to stability and adaptation as features of the developing cognitive system in older adults. Traditionally, the study of cognitive processing is concerned with issues such as attention and memory and brief reviews of findings in each of these areas will be given. It is, however, the phenomenon of intelligence that has been most frequently explored. Therefore, this area of investigation will be examined first.

Intelligence and its measurement

What happens to intelligence as one ages? This is not as simple a question as it first appears. For a start, what is meant by the term 'intelligence'? Some characterize intelligence as a single, unitary process, a general cognitive ability. Others construe it as a number of different, independent mental processes each of which is separately measurable by a standard test (e.g. the verbal and performance subscales of the Weschler Adult Intelligence Scale, 1955; see Chapter 7 for the requirements of a good psychometric test). Some psychometricians have gone further than this and proposed as many as 120 separate mental abilities.

It is, however, Thurstone's primary mental abilities and the concepts of fluid and crystallized intelligence that are most often used in discussions of intelligence and ageing. Thurstone (1938) proposed and devised psychometric tests to measure, seven primary mental abilities:

1. *Verbal comprehension*:* recognizing vocabulary.
2. *Word fluency*:* retrieving words.
3. *Number*:* doing simple arithmetic.
4. *Space*:* visualizing fixed or rotating spatial relations.
5. *Associative memory*: remembering paired items such as words.
6. *Perceptual speed*: grasping visual details.
7. *Inductive (general) reasoning*:* detecting a rule/relationship, e.g. in a number series task, and applying the rule to complete a sequence.

*Used by Schaie in his Seattle Longitudinal Study (SLS).

By contrast, Cattell (1963) and Horn (1970) have argued that all mental abilities can be subsumed under two components. *Crystallized intelligence*, which is measured by tasks such as reading, comprehension and vocabulary, is thought to be highly dependent on education and experience, but less dependent on central nervous system function. Thurstone's two primary mental abilities of verbal comprehension and word fluency are encompassed by this concept. *Fluid intelligence*, on the other hand, is measured by tests of response speed, memory span and non-verbal reasoning, that is, mental abilities that are not imparted by one's culture. It is thought to be dependent on the smooth working of the central nervous system. Thurstone's remaining five primary mental abilities correspond to fluid intelligence.

When does intelligence decline?

It appears that crystallized intelligence remains stable over much of the lifespan, while fluid intelligence shows decline. This raises the question, when does the decline begin? Early cross-sectional studies indicated a decline in this type of intelligence from as early as the mid-twenties, whereas longitudinal studies show declines to start much later, usually in the late fifties (see definitions in Box 22.1). However, owing to the problems associated with both cross-sectional and longitudinal methods (namely cohort effects and selective attrition, respectively) one is unable, from these studies, to arrive at a conclusion regarding when decline in fluid intelligence begins. This is where Schaie's cross-sequential method comes into its own. Participants were tested four times over a 21-year period on five different primary mental abilities. His findings are summarized as follows:

1. Fluid abilities tend to decline earlier than crystallized abilities.
2. Even in this study there is some uncertainty about when cognitive decline occurs. The data collected during the first three cycles of the SLS suggested that no reliable age decrements in fluid intelligence could be demonstrated before the age of 60. However, more recently, analyses from the last two cycles have revealed small but significant decrements for some birth cohorts during their fifties. By the age of 74, reliable decrements could be found for all five primary mental abilities tested.
3. At age 81, fewer than half of the participants had declined in ability over the last seven years (Schaie, 1989).
4. There are large individual differences at all ages. Substantial overlaps in the scores were found from young adulthood into at least the mid-seventies.
5. Generational (cohort) differences in psychometric abilities were demonstrated. There has been an improvement over historical time in inductive reasoning ability, with the more recent generations performing better on these tasks than older generations. What is less encouraging is the pattern for number skills. These peak for the 1917 and 1924 birth cohorts and decline thereafter!

Differences in intellectual functioning in older people

Various details of personal history, including health records, were collected for participants in the SLS. On the basis of these, Schaie proposes several reasons for the individual differences found. He lists the following variables as related to cognitive ageing.

Absence of chronic disease
As individuals move through the lifespan their intellectual functioning may be increasingly influenced by their physical health status (Siegler and Costa, 1985). Several studies have revealed a relationship between hypertension and cardiovascular disease and a decline in the mental abilities of older people (e.g., Schaie,

1989). Attention is now directed towards the link between other diseases, such as diabetes, and intellectual deficits during ageing (e.g. see Perlmuter *et al.*, 1987, for a review of the literature on diabetes).

High levels of education, occupational status and income
In addition to these obvious demographic variables, Schaie (1984) draws attention to the positive effects of exposure to stimulating environments, making use of educational resources throughout adulthood and having an intelligent spouse.

Personality
Self-efficacy (the belief in one's capabilities) and cognitive functioning were related, but this is hardly surprising and the relationship might be reciprocal (Lachman, 1983). High levels of mental flexibility in mid-life are predictive of numerical and verbal skills in old age (Schaie, 1984).

Speed of performance (i.e. reaction time)
Traditionally, this has been studied by measuring how long it takes a person to respond to the appearance of a stimulus. Other techniques include card sorting and providing as many words as possible that begin with a specified letter. Whatever the method used, these reaction times are seen as a convenient way of assessing how quickly the central nervous system is processing information. Reaction times tend to slow with age and this might explain why elderly people perform worse at timed intelligence tests than do young. However, this loss of speed does not account directly for all the age-related changes found. Practice can minimize reaction times and even when response speed is controlled for, age differences in test scores remain: old minds are not as efficient at mental processing as young minds. This suggests qualitative changes in cognitive functioning with age.

In addition to those variables identified by Schaie, the model of *terminal drop* (Riegel and Riegel, 1972) is often used to explain individual differences in the performances of elderly people and the differences found between age groups in both cross-sectional and longitudinal studies. (See Box 22.2 for more information on the concept of terminal drop.)

DISCUSSION POINT
To what extent do you think that the five primary mental abilities used by Schaie in the SLS provide adequate measures of the intellectual capabilities of his participants?

Ageing and attention

If a clear-cut deficit could be established in attentional processing in elderly people this could provide a parsimonious, single explanatory mechanism for the ubiquitous age-related differences found in cognitive functioning. However, the emerging picture is not so simple. Three types of attention having been investigated over the years, using cross-sectional methods.

BOX 22.2 **TERMINAL DROP**

This model proposes that there is negligible change in most people's cognitive functioning for most of their lives. A few months or a few years, however, before death, there occurs a marked decline or drop in their intellectual functioning. Several studies provide support for this notion (e.g. Palmore and Cleveland, 1976). Each successive older cohort will include more and more people likely to die within a few years and so this might explain some of the average and apparently gradual age deficits in cognitive processing. The way to check for this is to backtrack from the time of death for subjects in a longitudinal study to see how these individuals scored. Palmore and Cleveland did this and found evidence to support the model of terminal drop.

Jarvik (1983) developed this model to include the concept of *critical loss*: if declines on tests of intellect exceed certain levels then the probability of dying within a short time is greatly increased. Precisely what constitutes a critical decline, however, is not firmly established.

Another limitation of the terminal drop model is that it applies only to the young-old (those below 75 years) and not to the old-old (White and Cunningham, 1988). Stuart-Hamilton (1991) offers a plausible explanation for this. The young-old tend to die of specific illnesses or accidents. If this illness was in part caused by a sharp physical decline, then it is not surprising that psychological functions would also have been affected. The old-old, however, tend to die not so much from specific illnesses as from a gradual deterioration until one physiological system drops below a critical level. Because the decline happens slowly, it is unlikely to be mirrored in any sudden drop in psychological skills. As Stuart-Hamilton reflects, there is an exciting, if chilling, possibility offered by the terminal drop model (in spite of its present limitations): one day perhaps to be able to predict a terminal condition in a person from examining sudden changes in their psychometric scores!

---

1. *Sustained attention* is the term used to describe the ability to concentrate on a particular task over a period without being distracted. Salthouse (1982) reports that although there is some decline in this ability with age, it is not appreciable.
2. *Selective attention* involves the ability to focus attention on one task despite the presence of distractions. Evidence concerning the effects of ageing on this skill is inconclusive (see Rabbitt, 1979).
3. *Divided attention* describes the ability to attend simultaneously to more than one source of information. In many day-to-day activities we are called on to divide our attention, e.g. while preparing a meal and listening to the radio, while driving. Craik and Salthouse (1992) report the results of a meta-analysis of divided attention studies. This showed that there are age differences in the ability to carry out two or more tasks simultaneously. Such a conclusion helps to explain why elderly drivers have more accidents per mile driven than middle-aged drivers. These accidents take the form of sign, right of way and turning violations rather than speeding and other major offences (Sterns, Barrett and Alexander, 1985).

There are considerable differences of opinion among researchers in this area and these may be attributable to the different methodologies employed. Most, however, agree that age-related decrements do occur when multiple *complex* tasks are undertaken. The elderly, it appears, are victims of a loss of processing resources which limits their capacity to attend to as much as they did when younger (Salthouse, 1992).

DISCUSSION POINT
What are the implications of these findings on the attentional capacity of older people for the practising nurse?

Ageing and memory

(See Chapter 8 for a more detailed account of the memory process.)

Memory is usually thought of as a three-component process. It involves the encoding of information into the memory system, the storage of that information and the retrieval or recollection of that information. From time to time, we all experience problems with our memory. For instance, we forget a telephone number or an appointment. Seldom do these lapses cause concern – annoyance and embarrassment but not real alarm. Only when an 'appropriate' age is reached will an individual begin to wonder if experiences such as these herald the onset of old age or even senility. Age-based beliefs about memory may sensitize older people to be more aware of the same everyday memory failures that they have experienced all their lives. The stereotype of an elderly person often incorporates some notion of forgetfulness. How accurate a picture is this? Are memory deficits an inevitable consequence of the ageing process? Studies of ageing and memory have utilized different ways of modelling memory processes. A brief summary of some of the major models is given in Box 22.3.

The bulk of evidence suggests that short-term memory (STM) is relatively stable across adulthood, whereas certain aspects of long-term memory (LTM) are more prone to age-related decline (e.g. Craik, 1977). It has been suggested that where age deficits are found in STM, these may be due to the failure of elderly participants to use the best encoding and retrieval procedures spontaneously. Once aided or prodded to adopt more efficient methods, they perform as well as younger people.

General knowledge and memories about how to do things (see Box 22.3) are relatively unaffected by age. Such memories form part of crystallized intelligence. Where age changes in memory do occur these have been explained by some psychologists in terms of a decline in fluid intelligence. That is, a decline in the ability to process new information efficiently. However, Cockburn and Smith (1991) claim that such memory losses cannot always be satisfactorily explained in this way. Using 94 community dwelling people between the ages of 70 and 93 years, they showed that social and domestic activities provide a useful index for predicting verbal, visual and spatial memory performance, over and above the effects of fluid intelligence.

BOX 22.3 **SOME MODELS OF MEMORY**

The *dual memory theory* (Atkinson and Shiffrin, 1971) proposes a way of categorizing memories based on the length of time they are retained. Short- and long-term memory are seen as permanent structural components of the memory system. Short-term memory (STM) provides temporary storage of information. The majority of information held in STM fades rapidly. However, information to be retained can be transferred into long-term memory (LTM).

With their model of *working memory*, Baddeley and Hitch (1974) challenged the idea of a unitary STM. As a result of research designed to establish its function, they reached the following conclusion. STM acts as a working memory store that allows several pieces of information to be held in mind at the same time and to be used consciously. Working memory has a capacity based on time – about as many words as one can say in 2 seconds.

Tulving (1972) proposed that long-term memory could be divided into two types: episodic and semantic. *Episodic memory* (EM) is an autobiographical memory for events that happen in one's life. *Semantic memory* (SM) is one's store of general factual knowledge and is independent of personal experience. More recently, Tulving (1985) has added the concept of *procedural memory (PM)*. This term describes abilities such as motor skills or 'how to do' memories. EM is most vulnerable to central nervous system inefficiency and thus to ageing effects (see Chapter 8).

In relation to elderly people, there are two additional memory-related capacities which have attracted research interest. These are prospective memory and metamemory:

1. *Prospective memory* is one's ability to remember to remember (e.g. remembering to take medication). Several studies (e.g. Cockburn and Smith, 1991) have shown that this type of memory is vulnerable to ageing effects. This corresponds to the stereotyped image of the absent-minded older person. However, Moscovitch (1982) and Maylor (1990) have reported studies where older people were apparently better at remembering to carry out a future act previously agreed to. The key to their success seemed to lie in their taking more care than younger participants to set up reminders for themselves. It appears that while prospective memory abilities do seem to decline with age, older people often take measures to overcome this by active use of salient external cues such as calendars, lists, etc.

2. *Metamemory* refers to 'how much we know about what we know' (Lachman, Lachman and Thronesbery, 1979) and is an important aspect of memory, particularly in elderly people. Confidence in one's abilities will affect the amount of effort one devotes to trying to achieve certain goals. For example, if you believe that your memory is poor, you may rely heavily on passive memory aids such as lists and calendars, rather than employ active cognitive strategies, such as mnemonic devices.

Research findings on age differences in metamemory are mixed. Lachman and Lachman (1980), for instance, have found that older adults are as accurate in predicting what they can and cannot remember as younger adults. On the other hand, Murphy *et al.* (1981) found that older adults, compared with younger adults, tended to overestimate what they could remember. More recently, Rabbitt and Abson (1991: 148) reported on the metamemorial skills of 320 people aged between 50 and 79 years. Their data provide 'no evidence that . . . chronological age *per se* has any influence on optimism or accuracy of metamemory predictions'. Rather, they believe that the accuracy of individuals' assessments of their memory abilities declines with age-related changes in lifestyle and self-esteem. Such findings reinforce the belief of many that non-cognitive factors influence learning and memory in older people. Furthermore, Poon (1985) argues that by encouraging people to continue to use previously learned and demonstrably effective strategies and by promoting awareness of metamemory that we may enhance the memory performance of many older people.

DISCUSSION POINTS
If episodic memory is vulnerable to age-related deficits, how would you try:
(a) to slow down this process in a patient or client for whom you were caring?
(b) to help a patient or client overcome the effects of such deficits?
Use the information you have gained from this chapter, but also draw on your own experience, where possible.

Interventions using cognitive training

As we have seen, there is evidence for age-related decline in some areas of intellectual performance. To what extent can these declines be reversed by appropriate interventions? When considering the evidence on reversibility, one must also bear in mind the ethical issues that are raised, e.g. whether such reversal is always in the interest of the individual concerned or whether the high costs of training are the best use of limited resources.

Based on the disuse hypothesis of cognitive decline, cognitive training work has focused primarily upon psychometric abilities. Using participants from their Seattle Longitudinal Study, Schaie and Willis (1986) arranged training sessions for four groups of elderly adults, aged 64 to 95 years. Two groups had training in inductive reasoning and two had training in spatial reasoning. The majority of the participants showed improvement in both abilities. Willis (1989) claims that the results lend support to the idea that for many elderly people observed cognitive decline is attributable to disuse, and thus is remediable.

It is suggested that those people who showed no improvement lacked any reserve capacity to be actualized. Hayslip (1989) has scrutinized the findings from training in fluid intelligence tasks and concludes that individual differences are extensive in response to such programmes. Furthermore, he draws our attention to the need to explore their ecological validity.

Cognitive training interventions have interested psychologists for several reasons. Clearly, there is a desire to find ways of enhancing the cognitive performance of elderly people. Additionally, there is the potential for increasing our theoretical understanding of the cognitive ageing process. Further to this, Craik and Salthouse (1992) have summarized the empirical findings of cognitive training research under the three explanatory headings: limited processing resources; age-related slowing; and failure to inhibit.

Limited processing resources and explanations

This hypothesis proposes that there is a diminished pool of mental energy available to older adults, compared with younger adults. On this basis, the role of environmental supports to aid cognitive function is important. It has been suggested that information provided in pictorial format may help elderly adults, as complex picture recognition does not decline with age. Similarly, explicit explanations, not requiring subtle inferences to be made, are particularly beneficial to older people. Ways of limiting the processing requirements for elderly adults, especially when they are ill, requires more research attention.

Age-related slowing and information processing

With advanced age, the speed at which information is processed is reduced (Salthouse, 1985). Whatever the underlying cause, the effects of this phenomenon can be alleviated by permitting sufficient time for older people to absorb information. An alternative approach is to try, by means of cognitive training, to help elderly adults to speed up. Whichever approach is adopted, the result is unlikely to be the elimination of age differences in processing speed. Nevertheless, considerable improvement can be achieved for many.

Failure to inhibit

Rather than suffering from decreased processing resources, it has recently been proposed by Hasher and Zacks (1988) that elderly adults have faulty inhibitory mechanisms in working memory. That is, they are easily distracted by contextual irrelevancies and by internal musings which are only peripherally related to the task in hand. These distractions impede efficient processing of relevant information. Although findings are limited at present, this is a potentially fertile area for health professionals. Research in this area might inform the way in which advice, information and comfort are given to elderly patients and clients.

DISCUSSION POINT
How might knowledge about possible slowing, failure to inhibit and limited processing resources in elderly people influence the way a nurse might arrange to give advice, information or comfort to a patient or client?

This brings me to a note of caution sounded by Charness and Bosman (1990). It is often frail old people who most need cognitive interventions to help them understand instructions about medication, etc. However, most of what we know about cognitive functioning in elderly people is based on healthy samples. There is, therefore, a risk in generalizing findings from this population to the population most in need of help. One study has already established the kind of differences that can exist in cognitive functioning among elderly people depending upon their social and health status. Craik, Byrd and Swanson (1987) studied three groups of elderly adults: the active and affluent; the active and low income; and the less active and low income. The low income, less active group performed least well on memory, learning and word-generations tasks, and this same group benefited most from environmental supports. This finding is of practical importance for those who work with inactive or frail or ill people. Cognitive training work has tended to focus on healthy elderly individuals. What is needed now is a systematic evaluation of different supports and interventions with elderly people varying in their health status.

Ending on a positive note

In reading about age-related deficits and the need for cognitive supports and interventions, it is all too easy to form a pessimistic view of ageing. This would be unfortunate and unnecessary. Remember that Schaie's longitudinal study found few age-related declines in people's intellectual capacities before the age of 60 years. Most adults continue to use acquired knowledge in an effective manner throughout their later years. With increasing age, much of everyday experience depends less on fluid intelligence and more on specific domains of knowledge that are relevant to one's life at the time.

The role of expertise

Charness (1985) has shown that expert knowledge can compensate for general losses in processing speed and working memory. Older chess experts do not recall as many pieces from a briefly presented display of a game board as do younger chess experts, but they were found to be just as competent in choosing the best chess move from possible alternatives. Therefore, Charness concludes, older chess experts compensate for processing and memory deficits by bringing to bear retrieval structures that they have acquired over years of practice. The growth of these elaborate knowledge structures allows older experts to search for appropriate moves not just as deeply and quickly but also more proficiently than younger experts.

Salthouse (1984) has published comparable findings among typists. Older typists react more slowly, but overall typing speed is unaffected by age. This is the result of older typists compensating for decline in speed by looking further ahead and allowing themselves more time to plan what their next key stroke should be. These changes in ways of thinking and behaving can be construed as adaptational, rather than decremental. For practical purposes these adaptations equip most older adults to live independent and fulfilling lives.

Beliefs about development

Further evidence of the richness found in the thinking of many older adults comes from a study by Heckhausen, Dixon and Baltes (1989). They examined the belief systems of young, middle-aged and old adults about the nature of development. Three interesting findings emerged: (1) much inter-age consensus in expectations about the nature of adult development; (2) adult development perceived to be multidirectional, with both growth and decline in intellectual ageing; and (3) older adults held more elaborate views about development than younger adults, i.e. at increasing age levels, adults viewed development as increasingly multifaceted. The authors interpret this finding of increased differentiation concerning the nature of development as an index of 'continuing evolution of the knowledge system that adults acquire about the nature of lifespan development'. This can be seen as intellectual growth with age and can be set against the relatively small scale decrements found in psychometric studies.

Conclusion

In day-to-day activities, an elderly person need not be disadvantaged by some minor declines. The wisdom accrued by experience is more than sufficient to offset any slight reduction in speed of cognitive processing. It is when an elderly person faces the stress of illness or disability that these age-related decrements may become more significant. Well-informed nurses can use their knowledge about age-related cognitive changes to benefit elderly people in their care.

Summary

This chapter began by looking at the different ways in which age can be defined: biological, psychological, social, functional and normal versus pathological. After the procedures and limitations of the cross-sectional and longitudinal research methods were outlined, the cross-sequential method devised by Schaie was discussed.

Studies of cognitive ageing in three areas were summarized:

1. What happens to intelligence as we age? No reliable decrements can be seen before age 60.
2. Does ageing affect our ability to attend? Findings are mixed, but there appears to be some loss of attentional capacity.
3. Does memory deteriorate with age? Different types of memory are considered and reasons for some of the age-related memory decrements are considered.

The findings from some cognitive training programmes were outlined and theoretical explanations proposed. The chapter reached the conclusion that the minor declines experienced by some people after the age of 60 can easily be offset by experience and sensible planning so that daily living is not impaired.

Seminar questions

1. What skills have you noticed that older people possess that compensate for any loss of cognitive speed?
2. Under what circumstances, would you consider it appropriate to encourage an elderly patient or client to:
   (a) try to improve their active cognitive strategies for remembering?
   (b) rely on environmental aids to help memory?
   In addition to using lists and calendars, what other aids would you suggest to help a person living at home?
3. Do you think it is an appropriate use of resources to spend money on interventions to help the cognitive functioning of older people?

Further reading

Stuart-Hamilton, I. (1991) *The Psychology of Ageing: An introduction.* London: Jessica Kingsley. A book that succeeds in being both detailed and concise. Ageing and intelligence, memory, language and personality are covered in a highly accessible fashion.

A number of more demanding texts are available to those who feel they would like to tackle the complexities of this area. I recommend Birren, J.E. and Schaie, K.W. (eds.) (1990) *Handbook of the Psychology of Ageing.* London: Academic Press. This is the third edition of their handbook and provides an authoritative review of and reference source for the topic of ageing.

References

Atkinson, R.C. and Shiffrin, R.M. (1971) 'The control of short-term memory', *Scientific American* **224**, 82–90.

Baddeley, A.D. and Hitch, G. (1974) 'Working memory', in G.A. Bower (ed.) *Recent Advances in Learning and Motivation*, Vol. 8. London: Academic Press.

Birren, J.E. (1968) 'Psychological aspects of aging: Intellectual functioning', *Gerontologist* **8**, 16–19.

Birren, J.E. and Renner, V.J. (1977) 'Research on the psychology of aging: Principles and experimentation', in J.E. Birren and K.W. Schaie (eds.) *Handbook of the Psychology of Aging*, 2nd edition. New York: Van Nostrand Reinhold.

Birren, J.E. and Schaie, K.W. (eds.) (1990) *Handbook of the Psychology of Aging*, 2nd edition. New York: Van Nostrand Reinhold.

Botwinick, J. and Siegler, I. (1980) 'Intellectual ability among the elderly: Simultaneous cross-sectional and longitudinal comparisons', *Developmental Psychology* **16**, 49–53.

Bromley, D.B. (1988) *Human Ageing: An introduction to gerontology*. London: Pelican Books.

Cattell, R.B. (1963) 'Theory of fluid and crystallized intelligence', *Journal of Educational Psychology* **54**, 1–22.

Charness, N. (ed) (1985) *Aging and Human Performance: Studies in human performance*. New York: John Wiley.

Charness, N. and Bosman, E.A. (1990) 'Human factors and design for older adults', in J.E. Birren and K.W. Schaie (eds.) *Handbook of the Psychology of Ageing*, 3rd edition, London: Academic Press.

Cockburn, J. and Smith, P.T. (1991) 'The relative influence of intelligence and age on everyday memory', *Journal of Gerontology* **46**, 31–6.

Craik, F.I.M. (1977) 'Age differences in human memory', in J.E. Birren and K.W. Schaie (eds.) *Handbook of the Psychology of Aging*, 2nd edition. New York: Van Nostrand Reinhold.

Craik, F.I.M., Byrd, M. and Swanson, J. (1987) 'Patterns of memory loss in three elderly samples', *Psychology and Aging* **2**, 79–86.

Craik, F.I.M. and Salthouse, T.A. (eds.) (1992) *The Handbook of Aging and Cognition*. Hillsdale, NJ: Lawrence Erlbaum.

Cunningham, W.R. (1987) 'Intellectual abilities and age', in K.W. Schaie (ed.) *Annual Review of Gerontology and Geriatrics*, Vol. 7. New York: Springer.

Hasher, L. and Zacks, R.T. (1988) 'Working memory: Comprehension and aging. A review and a new view', in G.H. Bower (ed.) *The Psychology of Learning and Motivation*, Vol. 22. London: Academic Press.

Hayslip, B. (1989) 'Fluid ability training with aged people: A past with a future?' *Educational Gerontology* **15**, 573–95.

Heckhausen, J., Dixon, R.A. and Baltes, P.B. (1989) 'Gains and losses in development throughout adulthood as perceived by different adult age groups', *Developmental Psychology* **25**, 109–21.

Horn, J.L. (1970) 'Organisation of data on lifespan development of human abilities', in R.L. Goulet and P.B. Baltes (eds.) *Lifespan Developmental Psychology*. London: Academic Press.

Jarvik, L.F. (1983) 'Age is in: Is the wit out?' in D. Samuel, S. Algeri, S. Gershon, V.E. Grimm and G. Toffani (eds.) *Aging of the Brain*. New York: Raven Press.

Lachman, M.E. (1983) 'Perceptions of intellectual aging: Antecedent or consequence of intellectual functioning?' *Developmental Psychology* **19**, 482–98.

Lachman, J.l., Lachman, R. and Thronesbery, C. (1979) 'Metamemory through the adult lifespan', *Developmental Psychology* **15**, 543–51.

Lachman, R. and Lachman, J.L. (1980) 'Age and the actualisation of world knowledge', in L.W. Poon, J.L. Fozard, L.S. Cermak, D. Arenberg and L.W. Thompson (eds.) *New Directions in Memory and Aging*. Hillsdale, NJ.: Lawrence Erlbaum.

Maylor, E.A. (1990) 'Age and prospective memory', *Quarterly Journal of Experimental Psychology* **42**, 471–93.

Moscovitch, M. (1982) 'A neuropsychological approach to perception and memory in normal and pathological aging', in F.I.M. Craik and S. Trehub (eds.) *Aging and Cognitive Processes*, New York: Plenum Press.

Murphy, M.D., Sanders, R.E., Gabrieski, A.S. and Schmitt, F.A. (1981) 'Metamemory in the aged', *Journal of Gerontology* **36**, 185–93.

Palmore, E. and Cleveland, W. (1976) 'Aging, terminal decline and terminal drop', *Journal of Gerontology* **31**, 76–81.

Perlmuter, L.C., Tun, P., Sizer, N., McGlinchey, R.E. and Nathan, D.M. (1987) 'Age and diabetes-related changes in verbal fluency', *Experimental Aging Research* **13**, 9–14.

Poon, L.W. (1985) 'Differences in human memory with aging: Nature, causes and clinical implications', in J.E. Birren and K.W. Schaie (eds.) *Handbook of the Psychology of Aging*, 2nd edition. New York: Van Nostrand Reinhold.

Rabbitt, P.M.A. (1979) 'Some experiments and a model for changes in attentional selectivity with old age', in F. Hoffmeister and C. Muller (eds.) *Bayer Symposium VII: Evaluation of Change*. New York: Springer.

Rabbitt, P. and Abson, V. (1990) ' "Lost and found": Some logical and methodological limitations of self-report questionnaires as tools to study cognitive ageing', *British Journal of Psychology* **81**, 1–16.

Rabbitt, P. and Abson, V. (1991) 'Do older people know how good they are?' *British Journal of Psychology* **82**, 137–51.

Riegel, K.F. and Riegel, R.M. (1972) 'Development, drop and death', *Developmental Psychology* **6**, 306–19.

Rinn, W.E. (1988) 'Mental decline in normal aging: A review', *Journal of Geriatric Psychiatry and Neurology* **1**, 144–58.

Salthouse, T.A. (1982) *Adult Cognition: An experimental psychology of human aging*. New York: Springer-Verlag.

Salthouse, T.A. (1984) 'Effects of age and skill on typing', *Journal of Experimental Psychology: General* **113**, 345–71.

Salthouse, T.A. (1985) 'Speed of behaviour and its implications for cognition', in J.E. Birren and K.W. Schaie (eds.) *Handbook of the Psychology of Aging*, 2nd edition. New York: Van Nostrand Reinhold.

Salthouse, T.A. (1991) *Theoretical Perspectives on Cognitive Aging*. Hillsdale, NJ: Lawrence Erlbaum.

Schaie, K.W. (1965) 'A general model for the study of developmental problems', *Psychological Bulletin* **64**, 92–107.

Schaie, K.W. (ed.) (1983) *Longitudinal Studies of Adult Psychological Development*. New York: Guilford.

Schaie, K.W. (1984) 'Midlife influences upon intellectual functioning in old age', *International Journal of Behavioural Development* **7**, 463–78.

Schaie, K.W. (1989) 'Individual differences in rate of cognitive change in adulthood', in V.L. Bengston and K.W. Schaie (eds.) *The Course of Later Life: Research and reflections*. New York: Springer.

Schaie, K.W. and Willis, S.L. (1986) 'Can decline in intellectual adult functioning be reversed?' *Developmental Psychology* **22**, 223–32.

Siegler, I.C. and Costa, P.T. (1985) 'Health behaviour relationships', in J.E. Birren and K.W. Schaie (eds.) *Handbook of the Psychology of Aging*, 2nd edition. New York: Van Nostrand Reinhold.

Sterns, H.L., Barrett, G.V. and Alexander, R.A. (1985) 'Accidents and the aging individual', in J.E. Birren and K.W. Schaie (eds.) *Handbook of the Psychology of Aging*, 2nd edition. New York: Van Nostrand Reinhold.

Stuart-Hamilton, I. (1991) *The Psychology of Ageing: An introduction.* London: Jessica Kingsley.

Thurstone, L.L. (1938) 'Primary mental abilities', *Psychometric Monographs No 1*.

Tulving, E. (1972) 'Episodic and semantic memory', in E. Tulving and W. Donaldson (eds.) *Organisation of Memory.* London: Academic Press.

Tulving, E. (1985) 'How many memory systems are there?' *American Psychologist* **40**, 385–98.

Welford, A.T. (1966) 'Industrial work suitable for older people: Some British studies', *Gerontologist* **6**, 4–9.

White, N. and Cunningham, W.R. (1988) 'Is terminal drop pervasive or specific?' *Journal of Gerontology* **43**, 141–4.

Willis, S.L. (1989) 'Improvement with cognitive training: Which old dogs learn what tricks?' in L.W. Poon, D.C. Rubin and B.A. Wilson (eds.) *Everyday Cognition in Adulthood and Late Life.* Cambridge: Cambridge University Press.

CHAPTER 23

Wellbeing in later life

VALERIE FISHER

Chapter outline

> They know the literature but not the life
> Malcolm Cowley (1976: ix)

Introduction

Evidence shows that the mean age of the population in the United Kingdom is increasing. Evidence also shows that most older people's perception of their quality of life differs little from that expressed by younger age groups (Ryff, 1989a). However, old age is characterized negatively, especially by young people, and Skeet (1985) refers to 'deeply rooted discrimination against the elderly' occurring in some health care professionals. This chapter aims to demystify some of the commonly held negative stereotypes concerning ageing by examining the research which reveals the way ageing can be a positive psychological period of the lifecycle. In addition, contemporary approaches to nursing care involving empowerment and advocacy in relation to elderly people will be considered.

Aims of the chapter

This chapter addresses three issues: it will (1) explore the myths of ageing and examine successful ageing from a psychological perspective; (2) study health perceptions in later life by considering some of the recent research on the views of older adults; and (3) use current research and discussion about quality ageing to examine the role of the nurse and other health care professionals in managing adaptation and change in later life.

Demographic trends indicate a society in which older people will be increasingly numerous. By the year 2021, nearly 20 per cent of the population will be over 65 years compared with only 10 per cent in 1951, and this trend is set to persist (Central Statistical Office, 1993). However, the consequent demands on the health and social care systems are continuously portrayed as a negative 'add-on' to what should be considered to be a major social and individual achievement. What is often ignored in this scenario are the possible medical advances that may either delay the onset of many chronic illnesses suffered by older people or ameliorate the effects of illness and impairment. Added to this is an increased awareness among middle-aged and older people that their health potential in later life is, to some extent, within their control, making later life a time to be positively rather than negatively valued. Overall, life expectancy continues to grow: 'By the end of the century, we may regard anyone who dies before the age of 80 as having died prematurely' (Russell, 1989). This chapter will take a fresh look at the health potential of older people by using both the scientific evidence available, as well as drawing on the perceptions of older people themselves. It will also consider nursing strategies that in the future will be increasingly focused on the promotion of quality ageing rather than on the care of sick and dying individuals.

The experience of ageing is universal, but it is a period of life about which persistent myths and negative attributes abound (Wetle, 1991; see also Chapter 25). Past research on ageing has concentrated on the negative physical, mental and social loss which is characteristic of some individual's ageing process (Rowe and Kahn 1987), without reflecting on the positive and valued aspects of ageing expressed by elderly people themselves (Ryff, 1989a).

Myths of ageing

Common stereotypes applied to older people imply they are sick, sedentary, sexless, senile and impoverished. This collection of negative stereotypes, coined by Butler (1969) as *ageism,* is damaging, not just because we believe in them but because we behave as though they were true. These attitudes can permeate nursing care through actions (such as performing functions the older person is capable of achieving unaided) and omissions (such as talking about older people with accompanying relatives rather than addressing the older people themselves), both of which can undermine the confidence of older people and increase their dependence.

Wetle (1991) discusses these stereotypes as four common myths of ageing. In considering the evidence for these myths systematically it is difficult to understand why they should occur:

Myth 1: Elderly people are sick and sedentary

It is a fact that older people are not as healthy as younger people. However, the evidence does not suggest that older people are sick; rather, that the health problems of older people are inclined to be chronic (such as hypertension, arthritis or hearing loss), while the health problems of young people are inclined to be acute (such as infectious diseases). This is confirmed by GP consultancy rates in older age groups: in 1991 the average number of GP contacts per person per year was four for those aged between 16 and 64 years, and only two more for those over 65 years (Bridgewood and Savage, 1991). Chronic conditions of older people are not necessarily disabling and it is the individual's own perception of health that defines personal wellbeing rather than the criteria set by health care professionals. Indeed, Cartwright and Smith (1988) report that 60 per cent of elderly people regard their health as 'good for their age', while the research of van Maanen (1988) shows that 'the older the person, the more emphasis was placed on health as a state of mind, even in situations of a gradually failing body'. To compensate for physical impairment brought about by ageing processes, older people pace their daily routine.

Myth 2: Elderly people are sexless

There is a persistent myth that interest in sex and sexual activity disappears with age, whereas health statistics show the opposite. Kinsey's renowned reports on male and female sexuality (1948, 1953), which were based on the verbal sexual histories of more than 10,000 voluntary respondents, showed that most females maintained an interest in sexual relations until their 60s. Males in sound physical and mental health can expect adequate sexual performance beyond 80 years of age (Travis, 1987).

However, negative attributes are often given to men who express an interest in sexual matters (e.g. being labelled as 'dirty old men'). In addition, older women are often seen as undesirable and asexual. This labelling can result in both males and females being shamed into concealing their sexuality or sexual interest to the point where they begin to see themselves as quaint and ultimately as sexless individuals. The expression of love/emotional bonding, sexual activity and its enjoyment in later life, coupled with a desire for companionship and greater economic security, should lead to an increase in remarriage and cohabitation. However, statistics indicate a growing number of older people living in single households (Bridgewood and Savage, 1991) who therefore miss the benefits to health and wellbeing that positive relationships with a significant other can bring.

Myth 3: Elderly people are senile

There is a general lack of recognition that decline in intellectual ability which interferes with daily living is generally due to disease (e.g. stroke, Parkinson's disease, Alzheimer's disease) and is not due to ageing. The research on the effects of ageing on cognitive functioning, especially memory, remains inconclusive, although longitudinal studies produce more positive results, in terms of limited or reversible decline, than do cross-sectional studies (Craik and Jennings 1992; Rybash, Roodin and Santrock, 1991; see also Chapter 22).

Often, decline in memory is what troubles older people most. The majority of older people report that their memory is 'not what it was'; however, few report that any decline in memory interferes with daily living (Wetle, 1991). (See Chapter 22 for further discussion of memory changes associated with ageing.) Despite these findings, the prevalent lay view is that memory at least goes downhill with age, that memory decline is an inevitable part of the ageing process and that memory loss is uncontrollable and irreversible.

Another aspect of senility is depression. Although, statistically, depression increases with age, Costa, McCrea and Locke (1990) see it as puzzling that neuroticism does not, even though the two variables are highly correlated. They explain this by drawing attention to some common symptoms of depression that are the same as the physical and cognitive changes associated with ageing; for example, poor sleep patterns, decrease in appetite and a lack of concentration. The inference to be drawn is that depression in older people can be misdiagnosed if these and similar criteria are used.

Myth 4: Elderly people are impoverished

Despite radical changes in longevity, we continue to hold beliefs about old age that are more appropriate to the living conditions of an earlier, harsher industrialized society. With the spread of occupational pensions schemes, financial security in later life is being assured for an increasing number of individuals. On average, a quarter of a person's life is spent after occupational retirement and at present the majority rely on statutory provision (state/old age pension) as their main and only source of income. The level at which state pension is paid is crucial to wellbeing in later life and it is important that older people are financially cushioned against the negative effects of poverty on health (Whitehead, 1987).

Interestingly, despite economic indices showing that the income of older people in Britain compares badly with their European and North American counterparts (Hedstrom and Ringen, 1987), some studies demonstrate that their income is not a source of concern for many older people. Melanson and Downe-Wambold (1987) show that 96 per cent of their older respondents felt their income was adequate. This may be because all the respondents had the benefit of low home rental costs or had completed mortgage repayments. Another study by Kaplan et al. (1987) shows that although the relationship between low socioeconomic position and mortality and morbidity is strong in those below 60 years of age, for those over 60, there was no risk associated with inadequate income compared with very adequate income.

DISCUSSION POINT
Discuss the ways in which negative stereotypes applied to older people may affect their day-to-day life.

What is successful ageing?

Qualitative and quantitative criteria for successful ageing would include the following dimensions: length of life, physical and mental health, cognitive effectiveness, social capability and productivity, personal control and life satisfaction. Owing to the complexity of these dimensions, gerontologists, researchers and health care professionals often disagree about the direct causal relationship between variables and successful ageing. One thing that is usually agreed is that longevity in itself is not the ultimate definition of successful ageing. Furthermore, there is increasing evidence to suggest that the objective criteria of academics and professionals do not adequately address the subjective perception of successful ageing held by older people themselves (Heidrich and D'Amico, 1993; Ryff, 1989b; van Maanen 1988; see also Chapter 22). In addition, there has been an implicit negativism in many previous approaches to successful ageing. That is, research has been conducted with measures of illness, rather than measures of wellbeing (Ryff, 1989b). A related trend has been to equate positive functioning in later life with continuance of previous attitudes and behaviours, rather than the successful management of new experiences and challenges.

Ryff (1989b) in reviewing the literature on wellbeing describes six dimensions of positive functioning that are referred to repeatedly by various authors: *self-acceptance*, *positive relations with others*, *autonomy*, *environmental mastery*, *purpose in life* and *personal growth*. In exploring these dimensions one can recognize their applicability to the perceptions of older people concerning successful ageing:

1. *Self-acceptance.* The perception of later life as a period of tranquillity and calm, prominent in Eastern ideals of old age, is rarely emphasized in Western culture. Yet self-acceptance, a positive attitude towards the self, an acceptance of good and bad personal qualities and a positive feeling about past life, is shown to be important to older people's feelings of fulfilment, happiness and satisfaction (Ryff, 1989a, 1989b). For nurses and health care professionals, the recognition that older adults may benefit as much as younger adults from therapeutic counselling may facilitate the process of adjustment and acceptance required to achieve a tranquil old age.
2. *Positive relations with others.* Ryff (1989a) has investigated the personal perspective of older people about wellbeing. She demonstrated that older

individuals considered a person to be well adjusted if they were 'other oriented' (having positive relations with others, caring about others). Poorly adjusted individuals were reported by older people as being self-centred, cranky and complaining. Many older people value being seen as caring, being liked by others and feeling appreciated. Nurses and health care professionals, therefore, should use their interpersonal skills to enhance older people's feelings of self-worth and use their counselling skills to empower older people to ameliorate difficult or damaged relationships.

3. *Autonomy* includes self-determination, independence, the self-regulation of personal standards and a sense of control. Research in the area of autonomy and its loss show that a lack of control has adverse effects on emotional states, performance, subjective wellbeing and on physiological indicators (Rodin, 1986). The professional carer can help an older person to appreciate more autonomy by facilitating greater individual control of the physical, emotional and social aspects of their life. An older person should be given information about such items as local transport provision for older people, the use and availability of aids to daily living, without decisions being made for them. If nurses and health care professionals, through the best of intentions, usurp the decision-making responsibilities of older people, it will result in their clients being more concerned with the evaluation and judgement of others as well as increasing their dependence and decreasing their sense of control.

4. *Environmental mastery*. This dimension relates to the ability to manage a complex array of activities in the physical, mental and social realms. This mastery is typical in middle-aged people who manage a wide array of personal, occupational, family and social demands. With increased age the opportunity for this breadth of mastery diminishes, especially with the increase in chronic disability and general health impairment. However, with appropriate treatment most elderly people are able adapt and continue to live active and productive lives. Nurses and other professional carers can also assist by enabling the older person to understand and accept the current changes and developments in the 'wider' world by engaging in discussion with older people on topical news reports, social trends and contemporary mores.

5. *Purpose in life*. The individual who is functioning positively has goals in life, a sense of direction and positive intentions. Lack of purpose has a negative effect on mental health, intellectual efficiency and a sense of control (Lachman, 1986). If older adults can be enabled to reflect on their past life experiences, both positive and negative, they may be able to adapt to the challenge of defining new roles to take the place of those lost through time. The use professional carers make of older people as resources for, rather than recipients of, support, would encourage a mutual sense of interdependence between age groups. This could be achieved by encouraging older people, within the limits of their capacity, to become actively involved in functions that they see as valuable or meaningful to society (e.g. encouraging the use of past professional and occupational skills in community initiatives).

6. *Personal growth*. The ability of the professional carer to reduce feelings of personal stagnation, boredom and lack of interest in life which pervades the perception of some older people is a challenge which in practice is difficult to meet. However, even for older people, life is not a fixed state and personal growth can be appreciated in even the most simple of achievements. The skill of the professional carer is to enable older individuals to identify new and forgotten personal aspirations and to recognize and harness their individual potential for the achievement of appropriate goals.

In the future, one of nursing's goals will be the promotion and maintenance of the health and wellbeing of the older age group. In order to accomplish this goal, there is a need for nurses to understand how older adults perceive themselves and the world in which they live (Magnani, 1990). However, Biggs (1992) has identified a number of factors that might obscure practitioner's perception of old age. First, lack of personal experience of old age makes empathy more difficult to achieve – nurses and other health care professionals may have theoretical and professional understandings of ageing but this cannot be equated to personal experience. Second, power differences between service users and practitioners might influence whose agendas are addressed – scarcity of resources, including manpower, may make professional carers provide care based on their assessment of need rather than the expressed needs of older people themselves. Third, health care workers mainly have contact with those older adults who are requiring help, moving professional

---

BOX 23.1 EXERCISE ABOUT YOUR VIEWS OF OLDER ADULTS

Think of a person over 75 years of age with whom you have had recent contact. Make a list describing that person in terms of their abilities, signs of health, intellectual and emotional capacities and social activities. To give some weighting to these qualities, score each item on your list from 1 to 10 (where 10 equals excellent, and 1 equals poor).

Now make another list describing the person in terms of their illnesses, physical and mental impairments and chronic disabilities. Score each item as above.

Consider

- Which list was easier to compile and score?
- Did you score the older person more highly for positive or negative psychological and health attributes?
- How do you think the older person would have scored themselves?
- Was your list or score affected by negative stereotyping?

How do you think you will be at this age? Review your list as if you had reached 75 years of age and score yourself using the same criteria? If your score is different, what are the reasons for this?

understanding from a 'healthy' model of ageing to a 'sick' model of ageing; that is, towards an unrepresentative sample of the ageing population.

Before moving on reflect on what you have read, by completing the exercise in Box 23.1.

Health perceptions in later life

As previously discussed, lay beliefs hold that older adults suffer from numerous chronic illness and functional health limitations (Heidrich and D'Amico, 1993). General expectations among young elderly people (those less than 65 years of age), of poor physical health in old age may be partly due to negative stereotypes about old age. However, the health perception of older adults about themselves is not always negative and is linked with their general life satisfaction, social integration and mental health (Heidrich and D'Amico, 1993). This section will explore older people's perceptions about the continuum from health to illness. It will discuss how older people express satisfaction with their physical health, accepting positively the general physical impairment associated with age. In comparison, the concerns of older people about possible mental impairment in old age (derived from stereotypical images of senile dementia) will be reviewed and the effects of the commonly experienced psychosocial events associated with longevity that impact and impinge on mental health will be considered.

Older people's perception of their physical health and the effects of ageing

For most older people the adage 'you are as old as you feel' appears to be accurate. This view is frequently given in the literature concerning subjective views on health status in later life. The perception of health encompasses feelings, both positive and negative, as well as subjective definitions of personal fitness, illness, ailments, etc. Although self-perceived health and actual health status (based on a doctor's assessment) have had a high positive correlation, Magnani (1990) has asserted that too much weight may be placed on objective assessments and the conviction that subjective and objective assessments have to correlate in order for the subjective assessment to be valid. More recently, it has been recognized that how older people feel subjectively is equally, and at times even more, important than how they *should* feel objectively. Seedhouse (1986) in attempting to answer the question 'what is health?' states:

> People cannot be fully understood in isolation from what they do with their lives. Also people cannot be fully understood in only biological terms. . . . The idea that health is a specific, definable, fully describable state to which everyone can aspire equally is nonsense.

It is how individuals define or describe their health that should be the indicator of psychological wellbeing in older people, rather than an imposed medical or professional definition.

Heidrich and D'Amico (1993) sampled 37 over 80-year-olds who rated their health as generally good, reporting low levels of symptomatology and high levels of functional ability. The respondents were optimistic in terms of their health and anticipated future health to be about the same as their 'good' present health. A much larger study of the health perceptions of 889 older adults in senior citizens' public housing accommodation, demonstrated that only 6 per cent reported their health as poor (Melanson and Downe-Wamboldt, 1987). Another study by Schank and Lough (1990) demonstrated that in a sample of frail elderly women living independently, 70 per cent perceived their health to be good, 30 per cent fair and 80 per cent of the sample thought their health better than others of the same age. These findings do not imply that older people do not experience physical limitations and discomfort brought on by ageing, rather that their general optimism enables them to regard any health impairment as marginal to a broader experience of good health. However, the findings do exemplify the general perception of older adults that functional impairment is an acceptable part of growing old and is not seen as impinging on their 'health' in general. Furthermore, Cartwright and Smith (1988), in reporting that 60 per cent of elderly people regarded their health as 'good for their age', illustrate the widely held ageist view that 'health' itself declines with age (but see Chapter 6 on unrealistic optimism). The use of old age as a benchmark against which to derive standards of expected health is in itself a negative stereotype, with no other age range carrying this type of characterization.

Even with some functional impairment and age-related difficulties, many old people perceive life as satisfying, happy and meaningful. This suggests that it is not ageing *per se*, but perceptions about physical health and functioning, that are important factors in the quality of life of the older person (Heidrich and D'Amico, 1993). However, what appears to be a greater area of concern to young elderly people is their mental health in later life. They are influenced by the ageist stereotyping associating forgetfulness, emotional stress (e.g. resulting from bereavement) and mild depression as signs of incipient senile dementia.

Older people's perception of their mental health functioning and the effects of ageing versus traumatic life events

Older adults' views about the possible effects of age on cognitive ability is affected by commonly held misperceptions. Relatives, health care professionals and older people themselves tend to overestimate the magnitude and the significance of the memory problems experienced by the older adult. Lachman's (1986, Lachman and Leff 1989) research on personal control demonstrates that older people ascribed their forgetfulness to self-defeating or pessimistic causes over which they have no control, such as ageing or Alzheimer's disease. In contrast, younger people ascribed the same difficulty in more positive terms, such as to not paying attention, over which they do have control. With ageing, there may be a normal decline in the ability to remember information. This type of benign forgetfulness does not seriously affect older people's ability to function in everyday life and need not be perceived by them as a health problem nor as a sign of incipient loss of their senses (van Maanen, 1988).

A more significant feature of ageing, in terms of both physical and mental health perceptions, are the problems of loneliness and loss. Lonely older adults tend to report poorer health and are comparatively less happy and less satisfied with their lives than their non-lonely counterparts (Ribeiro, 1989). However, these mental health problems are the result of the loneliness and not the result of ageing *per se*. Indeed, loneliness is positively related to poor health and negatively related to happiness and spiritual wellness in *all* age groups (Ribeiro, 1989).

The most commonly experienced loss in later life, resulting in loneliness, is bereavement, and the rise in mortality and morbidity among bereaved individuals has been extensively reported over many years. Interestingly, the negative effects of bereavement on both physical and mental health seem to lessen with age (see Chapter 17). This is possibly because older adults expect to encounter grief and hence develop a readiness to cope with it (Rowe and Kahn, 1987). While older adults coping with bereavement show higher rates of reported ill-health, the measures of morbidity among bereaved elderly people do not show a significant increase in ill-health (i.c. changes in diagnosis patterns of major disease, increased doctor's visits or hospitalization). This suggests first, that older adults' ability to cope with existing ill-health or disability is lessened with the experience of loss, rather than the fact that ill-health itself increases following a bereavement; and second, that physical health perception is affected by mental wellbeing in elderly bereaved people.

Further commonly cited losses in later life are those associated with retirement and relocation. The associated loss of friendship and companionship, which is shown to have a detrimental effect on older adults' feelings of wellbeing and social worth (Rowe and Kahn, 1987; Ryff, 1989a), add to the emotional stress of ageing. However, despite these major life events, in general older adults perceive less stress in their lives than do younger adults. This is most probably due to their increased ability, gained though experience, to deal with the negative effects of life events (Ryff, 1989a). In summary, older people seem able to cope better, in terms of their mental health functioning, with the stress caused by major life events than their younger counterparts; and while the young elderly are concerned with deterioration in mental function in later life, any deterioration is usually well managed by older people themselves.

Although psychological stress may have less effect on the physical health of older people than young people, numerous studies have shown that poor health has negative effects on psychological wellbeing. This is regardless of age, and poor physical health has a greater impact on mental health in very old people than in other age group (Heidrich, 1993).

Heidrich's (1993) study revealed that those older people who rated their actual health as much worse than their ideal health had lower levels of psychological wellbeing, lower incomes, were less likely to be married and more likely to be living alone. Indeed, the study showed nearly a two-fold difference in the rating of general health indicators in those older people who were depressed. Depression emerged as a significant problem for 24 per cent of the sample and was strongly related to physical health problems. However, clinically depressed elderly people appeared to be quite different from the non-depressed or those experiencing stress, in terms of their physical health and functioning. Those who were reported a two-fold increase in health-related difficulties and health problems (Heidrich, 1993). Indeed, Heidrich (1993) suggests that a subjective assessment of physical health status by the very old may be for nurses a more reliable indicator of depression than other expressed symptoms, as very old people appear to have difficulty in identifying themselves as depressed.

In summary, as individuals age, increasing limitations are placed on their physical capacity and it could be expected that older people would be less optimistic and confident about their future wellbeing and life satisfaction. However, older people's perceptions of their health and the effects of ageing on them are mediated by a greater emphasis on affective definitions of wellbeing rather than cognitive and psychomotor. Van Maanen (1988) showed that, for Americans, health appeared to be 'a state of mind' with responses focusing on positive attributes, mainly in terms of psychological and social functioning. Changing perceptions of health, from cognitive and psychomotor definitions to a more affective definition commence in middle age. Ryff (1989a) revealed the importance that middle-aged respondents gave to self-confidence, self-acceptance and self-knowledge in defining wellbeing, with older people citing the acceptance of change as an important quality of positive functioning. It should be recognized that the psychological disposition of older people 'reflect the ability and inner strength to focus on positive attributes in a world of diminishing prospects' (van Maanen, 1988: 705).

In conclusion, it appears that the essence of health and wellbeing in later life is not necessarily the quantity and quality of physical impairments experienced but rather it is the ability of individuals to adapt effectively to the numerous and often unpredictable changes which occur as later life progresses.

DISCUSSION POINT
Discuss how older people might prepare themselves to manage the major changes in later life.

Managing adaptation and change in later life: the role of the nurse and health care professional

This final section explores health enhancement of older adults through the process of empowerment. It considers the dynamics of the communication process with and between older adults as a means of promoting wellbeing. The section concludes by considering a model for optimizing successful ageing from a psychological perspective. By focusing on those factors which contribute to quality ageing and by minimizing risk factors which lead to disease and disability in later life, it shows how health care professionals can enhance the opportunities for older people to experience the healthy, satisfying, productive time that old age can be.

Empowerment and advocacy

Power is associated with *autonomy* which, in today's society, as Drevdahl (1989) has shown, is related to financial security (a good proportion of older adults' income is at subsistence level); *productivity* (retirement means that older adults are not productive in relation to the wider economy); *knowledge* (the knowledge explosion, especially in technology, means much of the older adults learned wisdom is obsolete); *kinship* and *family* (with the death of peers, the older adult increasing has to rely on younger family members who have their own lives to lead); and *community life* (decreased mobility and physical impairment often means older adults cannot participate in community activity).

The role of the professional carer is to enable older individuals to have independence and control over decisions and directives that impinge on their quality of life. In undertaking this responsibility, the professional carer must focus on the personal beliefs and affiliations of the older adult as well as considering wider physical and psychological health care needs. For instance, an older person who has in earlier years been content with an introverted or reclusive lifestyle will not benefit or want to be socialized into a peer group with which he has no affiliation. Likewise, an older adult, who recognizes the benefit of regular exercise, but has never seen it as part of her lifestyle, will not want to be cajoled into undertaking activities to improve her mobility but which in the short term may cause fatigue and discomfort. The health care professional must be sensitive to the individual wishes, needs and constraints of the older person concerning health. Providing health information targetted at the age, sex and ethnicity of the individual will increase the knowledge and promote the choices available to individuals.

As advocate, the nurse's role is to 'open doors' for older people to enable them to continue to develop and use their potential as valued members of society. In acting as an advocate, a nurse must recognize that she does not make decisions for her clients but empowers them to make those decisions for themselves. By providing the information older people need and by informing them of various aspects to be considered, the professional carer allows older people to make informed decisions and to be more fully in control of their health and life. Projects have been developed by health care workers to teach assertiveness techniques to older adults and to enable them to protect and promote their own rights in decision-making, especially with regard to treatment of illness or disability when consulting general practitioners, nurses and other members of the primary health care team. An example of this type of strategy is Waterloo Pensioner's Health Group which uses role play between older people to increase their confidence in talking to their doctor. Many positive initiatives such as this have been set up by Age Concern as part of their Age Well campaign.

Communication, empowerment and advocacy

Effective communication is central to empowerment and advocacy in all age groups. In communicating with older people it is important for health care professionals to consider whether different communicative devices, commonly used by younger people when communicating with old people, affect the ability of older people to be self-determining. The effects of ageist attitudes demonstrated in the way professional carers over- or under-accommodate in talk, the problems and needs of older people will be discussed. However, communication is even more pertinent when responding to the health care needs of individuals who increasingly suffer impairment in their communicative ability, through hearing loss and forgetfulness.

As yet, ageism in language has not received the same public scrutiny that sexism and racism has incurred. Ageism permeates language to such an extent that reinforcement of ageist stereotypes can become a self-fulfilling prophecy in all but the most singular of individuals. However, ageism in language is not the prerogative of young people. Older adults commonly use stereotypical talk in defining themselves and their social situation. The telling of age is one of the many strategies by which older adults add age-related relevance to their talk. 'In my day . . .' is a common opening to topics in older adults' talk and phrases such as this support the personal interpretation of experiences, relationships and events through age. However, in the telling of age itself, it is significant how this tends to be consistently related to other topics of discussion, particularly issues of health and impairment. It is as though health 'complaints' are given greater validity through the assertion of old age; for example: 'I'm not very well these days too. I was seventy last October' (Giles *et al.*, 1992).

In health care interactions with older adults the listener/assessor of the older adults' talk (e.g. nurse, carer, social worker, doctor, etc.) is almost always a younger adult. Giles *et al.* (1992) found that younger adults state that they seek information from, and gain compliance of, older adults in ways that differ from how they would approach individuals in their own age group. These anticipated strategies are based on derogatory beliefs about the ways older adults communicate and talk. In the case of nurses, the communication strategies include over-accommodation of age-related topics (i.e. the recipient of talk puts greater emphasis on the age of the speaker in their replies when the speaker is older than they would do if the speaker was of average age – for example: 'You're doing very well for your age'). This can result in the reinforcement of older adults' perceptions concerning the debilitating nature of ageing (Williams *et al.*, 1990): 'Even when utterances, such as surprise in response to age disclosures, are seemingly supportive, they are in fact backhanded compliments. "Gosh, you don't look it", implies by rights you should' (Giles, 1992).

In addition, one study of nurses' interactions with elderly residents in long-stay hospital care showed how younger people can deflect and play down some of the seriously expressed concerns, thoughts, and feelings of older people (Grainger, Atkinson and Coupland, 1990) – an instance of under-accommodation to their apparent needs and rights (i.e. the dismissal or deprecation of an older person's expressed health needs on the grounds of 'that's what you must expect at your age'). This same scenario has been demonstrated when community nurses pay home visits to older adults, demonstrating that under-accommodation of expressed needs is related to interpersonal traits, rather than the circumstances in which the communication occurs. For example, when a client who completed the telling of a trouble by saying that at 87 she was too old to live, the health visitor responded, 'There you are, people live longer, don't they? Well, living conditions are so much better' (Fisher, 1988). Despite the often nurturing intentions of young people, over- and under-accommodation can impair communication, especially among cognitively alert and socially active older people (Giles *et al.*, 1992).

Stereotypes of older adults' intellectual competence or impaired sensory ability can lead to the 'Does he take sugar?' syndrome. This can be seen when health care workers either depersonalize older adults by directing conversation about the older person to a carer, or when they over-compensate with an older person by using patronizing or 'baby' talk.

It is important for nurses and health care professionals to reflect on their beliefs and attitudes concerning ageing and the way these may be demonstrated in verbal and non-verbal interactions with older people. The literature concerning the communication of nurses and older adults shows that younger people generally have negative assumptions about communicating with older adults and that they characterize intergenerational conversations as dissatisfying (Adelman, Greene and Charon, 1991; Nussbaum, Thompson and Robinson, 1991). Personal reflection by nurses and health care professionals on individual interactions with older people should enable the growth of understanding in their use of communication skills with the well elderly and thus facilitate more effective empowerment of their clients in this age group. Before you continue you may find it helpful to complete the exercise in Box 23.2.

Failure in intergenerational communication is not always the fault of the younger person, in this case the nurse or health care professional. In some instances, older people encourage and collude with others' perceptions of their helplessness. Giles *et al.* (1992) showed that in some circumstances older adults engage in self-stereotyping processes. This extends to acting out the characteristics (eg: behavioural: groaning on moving though it causes no pain; and communicative: making negative statements about age: 'You'll be like this when you get to my age'), which they believe are prototypical of old age. The negative results of this include, for instance, the self-imposition of ageist stereotypes as well as consequences such as the encouragement of dependence and the adoption of the sick role. However, older adults who have fulfilled the 'ageist prophecy' and live out the stereotype often indulge in 'victim narratives', continuing to talk about health and social

---

BOX 23.2 **EXERCISE TO HELP YOU MANAGE YOUR INTERACTIONS WITH OLDER PEOPLE**

Write a short descriptive account of your last professional encounter with an older person. What were the positive and negative features of the verbal or non-verbal interactions from your perspective and that of the older person?
Reflect on the following:

1. Your management of this encounter. Think through the processes that resulted in the positive or negative features.
2. Which of these features were the result of your actions?
3. What were the possible effects on your relationship with the older person?
4. How could you have better managed the interaction to promote the positive and diminish the negative features?

---

difficulties they perceive they are experiencing (Arntson and Droge, 1987). Professional carers can facilitate healthier attitudes by fostering a positive image of health potential in later life, especially within the areas of psychological and emotional wellbeing. Reference to appropriate role models with whom the older person has some affiliation, plus the encouragement of social exchange with more positive members of the older persons' peer group, will foster a healthier self-image and healthier attitudes.

In summary, it can be seen that motivation alone on the part of nurses and other professional carers will not enable them to empower older people or act as a successful advocate on their behalf. Attention to the content and context of interaction is important. Exerting a positive stance in conversation with older clients, developing a constructive approach to the clients' present situation, ensuring social engagement is meaningful and effective, and valuing and responding to clients' expressed needs will encourage older clients not to become 'victims' of old age: dependent, demoralized and lonely. In recognizing the negative, ageist talk about health characterized by some older clients, the professional carer will be able to elicit real health needs and effectively meet these needs without being overwhelmed by the 'potentially contagious talk of frailties, inabilities and ill health' (Giles *et al.*, 1992).

Enhancing quality of life

There is a major dilemma facing nurses and other professional carers when considering strategies to promote individual wellbeing in older adults. This dilemma centres on the rationalization of the objective, often academic, theory concerning the nature of successful human ageing with the subjective views of the experiences of older people themselves. Baltes and Baltes (1990) describe this dilemma thus:

'both the objective aspects of physical, psychological and social functioning and the subjective aspects of life quality and life meaning form a Gordian knot that no one is prepared to untie at this present time . . .' However, after considering her understanding of both the objective and the subjective perspectives, the professional carer has to decide what constitutes an effective nursing response to the health-related issues and problems presented by older clients in the practice situation.

An aid to the health care professional in intellectually synthesizing these understandings and deciding on appropriate effective action is a useful model of Baltes and Baltes (1990) given in Table 23.1. This model considers the psychological perspectives of successful ageing and includes both subjective (propositions about the nature of human ageing) and objective (individual strategies for successful ageing) indicators. To this can be added a possible nursing response appropriate to the enhancement of health in well older people.

First, the ageing continuum is defined: optimal ageing at one end of the scale and pathological or sick ageing at the opposite end. Optimal ageing, described by Baltes and Baltes (1990), is ideal ageing under development-enhancing and age-friendly environmental conditions. Normal ageing is ageing without biological or mental pathology. Sick or pathological ageing is determined by medical aetiology and syndromes of illness. Within these categories there is much individual variability depending on such factors as genetics, lifestyles and pathology.

Second, Baltes and Baltes believe that much of the movement from normal to optimal ageing can be achieved by older people themselves through engagement in healthy lifestyles which would reduce the probability of pathological ageing. The ability to engage in such lifestyes is seen by Gillis (1993) as being related to: (1) cognitive-perceptual factors (health, locus of control, health status and perceived benefits and actions); (2) self-concept and self-esteem; and (3) the related modifying factors of age, gender, marital status, etc. In encouraging health-enhancing activity, such as older people's engagement in physical activities, health care professionals must recognize the older adults' belief system, level of autonomy and ability to self-motivate. Only when health-promoting information or advice is delivered in a user-friendly and appropriate manner will it be adopted and internalized by the person to whom it was given. For a sick older person the movement from pathological ageing to normal ageing often needs the intervention and support of health care workers. In a psychological sense, this is more of a challenge to the nurse or other professional carer who, through communication and counselling skills can bolster the ego of the older person and provide then with a sense of control over their health and lifestyle.

Third, Baltes and Baltes describe a 'latent reserve' in cognitive functioning which is repeatedly demonstrated in studies on both older and younger people. This reserve of cognitive capacity allows, through proper utilization and training, the enhancement of those intellectual skills which can be shown to decrease with age. Indeed, Park and Smith (1991), in overviewing more than thirty research studies in cognitive functioning of older people, state that many problems associated with ageing are essentially behavioural not cognitive, and can be prevented through

Table 23.1   *Psychological perspectives on successful ageing: a model of successful optimization with compensation by the individual and nurse*

Propositions about the nature of human ageing	Individual strategies for successful ageing	The professional carer's response
1. There are major differences between optimal, normal and sick (pathological) ageing.	Engagement in a healthy lifestyle in order to reduce the probability of pathological ageing conditions.	Encourage and enable older adults to feel the benefit of health-enhancing activity such as individualized exercise and recreation plans.
2. There is much variability in ageing.	It is important to avoid simplistic generalizations and encourage individual and societal flexibility.	Relate to older adults as individuals and refrain from using stereotypical language. Use a positive approach to make the older adult feel valued and appreciated.
3. There is much latent reserve (i.e. the fully functioning potential of older individuals is not normally realized).	Strengthen one's reserve capacities, via education and health-related activities as well as the formation and nurturance of social networks.	Empower and facilitate older adults in their intellectual and social pursuits. Provide information on community activities where appropriate and encourage and facilitate peer group activity.
4. There is a loss near the limits of reserve (i.e. ageing becomes more pronounced as older individuals utilize their functioning potential and adaptation then becomes increasingly difficult).	Because of loss in adaptive capacity, particularly near the limits of capacity, older adults need special compensatory supports such as substitute and prosthetic devices, age-appropriate lifestyles and age-friendly environments.	Enable the appropriate disengagement from life tasks. Encourage partnerships in daily management and care between the older person and a caring relative or significant other. Ensure appropriate uptake of benefits through client advocacy. Enable access to welfare and voluntary agencies. Act as a catalyst for change in environmental provision.
5. Knowledge-based pragmatics and technology can offset age-related decline in cognitive mechanics.		
6. With ageing the balance between gains and losses becomes less positive.	Facilitate adjustments to 'objective' reality without loss of selfhood. Ageing is not a 'winning game'. In terms of absolute criteria of functional capacity, losses will occur.	Assist individuals in acquiring effective strategies involving change in aspirations and the scope of goals. Use positive role models from older adults' reference group to promote acceptance of limitations.
7. The self remains resilient in old age.		

Source: adapted from Baltes and Baltes (1990).

behavioural change. In empowering and facilitating older adults in their intellectual pursuits, health care professionals should recognize that behavioural change happens over time and that they will need to be resilient in their continued encouragement of the older person. For example, if an older, house-bound individual repeatedly rejects library books forwarded by the 'mobile library' service, this may be an indication of the individual making the same autonomous choices about book preference that an able-bodied person would do in an actual library, rather than a lack of motivation to read and enjoy books.

When the limits to this latent reserve are reached and cognitive abilities do suffer, the loss of adaptive capacity make older people more vulnerable to disengagement from normal daily activity and social intercourse. With current trends in community care and the rising number of very old people living alone (Bridgewood and Savage, 1991) health care professionals have a role in ensuring a safe and comfortable home and community environment for older people. By facilitating access to various voluntary and statutory welfare provisions, health care professionals must ensure that chronically disabled older people can make use of the facilities enjoyed by the rest of society. It can be a useful exercise for nurses and other health care professionals to consider carefully their own clinical environments for 'user-friendliness'. Often environments are adapted for disabled individuals (e.g. wheelchair-bound), rather than for those who are impaired.

The final stages of Baltes and Baltes' model demonstrates the resilience of older people in managing the balance between gains and losses. However, older adults need time and support in adjusting to loss at all levels and should be given the same form of counselling and other therapies that are afforded to younger adults. In assessing older individuals, professional carers must be astute in monitoring true signs of depression ensuring that troubles-telling, or overemphasis on illness and health problems in talk is not masking underlying mental health dysfunction. It should be accepted that not all support outcomes for older adults are positive. For example, if an older adult who is receiving support feels he cannot reciprocate, then feelings of inequality in the relationship may undermine both the support as well as the older adult's self-esteem.

Giles *et al.* (1992), in stating that 'older people are perhaps over-represented as recipients rather than resources of support', show the challenge facing nurses and other health care professionals in the psychological care of older adults. The required amount of involvement in the lives of older people for physical and social support may be easier to determine than the amount of support needed for psychological and emotional enrichment. In managing this fine line, nurses and health care professionals should develop a partnership approach with older people to enable the management of the required adaptation and change in later life. The initiatives and decisions of the older individuals themselves concerning their need for psychological and emotional support should always be the nurse's prime guide. In terms of nurses' 'counselling' involvement, older people have the right to accept or reject this type of support as would patients who form a 'captive audience'. This will enable an older person to take the lead in deciding the amount and type of psychological support and care required.

DISCUSSION POINT

Discuss the strategies you might use to enable older individuals and groups to enhance their feelings of self-worth and self-esteem.

Summary

While growing old inevitably entails both gains and losses, nurses in their day-to-day work deal mainly with the 'tip of the iceberg' – those 5 per cent who present as 'sick' elderly people. However, in the future nurses and health care professionals will be increasingly asked to meet the challenge of promoting health and preventing disability in the majority group of well elderly who view their life stage in pluses rather than minuses. Thus, the objective of this chapter has been to stimulate thinking about positive functioning in later life and to consider successful ageing from the perspective of older adults; various criteria for wellbeing have been presented and their relevance to the older adult and the professional carer has been discussed.

Promoting successful ageing could well become a leading challenge for nurses and health care professionals in the future. They can help older adults to remain autonomous and valued members of society and promote normal healthy ageing in three basic ways:

1. By helping older people to enhance their self-concept and positive perceptions of themselves and the ageing process.
2. By helping them to understand the importance of their positive psychological functioning.
3. By encouraging appropriate forms of activity.

There is much to be learned from and about older adults, but in order to learn we must listen to them and respect their individuality, their perceptions and their frailties.

As health care professionals, we have an obligation to promote both professional and general awareness of later life and what successful ageing has to offer. Only then can we continue to advance the art and science of gerontological nursing and assist older people to enjoy the success of surviving past 'three score years and ten'.

Seminar questions

1. How do the media portray older people? How does the portrayal of older individuals vary with their social status?
2. Are older people advantaged or disadvantaged by society's current attitudes to ageing?
3. What strategies could a nurse use in a residential home for elderly people to promote a positive self-image among its residents?

Further reading

Cowley, M.C. (1976) *A View From 80.* New York: Viking Press. A sensitive, personal account of the gains and losses of ageing. Cowley highlights the folly of professionals in interpreting old age through empirical research and literature: 'They know the literature, but not the life.' A charming and pleasurable insight into the incongruity between a failing body and a rich and reflective mind.

Biggs, S. (1993) *Understanding Ageing: Images, attitudes and professional practice.* A comprehensive, clearly written reader on the ageing process. Includes theories, general perspectives and health and social care practice mainly considered from a psychological perspective. Includes ageist, social and cultural perspectives.

References

Adelman, R.D., Greene, M.G. and Charon, R. (1991) 'Issues in physician–elderly interaction', *Ageing and Society* **11**, 127–47.

Arntson, P. and Droge, D. (1987) 'Social support in self-help groups: The role of communication in enabling perceptions of control', in T.L. Albrecht and M.B. Adelman (eds.) *Communication and Social Support.* Newbury Park, Calif.: Sage.

Baltes, P.B. and Baltes, M.M. (1990) 'Psychological perspectives on successful aging: The model of selective optimization with compensation', in P.B. Baltes and M.M. Baltes, *Successful Aging: Perspectives from behavioural sciences.* Cambridge: Press Syndicate of the University of Cambridge.

Biggs, S.J. (1992) 'Groupwork and professional attitudes to older age', in K. Morgan, *Gerontology: Responding to an ageing society.* London: Jessica Kingsley.

Bridgewood, A. and Savage, D. (1991) *General Household Survey: Social Survey Division.* London: OPCS.

Butler, R.N. (1969) 'Ageism: Another form of bigotry', *Gerontology* **9**, 243–6.

Cartwright, A. and Smith, C. (1988) *Elderly People, their Medicines, and their Doctors.* London: Routledge & Kegan Paul.

Central Statistical Office (1993) *Social Trends 23.* London: HMSO.

Costa, P.T., McCrea, R. and Locke, B.Z. (1990) 'Personality factors', in J.C. Cornoni-Huntley *et al.* (eds.) *Health Status and Well-Being of the Elderly: National Health and Nutritional Examination Survey–I.* Epidemiological follow-up study. Oxford: Oxford University Press.

Craik, F.I.M. and Jennings, J.M. (1992) 'Human memory', in F.I.M. Craik and T.A. Salthouse (eds.) *The Handbook of Aging and Cognition.* Hillsdale, NJ: Lawrence Erlbaum.

Drevdahl, D. (1989) 'Promoting power and control in the elderly client', *Journal of Post Anesthesia Nursing* **4**(1), 22–6.

Fisher, V.P. (1988) *Toil and Troubles: The conversational work of the health visitor versus the 'troubles-telling' of elderly clients.* Unpublished MSc dissertation, Surrey University.

Giles, H. *et al.* (1992) 'Intergenerational talk and communication with older people', *International Journal of Aging and Human Development* **34**(4), 271–97.

Gillis, A.J. (1993) 'Determinants of a health promoting lifestyle: An integrative review', *Journal of Advanced Nursing* **18**, 245–53.

Grainger, K., Atkinson, K. and Coupland, N. (1990) 'Responding to the elderly: Troubles-talk in the caring context', in N. Coupland, H. Giles, N. Coupland and J. Wiemann (eds.) *Communication, Health and the Elderly*, Fulbright Series No. 8. Manchester: Manchester University Press.

Hedstrom, P. and Ringen, S. (1987) 'Age and income in contemporary society: A research note. *Journal of Social Policy* **16**(2), 227–39.

Heidrich, S. M. and D'Amico, D. (1993) 'Physical and mental health relationships in the very old', *Journal of Community Health Nursing* **10**(1), 11–21.

Kaplan, G.A., Seeman, T.E., Cohen, R.D. *et al.* (1987) 'Mortality among the elderly in the Alameda County study: Behavioural and demographic risk factors', *American Journal of Public Health* **77**, 307–12.

Kinsey, A., Pomeroy, W. and Martin, C. (1948) *Sexual Behaviour in the Human Male.* Philadelphia: WB Saunders Co.

Kinsey, A., Pomeroy, W. and Martin, C. (1953) *Sexual Behaviour in the Human Female.* Philadelphia: WB Saunders Co.

Lachman, M.E. (1986) 'Personal control in later life: Stability, change and cognitive correlates', in M.M. Baltes and P.B. Baltes (eds.) *The Psychology of Control and Aging.* Hillsdale, NJ: Lawrence Erlbaum.

Lachman, M.E. and Leff, R. (1989) 'Beliefs about intellectual efficacy and control in the elderly: A five-year longitudinal study', *Developmental Psychology* **25**, 722–28.

Magnani, L.E. (1990) 'Hardiness, self-perceived health, and activity among independently functioning older adults', *Scholarly Inquiry for Nursing Practice: An International Journal* **4**(3), 171–88.

Melanson, P.M. and Downe Wamboldt, B. (1987) 'Identification of older adults' perceptions of their health, feelings towards their future and factors affecting these feelings', *Journal of Advanced Nursing* **12**, 29–34.

Nussbaum, J.F., Thompson, T. and Robinson, J.D. (1991) 'Communication, language and the institutionalised elderly', *Ageing and Society* **11**, 149–65.

Park, D.C. and Smith, A.D. (1991) 'Importance of basic and applied research from the viewpoints of investigators in the psychology of ageing', *Experimental Ageing Research* **17**(3), 79–102.

Ribeiro, V.E.D. (1989) *Loneliness in the Institutionalised Elderly: A Descriptive/exploratory study.* DNSc dissertation, Boston University.

Rodin, J. (1986) 'Aging and health: Effects of the sense of control', *Science* **233**, 1271–6.

Rowe, J.W. and Kahn, R.L. (1987) 'Human aging: Usual and successful', *Science* **237**, 143–9.

Russell, C.H. (1989) *Good News about Aging.* New York: John Wiley.

Rybash, J.M., Roodin, P.A. and Santrock, J.W. (1991) *Adult Development and Aging*, 2nd edition. Dubuque: Wm C. Brown.

Ryff, C.D. (1989a) 'In the eye of the beholder: Views of psychological wellbeing among middle-aged and older adults', *Psychology and Aging* **4**(2), 195–210.

Ryff, C.D. (1989b) 'Beyond Ponce de Leon and life satisfaction: New directions in quest of successful ageing', *International Journal of Behavioural Development* **12**(1), 35–55.

Schank, M.J. and Lough, M.A. (1990) 'Profile: Frail elderly women, maintaining independence', *Journal of Advanced Nursing* **15**, 674–82.

Seedhouse, D. (1986) *Health: The foundations for achievement.* New York: John Wiley.

Travis, S.S. (1987) 'Older adults' sexuality and remarriage', *Journal of Gerontological Nursing* **13**(6), 8–14.

van Maanen, H.M.Th. (1988) 'Being old does not always mean being sick: Perspectives on conditions of health as perceived by British and American elderly', *Journal of Advanced Nursing* **13**, 701–9.

Wetle, T. (1991) 'Successful aging: New hope for optimizing mental and physical wellbeing', *Journal of Geriatric Psychiatry* **24**(1), 3–12.

Whitehead, M. (1987) *The Health Divide.* London: Health Education Council.

Williams, A. *et al.* (1990) 'The communicative context of elderly social support and health: A theoretical model', *Health Communication* **2**(3), 123–43.

CHAPTER 24

Dementia in older people

D. JOHN DONE AND JUDITH THOMAS

Chapter outline

What is dementia?

Dementia refers to a disorder occurring in some 1 per cent of 65–74 year olds, and 10 per cent of 75+ year olds (Ineichen, 1987). The disorder is characterized by a decline in all aspects of cognition (i.e. memory, thinking, comprehension, problem-soving and general intellect) and is the result of a progressive destruction of brain tissue.

The question of whether we all experience a decline in cognition when we get old is addressed by Meldrum (this volume, Chapter 22). She draws the tentative conclusion that there does appear to be a decline, although this is probably true for only some cognitive skills and some people. This chapter deals with the group of elderly people who show such extreme cognitive deterioration in intellect and memory that it can be regarded as pathological. Members of this group are considered to suffer from *dementia*.

Since some noticeable cognitive decline often occurs as a normal function of ageing, society tends to hold a somewhat stereotyped view that any loss of memory is a natural part of ageing. It therefore becomes difficult to decide whether someone who is forgetful is in an early stage of a dementing illness or is experiencing something normally expected of someone of that age. As a result, there is often a tension, even among health professionals, about whether a person is suffering from dementia (thereby adopting the medical model) or simply forgetful and requiring supports such as a carer who provides reminders (thereby adopting a societal model).

Dementia does not only involve an impairment of intellect and memory, since just about every sphere of psychological functioning can also change or become disrupted in some way. Thus personality, emotional stability, behaviour towards others (e.g. becoming aggressive when previously passive and tolerant), speech and communication, and self-care may well change for the worse. But the pattern of deterioration varies considerably and its severity depends on whether the patient is at an early, middle or late stage of the illness, since dementia is normally a progressive disorder in which deterioration occurs over a period of time. One can consider there to be three stages of dementia: early, middle and late stages. In the *early stage* of dementia the most obvious disturbance is the impairment of memory. Difficulty in acquiring new information and retaining it over anything more than a few seconds is probably the most conspicuous sign. Recall of the sufferer's past life may be relatively well preserved compared with memory for recent events. This is often first noticed in the course of a daily activity. For example, a husband may return from a shopping trip without a significant number of important items which he had intended to buy and on being questioned about this by his wife he may not recall having written a shopping list.

The initial realization that something is not quite as it should be depends upon the *pre-morbid* abilities and the pre-morbid personality of the person . That is to say, there needs to be a degree of change which is noticed by a close friend or relative to be rather more than just absent-mindedness. The changes might not be noticed at first since sufferers often make excuses to hide these memory defects.

Changes of mood may also occur in this early stage and may involve anxiety, irritability and depression. Thinking becomes slow, impoverished in content and may well appear to become concrete. That is to say, dealing with abstract concepts (e.g. discussing a son's attitude towards his wife) may result in an upsettingly impoverished contribution from the dementing person. Judgement also becomes impaired.

At an early stage there may also be apparent changes in behaviour. Behaviour may become disorganized, inappropriate, distractable and restless and there may be few signs of interest or initiative.

It should be emphasized at this point that this early stage may be characterized by any combination of these changes, with some being more marked than others. Sometimes loss of memory is the most striking feature, whereas with others it may be an apparent change in personality, which is most noted when the person becomes antisocial, perhaps beoming sexually disinhibited or committing some petty crime.

| BOX 24.1 **WHAT'S IT LIKE TO BE A CARER?** |

Olive has been married to Fred for 35 years. Fred now suffers from Alzheimer's disease which has reached a moderate level of severity. This is an extract from Olive's report on how her husband's illness has affected her.

The children visit and talk on the phone, providing as much support as is possible, given that they have young children themselves. Friends are in scarcer supply. Olive thinks some friends would come over if she invited them, but she doesn't because Freddie's condition is simply too embarrassing. And so she lives without the job she loved, without any hope of a holiday, without trips to concerts and theatres, without adult conversation – and with Freddie. She is an intelligent, mild-mannered, articulate woman who tells the whole story evenly and unemotionally. Until you ask her, ever so gently, does she mind? Then her eyes flash and it pours out. 'Of course I mind! I resent it very much. I do not want to look after this . . . person. I've reached this age, I should be having an easier life, doing things I've never done. I'm no saint; you see articles where people say what a wonderful enriching experience it all is and I don't believe them.'

'. . . I can look at him and sometimes manage to remember it was someone I had fun with, or an affectionate relationship with. And at other times, he's like a stranger and I'm looking after him through circumstances beyond my control. I think, I do all this for him and all I get back is aggression – what's that speech, "Who will rid me of this troublesome priest?" – it runs through my head. You even get to the thought, well, perhaps he won't wake up tomorrow, and then you feel guilty about thinking it. I don't want to lose my life looking after him. It's like having a child without the joy. I've always been rather squeamish, and to have to do the things I have to do for him is . . . oh. . . .'

Olive believes Freddie still recognizes his own home and his dog: 'As long as he has that awareness I shall try to carry on. I can't think 10 years, I think just one more year . . . and at the end of that year I expect I shall think just another year. It's bloody awful, to be quite truthful.'

Ask Olive what she would really like and her requests are pitifully slight: a day care centre, specially geared to the needs of Alzheimer's sufferers, would be top of the list, or some alternative 'So I could have the house to myself. That's what I really long for.'

Source: The Sunday Times Colour Magazine, 26 May 1991.

Generally speaking the course of a dementing illness shows progression across this wide range of psychological functions. At a *middling stage* of progression sufferers will not be able to remember their date of birth, how old they are or be able to recall the names of certain significant others such as their wife, husband, the current prime minister or the monarch. Such forgetfulness becomes not only a social problem, but also a hazard as going out unaccompanied can result in forgetting arrangements to meet up and then forgetting one's own address. Speech at this stage is often very circumlocutory; that is, the speech becomes rambling, not getting to the point and failing to find informative words. Disorientation in time and space occur. Sufferers may forget where they are at the moment or even the current time of day, which may lead to inappropriate behaviour such as preparing dinner at an absurd hour for a family who left home years ago. This disorientation can lead to distress about where they are and concern that they should be somewhere else.

Another sign that may be observed at this stage is the blunting of emotions, i.e. there is little expression of either positive (happiness) or negative (sadness) mood, and sudden mood changes may occur without apparent cause (emotional incontinence).

In the *late stage* memory is very poor, sufferers not infrequently have difficulty in remember their own name, whether they are married or have children. Recognition of familiar others may not occur and emotions are blunted, and personality may not be expressed, through lack of communication or behaviour.

This gives a general picture of the decline in cognitive and other psychological functions during dementia. However, dementia is not a single disorder and so there may be considerable variation to this general picture.

Dementia is not a single disorder

Dementia is an umbrella term which covers all syndromes in which there is a marked cognitive decline. AIDS, Huntington's chorea, Parkinson's disease, Wilson's disease, multiple sclerosis and stroke can result in dementia, although this is not always the case. Other disorders that invariably result in dementia are Alzheimer's disease, Creutzfeld Jacob disease (CJD, more popularly known as 'mad cow disease'), and Pick's disease. Henderson (1983) points out that dementia can occur in 100 different diagnoses in which higher brain function is impaired.

Generally speaking, 45 per cent of cases of dementia are cases of Alzheimer's disease, 17 per cent result from arteriosclerotic causes (often referrred to as cases of multi-infarct dementia), 17 per cent are cases with both Alzheimer's disease and arteriosclerotic cause, and 19 per cent includes the rest, e.g. cases of Huntington's, Wilson's and Parkinson's disease who have become demented.

The focus of this chapter will therefore be Alzheimer's and multi-infarct dementias. Thus, whenever the term dementia is used, it will be referring to Alzheimer's and multi-infarct dementias.

What is Alzheimer's Disease?

A true diagnosis for Alzheimer's disease is achieved only after death when a post-mortem examination is undertaken. *Histopathology* of someone who suffered Alzheimer's shows the presence of *neurofibrillary tangles*, tangles of short and *neuritic plaques*. Both tangles and plaques can be seen under a microscope if the brain tissue has been suitably stained. Tangles consist of a dense aggregate of a particular kind of filament not seen in the normal brain, often referred to as 'paired helical filaments'. Plaques, on the other hand, are extracellular collections of degenerating dendrites and axons surrounding a core of protein known as *amyloid protein*.

However, tangles and plaques are found in the brain of 'normal' elderly people (Roth, 1994), and hence there was some debate about whether these abnormalities really are responsible for the psychological abnormalities of Alzheimer's disease. The debate was settled by the work of Roth, Tomlinson and Blessed (1966) and Blessed, Tomlinson and Roth (1968), who found that although tangles and plaques are found in the normal ageing population, when they occur in large numbers the person becomes clinically demented. They also found a direct correlation between the degree of cognitive impairment measured with the now famous Blessed Rating Scale and the number of plaques and tangles found in the post-mortem examination.

How is dementia diagnosed?

This is an important question. A test is required which will allow assessment of memory and intellect which will indicate that someone is demented. However, we return again to the problem that apparent cognitve decline is common in older people who do not have dementia. Someone who may have started pre-morbidly with a good memory may well be at an early stage of dementia but score higher on the test than someone who is benignly senescent, and always has had a mediocre memory. Thus fixed criteria, such as 'a score below 5 on a 10-item memory scale' will either be too strict and will miss those who used to have a good memory and are now at an early stage, or it will be too liberal and will label as 'demented' those who have always had a poor memory. As a result, a test of memory and intellect has to be judged in the light of (1) the person's pre-morbid abilities, and (2) how the average person of similar age would perform on the same test. Judgements about pre-morbid abilities are usually made by reference to occupation, number of years of full time education and social class. However, given that reading aloud remains surprisingly well-preserved in mild/moderate dementia, it is possible to derive a measure of pre-morbid ability from the National Adult Reading Test (Nelson, 1982). It may also be important to find out which type of dementia the person is suffering from, but this in general moves into the realms of medical diagnosis and will not be dealt with here.

Before leaving this topic, related conditions which can result in misdiagnosis should be discussed. Some elderly people who are depressed can have cognitive deficits, together with changes in affect and personality which appear very similar to dementia. This condition, when recognized, sometimes goes by the name of pseudodementia. In most such cases the symptoms of depression precede the onset of the signs of dementia, but in some cases the symptoms of depression begin at about the same time as the cognitive decline, which makes accurate diagnosis difficult. To complicate matters further, it is possible to suffer from both dementia and depression at the same time. Correct diagnosis is important since depression can be treated and the cognitive impairment thereby reduced, while dementia cannot be treated at present. Thus false diagnosis can have major implications.

Another medical disorder masquerading as dementia which will be mentioned here is *acute confusional state (delirium)*, the main features of which are disorientation and confusion. The state mimics dementia, but in fact results from physical causes, including drug intoxication, metabolic failure, withdrawal from alcohol and drugs and, in some cases, malnutrition (see Gelder, Gath and Mayou, 1989, for more details). It can arise over a 24-hour period, the person being normal one day and utterly confused the next. These conditions are reversible and thus accurate diagnosis is vital.

DISCUSSION POINT

Deciding whether an elderly person has dementia has important implications for patient management. How might you identify someone who is suffering from dementia? With reference to forming a care plan, why is it important to differentiate dementia from other disorders?

How long does dementia last?

In cases of dementia there may be periods in which there is no further deterioration of psychological functions. However, these will be followed by further decline, usually in a gradual progression. In multi-infarct dementia there may be a more step-like deterioration, i.e. a period of fairly rapid deterioration, followed by a period of stability.

Due to medical factors reducing the physical health of a dementia sufferer there does appear to be an association with premature death. Some studies show that this is true for early onset dementia, i.e. that occurring before the age of 70 (e.g. Henderson and Kay, 1984), but untrue for those who become demented in their eighties. In Kay *et al.* (1970) and Maule, Milne and Williamson (1984) the majority of sufferers had died within five years of the initial diagnosis, but survival time appears to be increasing (Christie, 1985), perhaps the result of advances in care. However, one can roughly estimate that the period between onset and death is in the order of some seven years, although this can vary from as little as 1–2 years to 15 years.

How common is dementia?

A review of the literature by Ineichen (1987) concluded that about 1 per cent of the 65–74 year olds and 10 per cent of the 75+ year olds become demented. These numbers might suggest that dementia is relatively uncommon, but of course the disorder is such that contact with hospitals and nurses is inevitable. In addition, the condition is likely to become more prevalent as the population of elderly people rises. The OPCS (1985) survey estimated that by the year 2001 there would be 9 million people in the United Kingdom over the age of 65 and 4.5 million over 75. But in some areas with a high density of elderly people, e.g. Bath, the increase in elderly people was predicted to increase by a third by 2001 (Ineichen, 1987).

What do we know about the causes of dementia?

Very recently there has been a number of breakthroughs that have suggested that Alzheimer's disease might be caused by the malfunction of genes; there is, however, also the possibility that environmental factors might trigger this malfunction.

It has been known for some time that there is a very high rate of Alzheimer's disease during early middle age in people with Down's syndrome (Oliver and Holland 1986). Down's syndrome is a genetic disorder which results from an abnormal division of chromosome 21. Molecular genetic research has led many (e.g. St. Clair, 1987) but not all (e.g. Harrison, 1993) to believe that genetic abnormality on this chromosome is central to the cause of Alzheimer's disease.

The psychology of memory and its contribution to understanding dementia

Memory is considered by many psychologists to be served by a number of different structures and processes. They consider that there is a need to separate out *encoding*, *storage* and *retrieval*. Encoding refers to the way information coming in from the outside world is transformed from sensory data into meaning; storage refers to a 'filing cabinet' of memories; retrieval refers to gaining access to the memory that was filed away. So, if you cannot remember what you did on your summer holiday last year it may be because (1) you spent most of the time inebriated with the result that you failed to encode much of what was happening around you, or (2) the memories you filed away have been replaced or faded away, or (3) memories are accurately stored, but without a prompt you cannot recall what happened. The loss of memory that occurs in dementia could result from impairments in any or all of the structures and processes responsible for encoding, storage and recall.

Generally speaking, this view of separate encoding, storage and retrieval processes is too simplistic. Godden and Baddeley (1975), for example, asked divers to learn and recall lists of words either on shore or under water. They found that what was learned under water was better recalled under water. Thus it appears that the situation you are in when trying to recall something can facilitate (or hinder) recall. In this case, encoding the situation at the time of recall influenced the ability to retrieve memories. Hence there can be considerable interaction between these three processes, so that treating them as separate processes is too simple. However, this provides a useful framework to aid the understanding of memory.

It is generally thought that there are three different types of memory store: sensory stores (which hold memories for a very short time, e.g. rather like an after-image); short-term memory stores (such as remembering the telephone number that a friend told you at lunch); and long-term memory (e.g. recalling events at the first school you attended) (see Eysenck and Keane, 1991).

Attempting to remember a telephone number for a few seconds illustrates two key features about short-term memory: (1) the limited capacity of this type of memory, and (2) items are lost quickly if you do not repeat them to yourself or if you are distracted. The limits to the capacity are best measured in terms of the number of *chunks* (a chunk being a familiar unit of information based on previous learning and experience). Thus, if I try to remember a list of names (say eight first names and eight surnames, making a total of sixteen names), I will remember only about eight if the individuals are unknown to me. However, if these were the names of personal friends, then I will remember the same number of units, i.e. eight, but the units this time will be a combination of one first and one surname.

In dementia the overall capacity (i.e. number of items that can be stored) is reduced, the rate of forgetting in short-term memory is increased and this is particularly so when there is distraction or competition from other memories. For example, if you tell a patient suffering from dementia your name and then ask him to say what he ate for breakfast, this increases the likelihood that the patient will forget your name within a few seconds.

Quite clearly there are profound deficits in long-term memory in dementia. Remembering people's names, or personal events in one's own life, or even recognizing objects or people can create problems. Psychologists have made a great play out of differences between different types of long-term memories. Some have suggested that there are differences between memories that might be for personal experiences (e.g. a visit to Brighton when aged 6) and those that are general knowledge, such as recognizing that an object is a spoon, not a knife. These different types of long-term memory have been referred to as *episodic* and *semantic* long-term memories, respectively. For these two types of memory there is a clear difference in content (you do not recall a scene and a series of personal events when asked to describe a spoon as you would if you were asked to describe a trip to the seaside as a child), and some patients with memory disorders (*amnesic* rather than demented patients) have deficits with episodic, but not semantic memory (Parkin, 1982). This is not the case for sufferers of dementia, for whom general knowledge about the world is impaired. Such impairments are typically held to demonstrate deficits in semantic memory. However, Nebes (1989) has suggested that semantic memory stores may remain intact in dementia sufferers. He argues that sufferers are simply unable to retrieve memories from intact memory stores, but when provided with relevant situational cues recall is possible. However Chertkow and Bub (1990) provided evidence to suggest that dementia sufferers not only have difficulty retrieving intact memories but also stored memories can be lost altogether or else severely corrupted. So the debate about the intactness of semantic memories in dementia continues, although increasingly the evidence is moving towards deficits in both access of memories as well as damaged memory stores.

There is yet another distinction between different types of long-term memory which is relevant to dementia. This is the distinction between the memory for the performance of a learned activity (e.g. using a knife, fork and spoon appropriately) as opposed to conscious recollection (e.g. being able to say what you use a spoon for). The distinction between these two types of memory has resulted in the labels *implicit* (memory for performance) and *explicit* (conscious recollection). Dementia sufferers can often perform activities (e.g. demonstrate the use of a corkscrew) but are unable to provide the name or give a verbal description (e.g. say that a cork-screw is used to remove a cork from a bottle). Thus sufferers of dementia show particularly marked impairments for explicit memory. Implicit memories at the early/moderate stages of dementia appear to be intact.

The application of psychology to improve communication with sufferers of dementia

If you want to communicate with someone who is demented, the first step has to be to get his or her attention. The psychology of attention shows that the most power-ful stimulus to attract attention is hearing someone speak your name. This can be facilitated by the provision of a sensory cue, e.g. giving a light touch. Simple as this may sound, there can be snags to this course of action. First, it is important to get the name right. A surprising number of people are not known by their given name. One often sees name labels on patients' beds with their nickname or familiar name in brackets, and it is obviously really important to discover what these are. Equally important is to establish whenever possible the mode of address preferred by each individual, as many people, particularly elderly people, are not at ease being called by their first name by those they do not know well. Ask them how they would like to be addressed and tell them your name.

A light touch on the arm, from the front or side so as not to startle, is usually a good accompaniment to saying someone's name, although there are those who dis-like being touched and one would need to be aware of this. Next remember to put the name before the message, as shown in Figure 24.1. (illustration by Wendy Ward).

The form of the communication

Before you embark on a communication exercise with someone who is dementing, consider the basic points in Box 24.2. We have mentioned that dementia sufferers have short-term memories which are limited in size such that they can store fewer items than normal, and they are also more prone to forgetting material, especially when there is a distraction. Therefore, the structure and content of orally given information needs to be in a form which pays due regard to these limitations. A few basic guidelines to avoid the more obvious pitfalls are:

Figure 24.1 *Remember to use a name before the message*

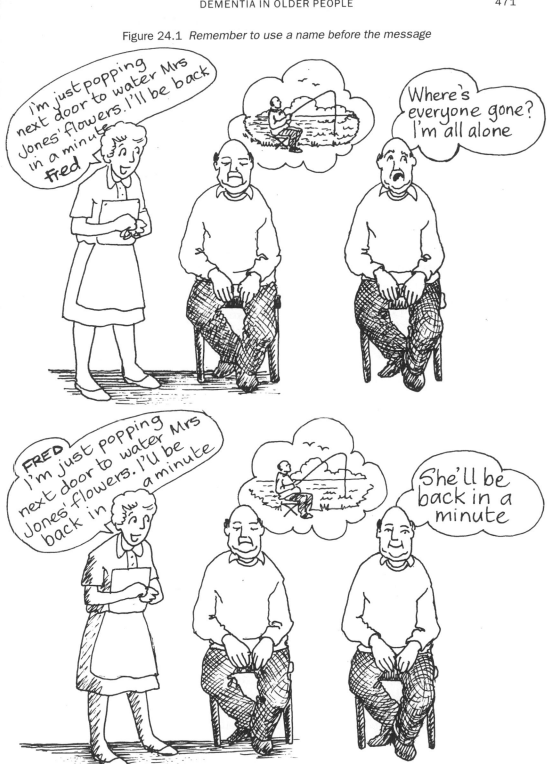

BOX 24.2 POINTS TO CONSIDER ABOUT COMMUNICATION

1. *Hearing aid*: Is one normally used? If so, is it in? Is it *correctly placed*? Check with family whether there is an aid at home that did not get brought in.
2. Check spectacles and dentures are in place.
3. Reduce surrounding noise as much as possible when communicating. Competing messages, or sounds which can attract attention, can refocus attention away from what you are saying, as well as impairing encoding of incoming message.
4. Speak a little more slowly than normal to give time for information to be processed.
5. Watch for signs that your message has not been understood and repeat or rephrase.
6. Give time for a response before you assume that repetition is needed.
7. Don't 'talk down' to the elderly dementing person.
   Simplifying language structure does not mean patronizing 'baby talk'.

---

1. Keep sentences short, so that information can be relayed in manageable 'chunks', e.g. 'Your wife will be a bit late. The bus from Poggleton has been cancelled. Your wife will be coming by train. She will be a bit late.' This is easier to analyze than 'Your wife won't be here just yet because the bus she usually gets isn't running today. But don't worry, she's going to come on the train instead so you'll get your visit, but maybe not for so long.'
2. Avoid using too many pronouns to link sentences; the sufferer may not be able to retain in short-term memory someone's name when additional information is given, e.g. 'Your friend John telephoned. John would like to see you. Would you like to see John?' is much easier to process than: 'Your friend John telephoned. He said he would like to come and see you. Does he live near you? Would you like to see him?'
3. Give information in a logical sequence so that the context developed at one stage facilitates the understanding of the next stage, e.g. don't say, 'Because Mr Smith is going home later today we are going to move you over by the window.' The fact that Mr Smith is going home may have no significance for the patient. But if you say, 'We are going to move your bed over by the window because . . .' the reason for the move will be understood.
4. Alert the sufferer to a change of subject or activity: 'Mary, now I want to talk to you about what the doctor said' or 'Mary, I need to give you some medicine.' This, too, provides some relevant context for the next communication or procedure. Box 24.3 provides a quick checklist of some of the common communication behaviours exhibited by dementia patients with carer strategies which could be tried.

Response to communication from the dementing person

Discussion so far has focused on the use of language to the dementing person. Equally important is responding to their communication attempts. Assuming that

---

BOX 24.3 STRATEGIES TO IMPROVE COMMUNICATION

Patient Behaviour	Carer Strategy
Poor auditory comprehension	Reduce complexity of utterance
	Reduce use of pronouns
Jargon output	Look for pragmatic clues (i.e. note context, watch for gesture, note tone of voice etc.
	Use 20 question technique
Lack of attention	Gain attention by alerting
Loses attention	Repeat alerters
	Reduce distractions
Unable to make choices	Avoid complex choices
	Use 'closed' questions
Perseveration (continued repetition of utterance)	Reply tactfully
	Distract attention
Word-finding problems	Intelligent guesswork
	20 question approach
Rambling, non-proposition speech (thought disorder)	Distract
	Ignore/Don't try to interpret

---

the words themselves are not obvious in meaning it is worth making a simple enquiry and asking for repetition. This may give the person a chance to reorganize their thoughts and convey the meaning better. Attending to the context in which the communication is made may also aid comprehension, noting accompanying gesture, tone of voice, facial expression, etc. It may be appropriate to try to clarify the subject with them, e.g. 'Are you talking about your slippers?' if she is pointing to the floor, and then watch her face for reaction to the question. Blankness or bewilderment may indicate that it has nothing whatever to do with slippers. If a complete blank is drawn, it may be advisable to try gently to change the subject, as it is possible that the original request/statement has by now been forgotten. One of the most difficult aspects of communication in dementia is how to cope with rambling and inappropriate statements/requests. This will be given further consideration in the next section.

Psychology and the reality orientation approach

'Reality orientation' approach

Reality orientation (RO) started in the United States in 1958 and was introduced into the United Kingdom in the mid-1970s. Alzheimer's disease sufferers have been

> BOX 24.4 **REALITY ORIENTATION TECHNIQUES**
>
> 1. On greeting in the morning, give basic information in a conversational way to orient the sufferer to the present, e.g. 'Good morning, Joe (Mr Smith). It's a lovely summer morning – a beautiful June day.' Or, 'What a cold Monday morning, not very nice for July.'
> 2. When someone has been dozing after lunch: 'Time to wake up after your nap. It's nearly three o'clock.'
> 3. 'The doctor will be here soon. Your doctor, Dr Roberts, always comes on Mondays, doesn't she?'

found to respond to RO and can be successfully taught to find their way round a ward, using signs. Some retraining programmes have been tried, after demonstrations that Alzheimer's patients have some learning ability.

Basically, the idea of RO is to keep the sufferer informed, in as natural a way as possible, of the current situation and circumstances, so that their place in it is understood. A large calendar on the wall depicting day, month and year is useful, provided that it *does* get changed daily and is not relaying confusing information. Other simple techniques can routinely be employed by nurses to put the sufferer 'gently on track', as given in Box 24.4. RO should ideally be a round-the-clock approach, gently reminding sufferers who they are, where they are and offering information about basic routines so that they feel they knew this information all the time for themselves.

We have already referred to the frequently experienced problem of rambling speech. It is quite important to distinguish between (1) purposeless rambling non-propositional, speech, which does not have any particular focus or theme and is not requesting any specific action, and (2) the endlessly repeated, inappropriate statements/requests, accompanied by anxiety, which are asking for action. With (1) it is likely to be fruitless to try to make sense of the rambling; the best strategy is either to distract, perhaps by suggesting a small task: 'Could you put this in the bin for me?', or, as there is not usually any anxiety, to ignore until a naturally occurring event distracts. In the case of (2) a gentle RO approach will sometimes be sufficient to allay anxieties and reorient the sufferer to the present. It is not usually appropriate to reinforce mistaken beliefs, as this will lead the person further down the path of confusion, but neither is it kind or helpful to deny abruptly their perceptions of what is a current situation and not help them to adjust to our reality. The old lady constantly anxious to get home to get the dinner on or meet the children, etc. and demanding a taxi, is more likely to be calmed by reassurance that everything is being taken care of, that her family knows where she is and that there is nothing she has to do at the moment, than by being told that there aren't any children, that her supper will be coming round later, etc.

Other strategies involve the presence of photographs of family and friends, with names underneath, to help preserve identity and also aid conversation. In addition, it helps to discover past hobbies and interests, as discussion on these subjects will be stimulating for a disoriented person, giving them a chance to participate and thus preserve a sense of worth and achievement.

Evidence suggests that a stimulated brain remains alert for a measurable time following cessation of the stimulus (e.g. Boddy, 1978) and the dementing patient is likely to be more responsive to subsequent events/information at least for a short time. Conversely, prolonged exposure to a continuing stimulus results in the habituation of the response. Habituation refers to the lack of response to a stimulus resulting from over-exposure to that stimulus. (Have you noticed how a strong smell noticed on entering a ward ceases to be apparent after 5 minutes?) A television permanently switched on and in the visual field of an immobile patient has just this effect. Selective viewing, however, can be useful to keep the patient up-to-date with current affairs. He can be shown the headlines in the newspaper to reinforce the auditory input and this also affords a second chance to absorb the information.

DISCUSSION POINT
How can knowledge of the cognitive disorders of dementia assist the nurse in using validation/reality orientation therapy?

Working with dementing people is never an easy option, but the nurse has the very privileged position of being the one closest to that person in everyday terms and therefore being entrusted with the difficult task of helping to preserve the value and worth of a life coming to a close in the cruel circumstances of a disintegrating mind.

Summary

Dementia results from a serious disorder of the brain, which affects every aspect of psychological functioning. The progression of dementia means that psychological and physical needs change over time. For both formal and informal carers this implies a need to be aware of the patient's current abilities and needs. Some psychological functions may be better preserved than others, but perhaps more important is knowing how to work with the client to make these psychological functions most effective. Here we have focused on communication and related psychological theory to techniques which can improve the communication between carer and sufferer.

Seminar questions

1. Imagine that you are nursing someone who is in a well-advanced state of dementia. Your patient cannot recognize you from one day to the next, and her

speech is often inappropriate and rambling. What could you do to engender and maintain your and your colleagues', motivation when caring for this patient?

2. How can psychological theory be applied to help in the management of a demented patient such that appropriate behaviour is elicited? Consider the following areas for discussion:

  (a) Responding to requests.
  (b) Restricting wandering.
  (c) Allaying anxiety.
  (d) Enhancing quality of life.

Further reading

Comer, R.J. (1992) *Abnormal Psychology.* New York: W.H. Freeman. Chapter 20 gives an overview of the clinical aspects of dementia.

Eysenck, M.W. and Keane, M.T. (1991) *Cognitive Psychology: A student's handbook.* Hove: Lawrence Erlbaum. For further developing your knowledge of theoretical psychology.

Huppert, F.A. Brayne, C. and O'Connor, D.W. (1994) *Dementia and Normal Aging.* Cambridge: Cambridge University Press. Contains a number of useful chapters which focus on the nature and causes of dementia.

Miller, E. and Morris, R. (1994) *The Psychology of Dementia.* Chichester: John Wiley. A contemporary book by two highly respected psychologists which covers the psychological dysfunctions of dementia sufferers.

References

Blessed, G., Tomlinson, B.E. and Roth, M. (1968) 'The association between quantitative measures of dementia and of senile change in the cerebral grey matter of elderly subjects', *British Journal of Psychiatry* **114**, 797–811.

Boddy, J.(1978) *Brain Systems and Psychological Concepts.* Chichester: John Wiley.

Chertkow, H. and Bub, D. (1990) 'Semantic memory loss in dementia of Alzheimer's type: What do various measures measure?' *Brain* **113**, 397–446.

Christie, A.B. (1985) 'Survival in dementia: A review', in T. Arie (ed.) *Recent Advances in Psychogeriatrics*, Vol. 1. Edinburgh: Churchill Livingstone.

Eysenck, M.W. and Keane M.T. (1991) 'Cognitive Psychology: A student's handbook. Hove: Lawrence Erlbaum.

Gelder, M., Gath, D. and Mayou, R. (1989) *Oxford textbook of psychiatry.* 2nd edition. Oxford: Oxford Medical Publications.

Godden, D. and Baddeley, A.D. (1975) 'Context-dependent memory in two natural environments: On land and under water', *British Journal of Psychology* **66**, 325–31.

Harrison, P. (1993) 'Alzheimer's disease and chromosome 14: Different gene, same process? *British Journal of Psychiatry* **163**, 2–5.

Henderson, A.S. (1983) 'The coming epidemic of dementia', *Australian and New Zealand Journal of Psychiatry* **17**, 117–27.

Henderson, A.S. and Kay, D.W.K. (1984) 'The epidemiology of mental disorders in old age', in D.W. Kay and G.D. Burrows (eds.) *Handbook of Studies on Psychiatry and Old Age.* Amsterdam: Elsevier.

Ineichen, B. (1987) 'Measuring the rising tide: How many dementia cases will there be by 2001?' *British Journal of Psychiatry* **150**, 193–200.

Kay, D.W.K., Foster, E.M., McKechnie, A.A., and Roth, M. (1970) 'Mental illness and hospital usage in the elderly: A random sample followed up', *Comprehensive Psychiatry* **11**, 26–35.

Maule, M., Milne, J.S. and Williamson, J. (1984) 'Mental illness and physical health in older people', *Age and Ageing* **13**, 349–56.

Nebes, R.D. (1989) 'Semantic memory in Alzheimer's disease', *Psychological Bulletin* **106**, 377–94.

Nelson, H.E. (1982) *National Adult Reading Test (NART).* Windsor: NFER-Nelson.

Office of Population Censuses (1985) *Social Trends*, 15.

Oliver, C. and Holland, A.J. (1986) 'Down's syndrome and Alzheimer's disease: A review', *Psychological Medicine* **16**, 307–22.

Parkin, A.J. (1982) 'Residual learning capacity in organic amnesia', *Cortex* **18**, 417–40.

Roth, M. (1994) 'The relationship between dementia and normal ageing of the brain', in F.A. Huppert, C. Brayne and D.W. O'Connor (eds.) *Dementia and Normal Ageing.* Cambridge: Cambridge University Press.

Roth, M., Tomlinson, B.E., and Blessed, G, (1966) 'Correlation between scores for dementia and counts of "senile plaques" in cerebral grey matter of elderly subjects', *Nature* **200**, 109–10.

St Clair, D. (1987) 'Chromosome 21, Down's syndrome and Alzheimer's disease', *Journal of Mental Deficiency Research* **31**, 213–4.

CHAPTER 25

The world of elders and health professionals

JULIE DOCKRELL AND GAIL WILSON

Chapter outline

Introduction
Systems theory and older people – the context
Nurses, older people and systems
  Societal values and beliefs
  National-level systems
  Local-level systems
  Personal-level systems
Systems as they affect nursing care for older people
Summary

Introduction

In this chapter we consider two major contributions which systems theory can make to gerontological nursing. First, it enables nurses and health professionals to gain some insight into the world of older people. In so doing health professionals can organize their behaviour and care packages into sets of interacting elements that are the first step towards the delivery of sensitive and appropriate services. Second, it helps health professionals to understand the ways in which they are consciously and unconsciously influenced in the care that they provide to older people.

Systems theory is a conceptual framework. It emphasizes the interactions and connections between elements in the social situation. In this chapter we have classified systems into four different levels: personal-level systems, local-level systems, national-level systems and societal values and beliefs. By considering systems in this way it is possible to identify both the explicit and implicit factors that affect our behaviour and the ways in which we behave towards older people. As Jerrome (1992) states in relation to staff working with older people: 'Relative youth . . . training in health care did not equip them to withstand the depressing effects of anxiety, confusion, loss and social marginality that their patients brought with them every day.' While social systems affect us all, their impact on older people and their carers can be particularly oppressive.

Systems theory and older people – the context

Social and organizational systems are rarely included when considering the later years of life (see Chapter 1 for discussion of the consequences for the individual of working in a complex organisation). Rather than consider the older person in relation to the social context in which they live, the tendency has been to concentrate on the characteristics of individuals, such as personality differences and cognitive change. If general social analyses are made, they often ignore and marginalize older people (see Chapter 22). There is a view that older people are no longer actively contributing to society. However, a focus on either the internal changes associated with ageing or the lack of role and status attached to growing older does not allow us to consider how some of the characteristic features of old age are produced. It also fails to address the effects of social context on the lives of older people.

The term *system* as used in psychology describes the ways in which people and ideas interact and affect each other. Systems are organized groups of individuals, services or ideas and they may occur at several different levels. Systems are not static. They are continually changing. Elements within a system alter each other. Individuals, families, communities and organizations all belong to and form systems.

General systems theory originated in the nineteenth century as a revolt against the more simple reductionist views held at the time. The theory recognizes the mutual dependencies between an individual and the environment. *The assumption made in describing any social organization as a system is that behaviour, events and social processes cannot be fully understood in isolation, but only in relation to each other.* As an example, consider the system that connects two cohabiting individuals. This relationship is continually changing as each partner develops and adjusts. This is a very simple social system which can be considered by itself, but which is also part of other wider systems, such as the local community.

According to systems theory, each system develops so as to function more efficiently *vis-à-vis* the outside world (Kaye, 1982). Such systems are open to outside influences and may increase in complexity with time. There are two criteria which characterize social systems. The first is that there is a *shared history* between members in the system – individuals grow and develop together and can learn to predict patterns of behaviour within the system. The second is that system members may work towards a *common purpose*. For example, a team improves in effectiveness as each member learns to anticipate the behaviour of the others. In the same way when system members are not in agreement, either explicitly or tacitly, effectiveness decreases. This means that approaches which focus on one aspect of a system are incomplete. They are attempting to understand or change behaviour by focusing on only one component, instead of taking account of the full range of interactions which make up a system. A medical approach which considers an elderly person only in terms of their presenting medical problem focuses only on a single component. If only a circumscribed medical model is used, much will be missed. An

individual's needs, personal and social histories, and the way that the social construction of old age affects both elders and those who care for them would not be
considered.

Systems theory, on the other hand, recognizes the mutual dependencies between
an individual and the environment. In the same way nurses and health professionals
provide care to patients and their families within specific contexts or environments
which form sets of systems. At an individual level the environment affects the way a
nurse or a patient functions and they in turn affect their environment. These
reciprocal relationships form the basis of systems. Higher level systems such as hospitals, local communities, the NHS and the value systems of society, affect individuals but the individuals themselves have much less impact on the way these systems
develop.

Elderly individuals encounter and interact with many different social and organizational systems. These systems impact on older people both directly and indirectly. For example, ways of delivering community care have a *direct* influence on
older people. Alterations in transport subsidies can have an *indirect* effect on the
diet of older people by restricting their choice of shops. This example shows that
social and organizational systems affect individuals in complex ways which must be
clarified before individual performance can be fully assessed and successful intervention planned.

Each individual has a personal life history and a set of strengths and needs, and
these will interact with surrounding systems. Traditionally psychology has emphasized individual strengths and limitations and these are discussed in Chapters 22–23
in relation to ageing. However, there is a growing movement within psychology
which emphasizes that individual behaviour needs to be considered within an extended framework that includes the shared beliefs which make up social reality.
This means that service providers must consider the *individual in society* instead of
individual traits alone.

A central assumption of studies investigating older people has always been the
expectation of a high degree of similarity between people who have reached old
age. This view has been challenged (see Maddox, 1987; Schaie, 1988; also Chapter
23, this volume). As an example, consider Baltes (1991), who draws a useful distinction between normal, optimal and pathological ageing. Normal ageing is defined as
growing old without serious or life threatening illness, be it mental or physical. Up
to the age of 70 or 80 this is a frequent event. Optimal ageing refers to ageing under
the best personal and environmental conditions, while pathological ageing refers to
the process of ageing where there is evidence of mental or physical pathology, such
as senile dementia (see Chapter 22). Thus, ageing is not a unitary process resulting
in homogeneous patterns of needs, wishes and behaviours.

Beliefs, ideologies and values also influence the opportunities afforded to individuals. Consequently, it is important to consider the impact of wider social systems. Davies (1982) has shown how social and organizational issues influence the
care provided to older people in long-term care. She found that staff managed
patients in a manner consistent with their underlying beliefs. Consequently, the

care patients received depended more on staff beliefs than on the patients' current functioning. For example, staff who held 'custodial' attitudes tended to feed patients, whereas those with 'rehabilitation'-oriented beliefs tended to encourage self-feeding. In other words, the needs of older people are interpreted in ways that reflect the organizational and personal values of their carers, rather than an unbiased measure of their capabilities.

In this chapter we shall outline the various systems that impinge on elderly service users and the health professionals who care for them, and discuss the ways in which these may enhance or inhibit life opportunities. Our aim is to show that a comprehensive perspective is necessary if appropriate services are to be offered to older people. The systems perspective identifies linkages and liaisons that occur between systems and older people. Adopting this approach should result in optimum independence for older people.

Nurses, older people and systems

There will be many cases where the nurse will not be a specialist in the care of older people and the contact with elders will be fleeting but frequent. For example, 40–60 per cent of patients in acute care are elderly and some will have additional complications and may take longer than average to discharge. However, even fleeting contact may draw on the nurse's gerontological expertise. The argument of Beckingham, van Maanen and McKnight (1992: 136) is becoming increasingly accepted:

> With the ageing of the population, the need for nurses well educated in
> gerontological care rapidly increases. However, their numbers are still relatively
> low, partially because (student) nurses tend to be unfamiliar with the challenges
> and rewards of a career path in gerontology. Since unknown makes unloved, it
> is important to expose students to gerontological education at an early stage in
> their programme.

It is also true that the placement of an older person in a long-term hospital is usually considered as a last resort when all other possibilities have failed. Hunter, McKeganney and MacPherson (1988) quote the psychogeriatrician who said: 'I see myself as catching those right at the bottom . . . when all other agencies can no longer cope. I have to take the one that I see as most urgent in view of the shortfall in beds.' Davies (1982) argues that in long-term care the goals involving maintenance of function and reduction in rate of deterioration replace those of cure and discharge.

The nursing systems that serve older patients reflect these different styles of care, whether they are hospital-based or community-based. Moreover, nurses working in a hospital ward belong to a different type of system from those working in community mental health, district nursing or health visiting. The organization and values of each system affect the way nurses order their work and interact with their patients (see Chapter 1). Thus, the context in which nurses encounter older people

Figure 25.1 *Four different levels of systems as they impact on the world of Elders*

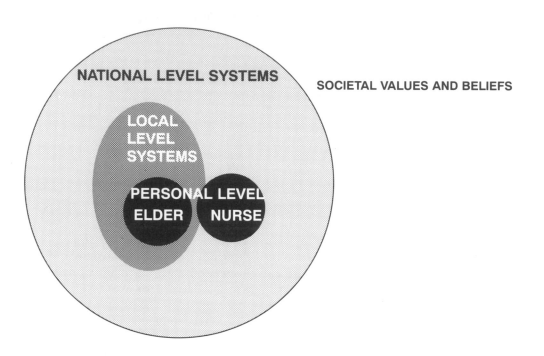

will place varying demands on their expertise and understanding. They will become involved with older people in a range of professional roles. They will frequently be faced with the difficult task of identifying the ways in which various systems impinge on the care needs and services provided for their clients. Any framework for care must acknowledge that:

- We are dealing with individuals.
- Individuals relate and interact with different people and organizations in different ways.
- Care is provided by professionals working within systems that enable and constrain their activities.
- Individuals and organizations are affected by system changes at societal, national and local levels.

Systems theory does not specify the processes by which effects occur. To be able to understand and use systemic approaches we have to be more precise about the ways we understand systems. To help with this task, we have considered systems at four different levels:

1. *Personal-level systems*: the individual's network of personal contacts.
2. *Local-level systems*: local/community groups and organizations.
3. *National-level systems*: the wider political economic framework.
4. *Societal values and beliefs*: the set of national cultures and subcultures.

These systems are presented in Figure 25.1. In the following sections we consider in greater detail the impact of systems on the nurse and older people. We begin by considering the wider social and national levels which affect us all, and end by discussing the specific details of personal systems which will relate to individual life histories.

Societal values and beliefs

Society is organized in ways that reflect its values. These values, in turn, are often translated into legislation. For example, as a society we are more concerned about children than older people and this concern is reflected in legislation and government action on child abuse. In contrast, there is no legislation, and only a slow growth of government concern about elder abuse (Bennet and Kingston, 1993; McCreadie, 1991). In this chapter we are concerned with the systems that are manifest in beliefs about old age, gender, social status or income, and race. These beliefs affect everyone. We may view them in three ways: (1) take them for granted as 'natural'; (2) recognize and accept them as part of the prevailing culture; or (3) oppose them. Whatever our view, they structure life chances and distribute power unequally in our society.

At this point you should consider your own views of older people. Box 25.1 presents an opportunity for you to decide whether misinformation affects your own attitudes about ageing. The box contains a list of statements about ageing that are either true or false. Many professionals who work with older people are not aware of the accuracy of these statements. Read each statement and decide whether it is true or false. Consider your errors. How might your views impact on the care you offer?

Ageism is the term used to describe beliefs about older people that devalue them and belittle their contribution to society. It affects older people themselves and those who work with them (McEwan, 1990; Victor, 1987; see also Chapter 23). Health professionals are affected by ageism in two ways. In the first place they may hold ageist beliefs and can easily slip into ageist attitudes which devalue older patients. In the second, professionals in contact with older people may feel less respected by society than those who care for people in the prime of life. It is important not to pass on this lack of respect to clients.

Ageism is responsible for the common beliefs that all older people are slow, unable to decide for themselves, out of date, unproductive and burdensome. It is only a short step to assume that therefore they can be provided with low quality care. They very rarely complain (Goldberg and Connolly, 1982). For one reason

BOX 25.1   FACTS ON AGEING

Before proceeding further, you are encouraged to try out this quiz to find out which facts you may be unaware of. Circle 'T; for True or 'F' for False.*

T   F   1 The majority of old people (past age 65) are senile (i.e. defective memory, disoriented or demented).

T   F   2 All five senses tend to decline in old age.

T   F   3 Most old people have no interest in, or capacity for, sexual relations.

T   F   4 Lung capacity tends to decline in old age.

T   F   5 The majority of old people feel miserable most of the time.

T   F   6 Physical strength tends to decline in old age.

T   F   7 At least 10 per cent of the aged are living in long-stay institutions (i.e. nursing homes, mental hospitals, homes for the aged, etc.).

T   F   8 Aged drivers have fewer accidents per person than drivers under age 65.

T   F   9 Most older workers cannot work as effectively as younger workers.

T   F   10 About 80 per cent of the aged are healthy enough to carry out their normal activities.

T   F   11 Most old people are set in their ways and unable to change.

T   F   12 Old people usually take longer to learn something new.

T   F   13 It is almost impossible for most old people to learn new things.

T   F   14 The reaction time of most old people tends to be slower than reaction time of younger people.

T   F   15 In general, most old people are pretty much alike.

T   F   16 The majority of old people are seldom bored.

T   F   17 The majority of old people are socially isolated and lonely.

T   F   18 Older workers have fewer accidents than younger workers.

T   F   19 Over 15 per cent of the US population are now age 65 or over.

T   F   20 Most medical practitioners tend to give low priority to the aged.

T   F   21 About 3 per cent *less* of the aged have incomes below the official poverty level than the rest of the population.

T   F   22 The majority of old people are working or would like to have some kind of work to do (including housework and volunteer work).

T   F   23 Older people tend to become more religious as they age.

T   F   24 The majority of old people are seldom irritated or angry.

T   F   25 The health and socioeconomic status of older people (compared to younger people) in the year 2000 will probably be about the same as now.

Source: E. Palmore (1977) 'Facts on aging: A short quiz.' Reprinted with permission, *The Gerontologist* **17**, 315–20, August 1977. Copyright the Gerontological Society of America.

* Answers at the end of Seminar questions, p. 494.

they are part of the ageist belief system. Most of them will have dreaded old age and looked down on 'the old' all their lives. This is one reason why people in their seventies and eighties will often say they do not want to mix with old people.

Gender-related prejudices also can have an effect on elder care. There are more older women than men, and the proportion of women rises as old age proceeds. Older women have been described as doubly disadvantaged (Norman, 1985): in the first place they are old and in the second female. High status in our society frequently goes with masculinity, youth and material possessions. Older women may therefore find themselves more devalued than older men and may often feel that they lack the ability to influence the systems they are in. Passivity and low expectations can result (Victor, 1987, 1991).

Nurses, too, may find themselves subject to the same forces. Nursing is still a predominantly female profession but traditionally professions were a male preserve. Nursing therefore has a heritage of gender-related subservience and a lack of professional recognition to live down (See, for example, Robinson, Gray and Elkan, 1992; Savage, 1987; Smith, 1992; Strong and Robinson, 1990). The image of female nurse as handmaiden to male doctor has not wholly disappeared, even though there are now male nurses and nearly half of all medical students are women.

Beliefs about differences in social status are often linked to paid work and income. Those groups of people who are not in the labour market, such as mothers of young children, the unemployed or pensioners, are not held in great social esteem. Retired people are often characterized as a burden on the working population. We forget that they have contributed to society all their lives, either as housewives and carers or as paid workers. They have paid taxes which financed health and social services. Many have done voluntary work and many are caring for frail spouses or for much older parents. The majority of older people live on or near the poverty line. The state pension allows a respectable, but very restricted existence. Poverty and the accompanying loss of social status that goes with it can be very disempowering (Victor, 1987). Health professionals too may feel that society does not value their services highly enough and that they are underpaid for the work they do.

Beliefs about the *value and abilities of people of different races* are widespread in our society. Most ethnic minority elders who were born in this country will have experienced racial discrimination all their lives (Norman, 1985). Others may have met it only when they arrived. In either case, the experience of racial prejudice, usually accompanied by ageism and low social status, makes any problems of old age more difficult to cope with.

Health professionals from ethnic minorities may find themselves coping with the same prejudices. They will be aware that their promotion prospects are still relatively poor, despite efforts by central and local government to reduce racial discrimination (GLARE, 1987; King Edward's Hospital Fund, 1990; Pearson, 1985). They will experience racism from patients (Wilkinson and Wilson, 1992) and are unlikely to have been offered training in the cultural needs of those they care for.

DISCUSSION POINT
At this point you should consider how far such values and beliefs:

- Influence your own working practice.
- Influence your organization's practice.

What can you do about it?

Now you should consider the contexts in which you have encountered older people in your professional capacity. List the older people you have cared for. Choose three patients and draw a chart listing:

1. Any additional requirements arising from the combination of age and medical problem.
2. Whether you altered your approach to individuals because of their age.
3. Whether an individual's physical appearance altered your contact with him/her.
4. Whether individual's personal characteristics altered your attitude towards him/her.

National-level systems

The belief systems mentioned above combine with others to produce the political, economic and social framework for national-level systems. From the perspective of elders and their carers, one key issue is the division between state, voluntary and private sector organizations. Political and economic considerations influence vitally important aspects of ageing such as the level of pensions, the age of retirement and the type of care which can be offered to those elders who need it. Such an analysis makes it clear that health professionals work within a system that is difficult to change and that indirectly influences the health of individuals (e.g. in terms of money available for nutrition and mobility). For example, the legal system provides a national framework that may have specific effects on certain groups. Nursing responsibilities for medication are backed by law, as are pension rights for retired people. Few individuals can change national-level systems, but national changes will affect local and personal systems in different ways.

Service provision has changed for older people (Henwood, 1992). A policy of rapid hospital discharge has a direct effect on the lives of many older people but it is set at the level of national government. As a further example consider the introduction of market forces in health and social care as exemplified through the purchaser/provider split. Nursing professionals in NHS trusts now find themselves in direct competition with nurses in other trusts. As for the impact on the older people themselves, the decrease in national provision has meant there has been a steady growth in private nursing homes and places are paid for by the resident of the nursing home, by relatives or by the local authority.

The value of state pensions fell in the 1980s (Johnson and Folkingham, 1992). This has made most older people who rely on state pension or on welfare benefits poorer in relation to the rest of the population. Simultaneously, private pensions rose and many newly retired people find themselves able to live quite comfortably.

However, most private pensions lose their value over time and people over 70 are still likely to have difficulty paying for a healthy lifestyle unless they budget very carefully. If they fall ill or become disabled, the increased costs may mean that they have to economize on food or heating.

Changes in policy and the accompanying legislation have also affected the National Health Service. The aim has been to reduce expenditure and to shift the long-term care of older people out of hospital and into the community or private nursing homes. In practice, this has meant that relatives (usually women) have to care for older people at home for longer periods, consequently making greater demands on community nursing services. These system changes are likely to have a growing impact on nursing opportunities in the future (Henwood, 1992).

The NHS and Community Care Act 1990 also changed the basis of local government services for older people. Local social service or social work departments have the lead responsibility for assessing individuals who need care. They are required to buy most of the care they need from private or voluntary providers or from community health services. Also general practitioners are now able to buy social and community care for their elderly patients. Most nurses will find themselves as part of provider teams rather than as purchasers. It will be some years before the new systems settle down and all parties, professionals and older people, have enough information to make the best use of what is available.

There is a danger that care of older people, and those who work in this area, because of the prejudices outlined above, will be further devalued by the changes. Ageist beliefs, the high cost of older patients, who may block beds in acute care wards, and the high priority given to children's problems may combine to lower standards of care for older people. Community nursing teams may find that they are unable to give enough support to older patients and their carers. Nurses working in homes may find that standards are being driven down as competition for residents increases. Ethnic minority elders, like all those who need specialized services, will be less likely to receive what they need. This will be especially true of most Chinese older people, for example, who live in small scattered groups.

The division of health service personnel into professions or grades is another aspect of the way legislative systems impinge on care. Tradition and custom have resulted in professional divisions which may not be in the best interests of clients (Wilson and Dockrell, 1994). There are, for example, many tasks that could be done by nurses which are now reserved for doctors only. Similarly, many nursing activities can be and are performed by untrained relatives or by social service staff. Often existing divisions are reinforced by the legal system and change may be outside the competence of individuals.

DISCUSSION POINT

At this point you should consider what makes a nurse distinct from other professionals. You should include professional skills and wider characteristics such as dress and language. To what extent could these characteristics become a barrier to successful interdisciplinary elder care?

Local-level systems

Local-level systems are formed by the interactions between the older person and service providers and associations. Local-level systems are effectively the impact of organizations on the life of the older person. They refer to associations or groups in the local community and to voluntary and statutory services catering for the needs of older people (see Anderson and Carter, 1984, on organizations). After retirement older people, especially older men, may lose their workplace-based social systems. This loss may be balanced by gains as they make new friends or have more time to spend with relatives (Jerrome, 1990). Religious groups may also provide valuable care and support to their members.

Local associations and support networks can be a valuable resource to the frail elderly, but often these informal support systems are weakest in areas where the need is greatest (Bulmer, 1986). Poor housing, poverty and the presence of social tensions make successful community action difficult. In rural areas, transport is often the key to strong support systems (Wenger, 1984). Voluntary organizations – for example, Age Concern or Crossroads – can also help out when nursing resources are stretched.

The second set of local systems that older people may come into contact with are statutory services. Health and social service clients are often confused about what is on offer (Allen, Hogg and Peace, 1992). They may be unaware of what is available or of their eligibility for it. As one client in the study by Allen, Hogg and Peace said, 'You hear of things. It's like this – people gossip. You have to keep your wits about you. I'm quick on the uptake' (p. 80). Service users in this study generally felt that they were not well informed. They failed to receive information about the services available and lacked specific information about their own health status, particularly from GPs. GPs are centrally placed in the health care systems of most older people, but Allen, Hogg and Peace, like other researchers (e.g. Goldberg and Huxley, 1980), question whether they can adequately fulfil such a central role. Community nurses who collate information on sources of help may be more effective. Disability or expenditure cuts leading to a reduction in access to health and social care services mean that problems get worse when prompt attention might have avoided or minimised them.

Successful interagency and interprofessional work requires personal contact – getting to know the other agency and its staff. Other agencies are part of the same care system and so worthy of cooperation and respect (Dockrell and Wilson, 1994). Nurses who feel threatened are not likely to respect social workers or home helps. They may patronize volunteers. Such attitudes are understandable, but they do not result in good client care. Setting the boundaries of nursing competence and understanding the boundaries of other professionals and agencies is the first step to good relations. It should bring confidence and lead to flexibility and putting the needs of the client first. Once boundaries and needs have been identified, it becomes possible to negotiate who will do what and when. Clearly, such negotiations are most important in community nursing but, as the staff mix in hospitals changes, the issues are the same.

Government policies create systems that sometimes conflict with each other. When this happens individuals, whether patients or professionals, may find themselves caught between competing systems and their welfare may suffer. To take one example, government policy on reducing public expenditure may be seen as beneficial to the population as a whole. However, at the local level, it can lead to cuts in service that threaten professional values and leave older patients with unmet needs.

Health professionals work in local systems that vary in terms of size, dominant values, power structure and professional values, to list but a few attributes. The NHS, for example, is a big and bureaucratic organization. Career opportunities, and even pay, may be better in the NHS than in the smaller private or voluntary organizations that employ nurses. However, small systems may offer more opportunity for face-to-face negotiation and for more flexible working practices (Anderson and Carter, 1984). Therefore, these local systems may be very different from each other and have very different effects on their staff and clients. A basic division is between residential and non-residential systems. Hospitals and nursing homes are systems that affect very large areas of life – more for their residents than their staff, but staff too can become institutionalized (Goffman, 1963). The values and beliefs and the impact of legislation outlined in the previous sections often make it hard for staff to respect the dignity of elderly residents if they are short staffed or poorly managed. Residents themselves may be unhappy with their condition and be uncooperative. In such circumstances, the nursing task is as much about establishing minimum levels of emotional welfare as about physical care. A strong commitment to patient autonomy is essential.

It is often easy to forget that long-term care patients can have social systems outside the institution. This mistake is less likely in acute care and community nursing. In these cases, successful discharge or maintenance in the community may depend on mobilizing informal care in a partnership with nursing services. Community practitioners have more freedom of action than hospital-based nurses. Their own system is more flexible than is possible in a residential setting. On the other hand, they are more vulnerable to actions and decisions taken in other local care-giving systems. Cuts in one service can cause unforeseen problems for others. For example, cuts in hospital budgets mean that more frail elderly people with a high need for nursing care are discharged into the community, so altering the skill mix needed by community nurses.

Personal-level systems

Everyone has a close personal system. Nurses and other health professionals will each have their own personal systems, but from a professional point of view it is the personal-level systems of older people that need to be understood. Personal systems impinge directly on the older person at a day-to-day level. These refer to the activities, roles and interpersonal relations of/experienced by an older person in a given setting. Such situations include interactions with carers, friends and partners. When a nurse has direct contact with an elderly person or carer, she will have become part of the individual's personal system. Good nursing practice will take account of the personal systems of each patient, including close relatives and friends. Very often, particularly in community nursing, good care depends on how effectively nursing systems link in with the personal systems of patients (Jones and Vetter, 1984; NHSME, 1993).

Research suggests that being embedded in a social network is vital for general wellbeing. At the personal level, this network includes individuals who have direct contact with the older person. These may be informal networks, such as family, friends and neighbours, or contacts that are formally established, such as visits by the district nurse. Formal contacts would include meetings with the district nurse or health visitor, as well as with the driver for the meals-on-wheels service. Informal networks often involve a long history of contact with the older person, but many older people have very few informal networks (Allen, Hogg and Peace, 1992) and some have no informal support available at all. There is a myth that Black and Asian older people live in extended families who look after them. But in reality many ethnic people do not live in extended families (Ebrahim and Hillier, 1991). Even when they do, overcrowding and low incomes may mean that they and their carers urgently need appropriate services.

Personal-level systems are important sources of support throughout the lifespan. For many older people these systems change with time. Some of these changes, such as retirement are predictable; others, such as time of bereavement or illness, are often unforeseeable. Every change that occurs in the life course requires adjustment. A special problem for older people is the likelihood of unwanted changes in their personal systems. There are three common types of change that can influence an individual's personal system: (1) retirement, (2) disabilities, and (3) bereavements. It is important to consider how some of these developmental changes might alter an individual's personal network.

Retirement
Retirement has frequently been associated with decreased activity and interaction. However, most retired people see retirement as an active independent state of affairs (Atchley, 1974). Financial considerations are an important element in actualizing retirement as a positive phase and, as we have already outlined, inadequate income is frequently a serious problem for retired individuals. Irrespective of the nature of retirement, personal contacts will change. There will no longer be the structured interaction with others in the workplace. Partners, friends and acquaintances may fill the space. Cohabiting partners will find that they have more time to spend together and will need to readjust. Often, there is a change in gender roles leading to a shift in power and dominance. This may be due to illness or to the female partner continuing to work when the male has retired.

Disabilities
The onset of disability can affect both partners and result in role reversal. Men may become carers (Arber and Gilbert, 1989) and women may find themselves managing the finances or changing fuses. The needs of men and women will differ, but not necessarily in the ways currently recognized by professionals. Jones and Vetter

(1984) found that fewer than one in ten older people living at home in South Wales who required help had access to a statutory helper. By far the biggest group of helpers were informal carers. These carers are children, partners and neighbours. The quality of informal care and the length of time that care is provided for depends on the relationship between carer and patient. Those looked after by a husband or a wife tend to stay at home longer than those being cared for by other relatives or friends and neighbours. Caring becomes especially stressful if individuals become frail and dementia is involved (Gilleard *et al.*, 1984). Mental frailty can pose special problems for relationships. If your partner or parent is unable to recognize you, it becomes difficult to accept that they are still the person you are concerned about and care for (see Chapter 24). Disabilities can restrict individual access to previously established personal networks. Problems can arise from restrictions caused by decreased mobility or a move into residential care. Access to partners and friends and relations may be curtailed.

Disability is not the only influence on access. Financial constraints, tiredness and time required to complete an activity all have their effects. For those who have a car, the change from driving to not driving is an important one. In Britain, once a person reaches the age of 70, the driver's licence must be renewed every three years. The loss of the licence can have a marked effect on both the maintenance of personal networks and the health and wellbeing of an individual. The inability to reach high street shops can result in both expensive and poorly balanced meals.

Bereavement

Bereavement is a common occurrence as individuals age (see chapter 17). Later life is frequently characterized by multiple losses and the loss of friends and loved ones through death. A significant proportion of older women are widowed, rising to approximately two-thirds over the age of 80. Responses to these personal losses vary. Grieving may invoke multiple, contradictory emotions: despair, anger, detachment, sadness, denial, guilt and depression. The pattern of personal relationships which remains following a bereavement will contribute to an individual's subsequent ability to cope. It is important to realize that changes in an individual as a result of dementia may result in the partner experiencing a grief reaction similar to that which occurs with death. There is a loss of the person who was known and loved.

Society requires older people to resign roles and activities. Health professionals need to acknowledge these losses and to help the grieving process. However, it is wrong to assume that all older people wish to become observers of life rather than participants. When the opportunity arises many older people choose continued activity and involvement.

Systems as they affect nursing care for older people

The use of systems theory in understanding elder care has two immediate and important implications for the nurse practitioner. In the first place an individual's

| BOX 25.2   **ELDERLY PEOPLE IN NEED OF CARE** |

Mr C is 87 and recently broke his hip. He has been discharged from hospital early to free a bed.

Relevant background
- Mr C is white and lives with his 72-year-old wife in their own home in a pleasant suburb; there is no downstairs toilet.
- He has a good private pension paid by his former employers as well as his state pension.
- When he retired from his job as a bank manager he was very happy playing golf and bowls and keeping the garden tidy.
- Their only daughter lives at some distance but visits every weekend, grandchildren permitting.
- They have a private home help.
- He has been incontinent of urine for the last seven years.
- Recently Mr C has become frail and a bit confused.
- He can no longer drive.
- Mrs C never worked outside the home. She has always had problems with her nerves and takes daily medication for this and to sleep at night.

Mrs A is 78 and recently broke her hip. She has been discharged from hospital early to free a bed.

Relevant background
- Mrs A is Afro-Caribbean and lives on her own on an inner city council estate which is badly run down and troubled by vandalism.
- Mrs A has lived most of her adult life on the estate and remembers it in better years. She is very proud of her clean and tidy house.
- Mrs A worked all her life but did not qualify for a pension because she was in part-time work. Her state pension is therefore low and she receives income support.
- Her husband left her 30 years ago and she brought up her son and daughter on her own. Her son has moved to Jamaica and her daughter has a family of her own in the suburbs.
- She is diabetic and her poor balance is beginning to hamper her mobility.
- She finds it hard to cook, but does not like the meals-on-wheels that are delivered to her.
- She is very involved in the local church and this is her main social contact now that her friends have died or have moved away.
- Until recently Mrs A had a 'wonderful' home help, but she did not qualify as high need and the service was withdrawn after budget cuts. No new assessment has been made.

behaviour can never be viewed or understood in isolation. This is important both for developing care plans and for service initiatives. Second, the nurse herself must realize that there are other systems that impinge of her own working practice.

The two case studies in Box 25.2 will help highlight some of these system effects on the lives of older people. Mr C and Mrs A are typical examples of older people who come into contact with services when they are discharged from hospital. Let us consider the ways in which the different systems levels impact on Mr C. The *national systems* level has led to the early discharge of Mr C into the care of his wife. Mrs C's lifestyle reflects the wider *societal attitudes and beliefs*. She has never worked outside the home. She has been the homemaker and carer and is now expected to continue in that role caring for her frail husband. Mrs C clings to a commonly held belief about the need to cope with one's family on one's own. After all, Mrs C successfully raised a family, ran a home and has cared for her grandchildren.

The *local support systems* have failed this couple. Discharge has occurred prior to establishing their eligibility for home care assistance. At any rate, additional help would place demands on their savings. Liaison between the GP, district nurse, social services and the hospital was negligible. Mr C was discharged on the day that these professionals were written to. The hospital staff were not unduly concerned, as Mrs C seems to be a competent woman.

Caring for her husband has led to restrictions in her *personal network*. She cannot leave her husband alone to go to church or visit her friends. Yet she is unwilling to have her friends and great grandchildren into the house. Mr C can no longer make his weekly visits to the Masonic Lodge, so Mrs C has no time on her own. Unfortunately, Mrs C's relationship with her husband has changed. The excessive demands of coping with an incontinent, slightly dementing male, who, like some other older people (see Wilson, 1994), abuses her by hitting her is depressing. She regards herself as a private person with self-respect and is therefore unwilling to report these difficulties. There are no local help lines for elder abuse; in fact, Mrs C has never heard the term – a reflection of *societal attitudes and beliefs*.

As this case illustrates, Mr and Mrs C are influenced by the interactions and connections between elements in their social situation. They are both part of and affected by the different system levels that characterize the lives of elders in our society.

At this point you should consider Mrs. A's case (see Box 25.2) and:

1. Identify the different system levels which will impact on Mrs A.
2. Specify which factors at each level you think will affect the delivery of services.
3. Explain why these effects might occur.

Summary

This chapter has shown that nurse practitioners need to identify a range of systems at a number of different levels. These systems will be their own and those of their patients. Systems affect us all in ways that are often hard to identify. This is particularly true of the social beliefs which can easily be taken as 'natural' when in fact they should be questioned. In this chapter, we have been concerned with the impact of systems on nurses and health professionals and on their older clients.

Good practice means an ability to identify systems, particularly the systems which will enhance the quality of life of clients and support their nursing care. Increasingly, health professionals will have to take a wider view of both their clients and of their place in a subset of local systems. The NHS and Community Care Act 1990 highlights the need for more interprofessional and interagency cooperation. Such work across specialties and nursing disciplines has always been essential in elder care. The problems it creates are not new. Services and professions have traditionally drawn boundaries round their areas of competence. One way forward is to identify the boundaries between services, such as hospital and community, or district nursing and home care, and to negotiate how work is distributed across them.

The success of interprofessional work will also depend on the nature of the organizations involved. Nurses will come in contact with other professionals or even, in the voluntary sector, with non-professionals, who are committed to elder care. Their cooperation is vital for good quality services. Understanding these local systems is a key to high quality care.

High quality nursing care for older people is impossible unless the ageist beliefs that pervade society are acknowledged and addressed. This is a first step in understanding nursing in the world of elders.

Seminar questions

1. Using the statements in Box 25.1 consider the ways in which the negative views of ageing could be altered in our society. Consider changes at each of the four different system levels.
2. Devise a care plan for Mr C. Outline medical, social and psychological factors that you consider central in devising this care plan. Consider how you would help Mrs C cope with the changes that have occurred in her life. Would you help her to make contact with any carers' support groups? Give the reasons for your decisions. Discuss the repercussions of your care plan for wider issues of service provision for elders, considering factors such as liaison between professionals, appointing an advocate.

Answer to Box 25.1
All the odd numbered statements are false; all the even numbered statements are true.

Further reading

Anderson, R.E. and Carter, I. (1984) *Human Behavior in the Social Environment*, New York: Aldine Publishing. Chapter 3, 'Culture and Society', has an interesting discussion of the way that values systems influence behaviour. Chapter 5, 'Organization', is stimulating on local systems. The authors suggest reading N. Mailer (1979), *The Executioner's Song*, as a way of understanding how personal systems are affected by wider structures.

Bennett, G. and Ebrahim, S. (1992) *Health Care of the Elderly*. London: Edward Arnold. This book covers a range of medical, practical and psychological issues related to caring for elders. There are three major sections – medical gerontology, the medical needs of elders and services for elderly people. Each of the major sections is divided into short succinctly written chapters of 2–4 pages. Each chapter provides a balanced analysis of the topic.

Iveson, C. (1993) *Whose Life? Community care for older people and their families*. London: Brief Therapy Press. Chris Iveson is a family therapist and the cases he presents in this book are discussed from a systemic point of view. The book will challenge many of the assumptions that are generally held about how to help older people. Readable and provocative.

Twining, C. (1988) *Helping Older People: A psychological approach*. Chichester: John Wiley. Twining shows, in straightforward language, how the application of psychological principles can help those working with older people to meet their clients' needs. Based on research, the book covers a wide range of topics related to the psychological wellbeing of older people.

References

Allen, I., Hogg, D. and Peace, S. (1992) *Elderly People: Choice participation and satisfaction*. London: Policy Studies Institute.

Anderson, R.E. and Carter, I. (1984) *Human Behavior in the Social Environment*. New York: Aldine.

Arber, S. and Gilbert, N. (1989) 'Men: The forgotten carers', *Sociology* **23**(1), 111–8.

Atchley, R.C. (1974) 'The meaning of retirement', *Journal of Communications* **24**, 97–101.

Baltes, M.M. and Baltes, P.B. (eds.) (1986) *The Psychology of Control and Ageing*. Hillsdale, NJ: Lawrence Erlbaum.

Baltes, P. (1991) 'The many faces of human ageing: Toward a psychological culture of old age', *Psychological Medicine* **21**, 837–54.

Beckingham, A., Van Maanen, H. and McKnight, J. (1992) 'Curriculum innovation for gerontological nursing in Canada: A health for all systems-based approach', *International Journal of Nursing Studies* **29**, 135–49.

Bennet, G. and Kingston, P. (1993) *Elder Abuse Concepts, theories and interventions*, London: Chapman & Hall.

Bulmer, M. (1986) *Neighbours: The work of Philip Abrams*. Cambridge: Cambridge University Press.

Davies, A. D. M. (1982) 'Research with elderly people in long-term care: Some social and organizational factors affecting psychological interventions', *Ageing and Society* **2**, 285–98.

Dockrell, J. E. and Wilson, G. (1994) 'Interprofessional management issues in services for older people', in K. Soothill, L. Mackay and C. Webb (eds.) *Interprofessional Relations in Health Care*. London: Edward Arnold.

Ebrahim, S. and Hillier, S. (1991) 'Ethnic minority needs', *Review of Clinical Gerontology* **1**, 195–9.

Gilleard, C.J., Bedford, H., Gilleard, E., Whittick, J.E. and Gledhill, K. (1984) 'Emotional distress amongst the supporters of the elderly mentally infirm', *British Journal of Psychiatry* **145**, 172–7.

Goffman, E. (1963) *Asylums*. Harmondsworth: Penguin Books.

Goldberg, D. and Huxley, P. (1980) *Mental Illness in the Community*. London: Tavistock.

Goldberg, M. and Connolly, N. (1982) *The Effectiveness of Social Care for the Elderly*. London: Heinemann.

GLARE (Greater London Action for Race Equality) (1987) *No Alibi, No Excuse: A progress report on the development of equal opportunities in London's Health Authorities.* London: GLARE.

Henwood, M. (1992) *Through a Glass Darkly: Community care and elderly people.* Research report No. 14, London: King's Fund Institute.

Hunter, D.J., McKeganney, N.P. and MacPherson, I. (1988) *Care of the Elderly Policy and Practice*. Aberdeen: University of Aberdeen Press.

Jerrome, D. (1990) 'Intimate relationships', in J. Bond and P. Coleman (eds.) *Aging in Society: An introduction to social gerontology*. London: Sage.

Jerrome, D. (1992) 'A personal experience of counselling older adults', *Clinical Psychology Forum* **43**, 28–34.

Johnson, P. and Folkingham, J. (1992) *Ageing and Economic Welfare.* London: Sage.

Jones, D.A. and Vetter, N.J. (1984) 'A survey of those who care for the elderly at home: Their problems and their needs', *Social Science and Medicine* **19**, 511–14.

Kaye, K. (1982) *The Mental and Social Life of Babies*. Chicago: University of Chicago Press.

King Edward's Hospital Fund for London (1990) *Racial Equality: The nursing profession: Task force position paper*. London: King Edward's Hospital Fund.

Maddox, G.L. (1987) 'Aging differently', *Gerontologist* **27**, 557–64.

McCreadie, C. (1991) *Elder Abuse: An exploratory study*. London: Age Concern, Institute of Gerontology.

McEwan, E. (ed.) (1990) *Age: The unrecognised discrimination*. London: Age Concern.

Norman, A. (1985) *Triple Jeopardy: Growing old in a second homeland*. London: Centre for Policy on Ageing.

NHS Management Executive (1993) *New World, New Opportunities: Report of a task group on nursing in primary health care*. London: HMSO.

Pearson, M. (1985) *Equal Opportunities in the NHS: A handbook*. Leeds: Training in Health and Race.

Robinson, J., Gray, A. and Elkan, R. (eds.) (1992) *Policy Issues in Nursing.* Milton Keynes: Open University Press.

Savage, J. (1987) *Nursing, Gender and Sexuality*. London: Heinemann.

Schaie, K.W. (1988) 'Variability in cognitive function in the elderly: Implications for societal participation', in A. Woodhead, M.A. Bender, and R.C. Leonard (eds.) *Phenotypic Variation in Populations*. New York: Plenum Press.

Smith, P. (1992) *Emotional Labour in Nursing: Its impact on interprofessional relations, management and the educational environment*. Basingstoke: Macmillan.

Strong, P. and Robinson, J. (1990) *The NHS: Under new management*. Milton Keynes: Open University Press.

Victor, C. (1987) *Old Age in Modern Society*. London: Croom Helm.

Victor, C. (1991) *Health and Health Care in Later Life*. Milton Keynes: Open University Press.

Wenger, G.C. (1984) *The Supportive Network*. London: George Allen & Unwin.

Wilkinson, R. and Wilson, G. (1992) 'Pressure points'. *Social Work Today* **23**(39), 11 June, 16–17.

Wilson, G. (1994) 'Abuse of elderly men and women among clients of a community psychogeriatric service', *British Journal of Social Work*, **24**, 681–709.

Wilson, G. and Dockrell, J. E. (1994) 'Interprofessional issues in the care of older people', in P. Owens, J. Carrier and J. Horder (eds.) *Interprofessional Issues in Health and Community Care*. London: Macmillan.

Author Index

Subject Index